Women and the Menstrual Cycle: From Adolescence to Menopause

Women and the Menstrual Cycle: From Adolescence to Menopause

Editor: Daisy Robinson

MURPHY & MOORE
www.murphy-moorepublishing.com

www.murphy-moorepublishing.com

MURPHY & MOORE

Cataloging-in-Publication Data

Women and the menstrual cycle : from adolescence to menopause / edited by Daisy Robinson.
p. cm.
Includes bibliographical references and index.
ISBN 978-1-63987-573-3
1. Menstrual cycle. 2. Menstruation disorders. 3. Sexual cycle. 4. Women--Physiology.
5. Endocrine gynecology. I. Robinson, Daisy.
RG161 .W66 2022
618.172--dc23

Murphy & Moore Publishing,
1 Rockefeller Plaza,
New York City, NY 10020, USA

ISBN 978-1-63987-573-3 (Hardback)

Contents

Preface

This book was inspired by the evolution of our times; to answer the curiosity of inquisitive minds. Many developments have occurred across the globe in the recent past which has transformed the progress in the field.

The series of changes in hormone production and structures of the ovaries and uterus of the female reproductive system which occurs naturally and makes gestation possible is known as the menstrual cycle. The ovarian cycle regulates the formation and release of eggs. It also regulates the cyclic release of estrogen and progesterone. The uterine cycle controls the production and maintenance of the lining of the womb to receive a fertilized egg. The median length of a complete menstrual cycle is 28 days, but it can last for 21 to 35 days in adult women. Menstrual cycle typically begins in the preadolescent or adolescent phase of a girl's life. Menopause is the time when menstrual cycle permanently stops in a woman and she is no longer able to conceive. From theories to research, case studies related to all contemporary topics of relevance to this field have been included in this book. It is compiled in such a manner, that it will provide in-depth knowledge about the clinical research on menstrual cycle and menopause. This book will serve as a valuable source of reference for graduate and post graduate students.

This book was developed from a mere concept to drafts to chapters and finally compiled together as a complete text to benefit the readers across all nations. To ensure the quality of the content we instilled two significant steps in our procedure. The first was to appoint an editorial team that would verify the data and statistics provided in the book and also select the most appropriate and valuable contributions from the plentiful contributions we received from authors worldwide. The next step was to appoint an expert of the topic as the Editor-in-Chief, who would head the project and finally make the necessary amendments and modifications to make the text reader-friendly. I was then commissioned to examine all the material to present the topics in the most comprehensible and productive format.

I would like to take this opportunity to thank all the contributing authors who were supportive enough to contribute their time and knowledge to this project. I also wish to convey my regards to my family who have been extremely supportive during the entire project.

Editor

1

Premature Ovarian Insufficiency

Abdelhamid Benmachiche and
Amel Dammene Debbih

Abstract

Premature ovarian insufficiency (POI) is a heterogeneous disorder, affecting approximately 1% of women before the age of 40. Heterogeneity of POI is reflected by various causes. The known causes are genetic defects, autoimmune ovarian damage, metabolic, iatrogenic following surgery, cancer therapy, and environmental factors. However, in most cases, the cause remains unknown (idiopathic POI). The main symptom is the absence of regular menstrual cycles, and the diagnosis is confirmed by the raised gonadotropins and low estradiol. The disorder usually leads to infertility and has long-term comorbidities such as cardiovascular diseases, osteoporosis, and cognitive impairments. Management includes the use of hormone replacement therapy till the age of natural menopause. In women having fertility issues, the spontaneous conception varies between 5 and 10%, and in vitro fertilization with donor oocytes remains the treatment of choice. Moreover, fertility preservation options can be offered to some patients with cancer and those at risk of early menopause, such as those with familial cases of POI. Further research is clearly needed, to identify new mechanisms which may improve the prediction of the early onset of the disease.

Keywords: premature ovarian insufficiency, irregular menstrual cycle, estrogen deficiency, hormone replacement therapy, infertility treatment

1. Introduction

Premature ovarian insufficiency (POI) is a heterogeneous condition defined by the presence of menopausal-level serum gonadotropins in repeated blood tests with menstrual disturbance (oligomenorrhea or amenorrhea) in adolescent girls or women under 40 years of age [1]. Several different terms have been used to describe this condition, such as premature menopause, premature ovarian insufficiency (POI), or premature ovarian failure (POF). Confusion exists concerning nomenclature, namely, the use of POF or POI. The term POI has been adopted recently by the European Society of Human Reproduction and Embryology (ESHRE) consensus instead of "failure" [2]. Because it was found to more accurately describe the fluctuating nature of the condition. The POF is best considered as the only final stage of POI [3, 4]. The incidence of spontaneous POI has been estimated to affect 1 in 100 women before 40 years of age and 1 in 1000 women before 30 years of age [1, 5]. Although the incidence of spontaneous POI appears to have remained stable, of increasing concern is the rising incidence of iatrogenic POI [6]. Improved survival following malignant diseases has led to increasing numbers of women experiencing the long-term effects of cancer treatments. A recent cohort study estimated the incidence of POI, both spontaneous and iatrogenic, at 7.4% [7]. The risk of POI varies by ethnicity, ranging from 0.1% in Japanese to 1% in Caucasian and 1.4% in African American and Hispanic groups [8]. Environmental factors such as cigarette smoking and poverty were associated with an increased risk of idiopathic POI. In contrast, certain factors related to ovulation, such as late menarche, irregular menstruation, and longer breastfeeding seem to reduce the risk of POI [9]. The familial form of POI is rare, representing 4–31% of all cases of POI [10–12]. Morris DH et al. (2011) reported that women were around six times more likely to have early menopause if their mother (odd ratio [OR], 6.2; $p < 0.001$) or older sister (OR, 5.5; $p < 0.001$) also experienced early menopause [13].

2. Objective

In this comprehensive review, we aim to provide an overview of the current knowledge of the identifiable causes leading to POI development and the recent advances in the management of its consequences in terms of long-term complications as well as in terms of infertility concerns.

3. Methods

Literature search strategy: Using the MEDLINE database and Google Scholar, we conducted a comprehensive literature search to identify relevant publications on menstrual cycle disorders associated with premature ovarian insufficiency. The keyword combinations include "premature ovarian insufficiency," "primary ovarian failure," "hypergonadotropic amenorrhea," "hypergonadotropic hypogonadism," and "early menopause."

Selection criteria: The search was restricted to articles that were published up to May 2018 in English language and that assessed at least one of the following aspects of the condition: "epidemiology," "diagnosis," "etiology," "long-term consequences," "hormonal replacement therapy," "infertility management," and "prediction."

Data synthesis and analysis: The conclusions and the interpretation of the findings were based on our personal experience. In addition, we provided some clinical recommendations and guidelines about the management of patients experiencing premature or early menopause based on the expertise of prestigious scientific societies such as the European Society for Human Reproduction and Embryology (ESHRE) and the American Society for Reproductive Medicine (ASRM). Statistical testing was not conducted.

4. Diagnosis

Current studies have failed to determine specific biomarkers or signs/symptoms of POI that will accurately predict when menopause will occur. Some women with POI may not experience any specific symptoms particularly in the idiopathic form of the largest etiology, which may delay the establishment of the diagnosis.

One study reported that over 50% of patients with POI had seen at least three clinicians before the diagnosis was made, and in 25% the diagnosis took more than 5 years [14]. Before puberty, the clinical picture is characterized by absent menarche, and pubertal delay results in absent sexual maturation. After puberty, the typical disorder is characterized by the loss of menstrual regularity (oligomenorrhea or amenorrhea) in young women for 3 or more consecutive months and often associated with symptoms of estrogen deficiency such as vasomotor symptoms which are similar to those observed with the onset of menopause, such as hot flushes, insomnia, nervousness, irritability, loss of libido, vaginal dryness, dyspareunia, etc. Female infertility is a common concern, as only 5–10% of the patients will conceive spontaneously [15]. POI may be part of other syndromic features: autoimmune polyendocrinopathy-candidiasis-ectodermal dystrophy, blepharophimosis-ptosis-epicanthus inversus syndrome, carbohydrate-deficient glycoprotein syndromes, galactosemia, Turner syndrome, and PHP I [16].

Additionally, patients can experience long-term consequences of hypoestrogenism, including low bone density (osteoporosis) [17], cardiovascular diseases [18], and neurocognitive disorders [19]. For the biochemical confirmation, follicle-stimulating hormone (FSH) levels are used as the gold standard in establishing a diagnosis of POI. Two serum FSH levels in the menopausal range should be obtained at least a month apart (**BOX 1**) [27]. However, there is a lack of consensus on adequate cutoff levels used to define hypergonadotropism. No follicles were found in ovarian biopsies when FSH levels are above 33 and 40 mIU/ml in women with primary and secondary amenorrhea, respectively [20]. Some women with POI express FSH levels lower than these proposed cutoff values, particularly women with autoantibodies. La Marca et al. (2009) found that women with POI due to steroidogenic cell autoimmunity had significantly lower FSH levels (n = 26, median 37 mIU/ml) compared with idiopathic POI (median 99 mIU/ml) (P = 0.001) [21]. Furthermore, estradiol (E2) levels are typically low, with a level of 50 pg/ml in women with absent or nonfunctioning follicles [22]. Antimullerian hormone (AMH) is currently the most convenient predictor of ovarian reserve. Very low AMH levels seem to play a role in predicting age at menopause [23, 24].

Younger than 40 years of age

Oligo/amenorrhea for at least 4 months

Two FSH levels in the menopausal range, obtained at least a month apart

Data from [27].

Box 1. Criteria to establish the diagnosis of premature ovarian insufficiency.

Test	Implications	
	Positive test	**Negative test**
Genetic/Chromosomal		
Karyotyping (for diagnosis of Turner syndrome)	Refer to endocrinologist, cardiologist and geneticist	A second analysis of the karyotype in epithelial cells (in case of high clinical suspicion)
Test for Y-chromosomal material	Discuss gonadectomy with the patient	
Fra-X	Refer to geneticist	
Autosomal genetic testing[1]		
Antibodies2		
ACA/21OH antibodies	Refer to endocrinologist	Re-test in case of clinical signs
TPO-Ab	Test TSH every year	or symptoms

[1]not at present indicated in women with POI, unless there is evidence suggesting a specific mutation (e.g. BPES).
[2]POI of unknown cause or if an immune disorder is suspected.
Data from [25].

Table 1. Summary of diagnostic workup.

The differential diagnosis is based on the exclusion of other causes of primary and secondary amenorrhea, for example, pregnancy, polycystic ovarian syndrome, hypothalamic-pituitary disease (pituitary tumors, hyperprolactinemia, Kallmann syndrome), hypothalamic amenorrhea (induced by stress, intensive exercise, anorexia, weight loss, fasting, and severe diseases), endocrine disorders (hyperthyroidism, hypothyroidism, and Cushing syndrome), and vaginal/uterus anatomical abnormalities, such as Rokitansky syndrome or Asherman syndrome. Once the diagnosis has been confirmed, second-line investigations to look for an underlying cause should be considered which may have implications for the individualization of the management **Table 1** [25].

5. Etiology

Three potential mechanisms can be associated with POI, that is, a congenital decrease in primordial follicles, accelerated follicular atresia, and an inability to recruit primordial follicles [26]. The known causes of POI are wide ranging and can be divided into spontaneous and iatrogenic categories.

5.1. Spontaneous POI

Most cases of spontaneous POI are idiopathic despite the diagnostic advances [27] but may be also due to genetic causes, autoimmune disorders, metabolic dysfunction, enzyme deficiencies, toxins, or infections [27–29].

5.1.1. Genetic causes of POI

The normal ovarian function requires the presence of many intact genes functionally normally and in a coordinated fashion. Chromosomal abnormalities are found in around 10–12% of women with POI, of which the majority is X chromosomal abnormalities [30]. An increasing number of studies have documented autosomal involvement. The incidence of chromosomal abnormalities is higher in women with primary amenorrhea (21%) than in those presenting with secondary amenorrhea (11%) [31].

5.1.1.1. X Chromosome defects

Both the short and long arms of the X chromosome appear to play important roles.

X Chromosome defects usually involve either complete deletion of one X (Turner syndrome) or partial deletions, duplications, and balanced translocations between the X and autosomal chromosomes. Females lacking an X chromosome as well as those showing an extra X chromosome are predisposed to developing POI. Monosomy X (45X), known as Turner syndrome, is due to the loss of the second sex chromosome and affects 1 in 2500 live-born female infants and has a frequency of 4–5% in POI [32]. In phenotypic women, Turner syndrome is associated with short stature, gonadal dysgenesis, and primary amenorrhea. In women with Tuner syndrome, oocyte loss usually begins early in childhood as a result of accelerated follicle atresia [33]. The vast majority of pregnancies with this karyotype end in spontaneous miscarriage, and it is argued that the surviving individuals most likely carry some degree of mosaicism [34]. In mosaic Turner syndrome (45X/46XX), patients have a milder phenotype and may present later with secondary amenorrhea and hypergonadotropic hypogonadism. Trisomy X (47XXX) is caused by nondisjunction of the X chromosome during meiosis. It is the most common form of aneuploidy, occurring in 1:900 women. About 1.5–3.8% patients with POI had the triple X [30, 35] and may manifest in many mosaic forms, that is, 45X/47XXX, 46XX/47XXX, or 47XXX/48XXXX [36]. The presence of three X chromosomes presumably leads to meiotic disturbance and, secondarily, ovarian failure. X Chromosome deletions associated with POI are more common than translocations. At present, the microdeletions are not normally identified by conventional karyotyping and so often go unrecognized. Krauss et al. reported in 1987 a family in which one woman and two girls, with early menopause, had a deletion of the long arm of the X chromosome (Xq21–Xq27) [37]. Cytogenetic and molecular analyses of POI women carrying a balanced X-autosome translocation allowed the identification of a "critical region" for the ovarian development and function on the long arm of the X chromosome from Xq13.3 to q27. Various deletions or translocations occurring within this region and also on the short arm of the X chromosome have been associated with POI [38, 39]. POI can also be associated with the Xq isochromosome which occurs when the centromere splits abnormally in the transverse plane instead of the longitudinal plane. The resulting chromosome pair contains structurally identical arms with identical genes. The isochromosome for the long arm (q) is the most common X structural abnormality. These patients present with streak gonads and Turner-like characteristics which are rare causes of POI [40].

5.1.1.2. *Single-gene defects*

The fragile X syndrome is an X-linked dominant genetic disorder that is a leading cause of mental retardation and autism. Women exhibiting extended repeats of the CGG trinucleotide sequence may be classified as having the permutation (55–199 repeats) or the full condition (>200 repeats). There is an association, although nonlinear, between the number of repeats and the severity of the condition. The fragile site of the X chromosome contains a (CGG) repeat in the 5′ region of the gene. In normal variants, the trinucleotide repeat ranges from 6 to 55 repeats.

The syndrome occurs when the number of the repeats exceeds 200, being denominated as full mutation alleles. The fragile X mental retardation 1 (FMR1) gene premutation, mapped at position Xq27.3 on the X chromosome, is the most frequently identified single-gene mutation associated with POI outside the Xq POI critical region. It has been shown that females carrying a premutation have up to 23% rate of POI and experience menopause 5 years earlier than average [41]. The FMR1 premutation has been identified in 11% of familial POI and 3% of sporadic cases [42–44], and therefore, screening for the FMR1 premutation is usually recommended in women diagnosed with POI to identify those patients and family members who may be at risk of having children with fragile X syndrome. Those with identified premutation should be referred for family genetic counseling. *The bone morphogenetic protein 15 gene* (BMP15) *is a member of transforming growth factor beta (TGF-ß) superfamily and is located on the short arm of the X chromosome (Xp11.2) within the Xp POI critical region* [45, 46]. It is an *oocyte-specific folliculogenesis growth differentiation factor (GDF) and appears to have a vital role in folliculogenesis and granulosa cell growth.*

Approximately 1.5–12% of POI is associated with *BMP15* gene mutation [47–50].

Fragile site, folic acid type, rare (*FRAXE*)/fragile site mental retardation 2 gene (*FMR2*) has been described in patients who have the cytogenetic changes of fragile X syndrome but who are *FMR1* mutation negative. It was found at Xq28 and found to be folate sensitive [51].

5.1.1.3. *Autosomal genetic defects*

While several genes relevant to ovarian function lie on the X chromosome, autosomal genes also appear to be involved in the development of POI [26].

In recent years, attention has focused on genes that are known to play a role in folliculogenesis and ovarian function. Oocyte-specific gene expression is necessary for primordial follicle formation and their subsequent differentiation into primary follicles. A number of autosomal genes have been suggested as a causative factor of POI. For some of these genes, mutations are identified, while others are listed as candidate genes with a need for further investigation. The genes with identified mutations that could result in POI are genes involved in folliculogenesis (NR5A1, NOBOX, FIGLA, and FOXL2), folliculogenesis growth factors (GDF9 and inhibin A), sex hormone function (*CYP17A1, CYP19*, FSH/ luteinizing hormone (LH) receptors, and *NR5A1*) [26, 38], or genes identified in syndromes often associated with POI such as Bloom syndrome BLM 15q26.1 [52], Ataxia telangiectasia,

A-T. ATM 11q22-q23 [53], Werner syndrome WRN 8p12 [54], and Rothmund-Thomson syndrome RTS 8q24.3 [55]. Given that the conventional approaches have had limited success in finding causative genes, further research and new techniques on the genetic background of POI including genome-wide analysis in affected families may change this recommendation in the near future.

5.1.2. Autoimmune causes of POI

Anti-ovarian antibodies are reported in POI by several studies, but their specificity and pathogenic role are questionable. Autoimmune diseases are estimated to be involved in the pathogenesis of up to 5% of POI cases. Adrenal autoimmunity is thought to account for 60–80% of autoimmune POI [56], and there is a strong association between the presence of adrenal antibodies and a diagnosis of autoimmune lymphocytic oophoritis [57]. The evidence of oophoritis is rare (<3%) in POI in the absence of adrenal involvement [16]. The presence of many other autoantibodies has been investigated such as ovarian and other steroidogenic cell autoantibodies; however, reliable markers to diagnose non-adrenal autoimmunity are yet to be identified [56]. POI can be associated with endocrine (thyroid, hypoparathyroid, diabetes mellitus, and hypophysitis) and non-endocrine diseases (chronic candidiasis, idiopathic thrombocytopenic purpura, vitiligo, alopecia, autoimmune hemolytic anemia, pernicious anemia, systemic lupus erythematosus (SLE), rheumatoid arthritis, Crohn's disease, Sjogren syndrome, primary biliary cirrhosis, and chronic active hepatitis) (**Table 2**) [16, 58, 59]. POI may be part of the autoimmune polyglandular syndromes (APS) when accompanied by other autoimmune endocrinopathies. POI is more common with APS types I and III than with APS type II [60].

5.1.3. Metabolic causes of POI

A number of inherited enzymatic pathway disorders have been associated with ovarian follicular dysfunction leading to POI such as galactose-1-phosphate uridylyltransferase deficiency (galactosemia) [61], 19, carbohydrate-deficient glycoprotein deficiency [62], 17α-hydroxylase/17,20 desmolase deficiency [63], and aromatase mutations [64] where there is biochemical damage of the ovary and autoimmune regulator which triggers autoimmune damage. However, the strength of evidence linking each anomaly with POI is variable.

Endocrine	Hypo/hyperthyroidism, Hypoparathyroidism, Diabetes mellitus type II, Hypophysitis, Addison's disease.
Non-endocrine	Idiopathic thrombocytemic purpura, Chronic candidiasis, Vitiligo, Alopecia, Hemolytic or Pernicious anemia,
	Systemic lupus erythematodes, Rheumatoid arthritis, Cirrhosis, Sjogren's sy, Primary biliary cirrhosis, Chronic hepatitis etc.

Data from [16, 58, 59].

Table 2. Endocrine and non-endocrine diseases associated with premature ovarian failure.

5.2. Induced POI

The induced POI may result from damage to the ovaries, such as that caused by iatrogenic agents like chemotherapy, radiotherapy, pelvic surgery, and also environmental toxic agents.

5.2.1. Cancer therapy

There is an overall increase in cancer prevalence followed by an increase in long-term survival of the affected patients these days compared to the past. The 5-year survival rate for childhood, adolescent, and young adult cancer currently exceeds 80% [65]. Medical treatment for neoplastic conditions can be associated with POI. Chemotherapy and radiotherapy are well-documented causes of POI.

Chemotherapy induces apoptosis of mature ovarian follicles, and histological studies have shown fibrosis, vascular damage, and reduced follicle numbers. The gonadotoxic effect of chemotherapy is drug and dose dependent [66]. Alkylating agents have been shown to be gonadotoxic [67]. The prepubertal ovary is relatively resistant to this form of gonadotoxicity [67]. The risk of developing POI after radiotherapy is dependent on the radiation therapy field (abdominal pelvic, total body irradiation) and on dose and age [68–70]. Transposition of the ovaries in young women requiring pelvic irradiation helps in preserving their ovarian function.

5.2.2. Pelvic surgery

Aside from surgical menopause due to bilateral oophorectomy, limited evidence suggests that pelvic surgery is maybe associated with POI such as hysterectomy [71], tubal sterilization [72], or both ovarian surgery for endometrioma and endometriosis [73] presumably due to damage to ovarian blood vessels as a result of the surgical procedure. Research has now also linked ovarian drilling for polycystic ovary syndrome and removal of endometriotic cysts to an earlier age at menopause [74, 75].

5.2.3. Toxins

The increasing prevalence of POI in recent years might be also due to an increase in presently unidentified environmental toxic agents. However, studies examining the cause and effect of the chemical substances and POI in humans are rare.

Chang et al. (2007) found that cigarette smoking was associated with an increased risk of POI (OR = 1.82 [1.03–3.23]) [76]. Many other endocrine-disrupting substances have been also suggested to be ovotoxic and influencing the age of menopause such as 2-bromopropane [76], vinylcyclohexene diepoxide (VCD) [77], polycyclic aromatic hydrocarbons (PAHs) [77], etc., but they are not readily considered as diagnosable causes of POI. Further research is warranted to clarify in which toxicants affect human reproduction and how insufficiency with FSH values is found in the menopausal range [78].

5.2.4. Infections

It has been indicated that many viral infections can be followed by POI, but only mumps oophoritis has been directly linked to POI, explaining 3–7% of POI cases [79]. Other potential causes of POI include tuberculosis, malaria, varicella, and *Shigella* [80]. More recently, there has been suggestion that human immunodeficiency virus (HIV) infection (or antiviral therapy) can lead to POI. However, a recent systematic review revealed nonconclusive evidence due to a significant methodological limitation with available data [81].

6. Management

Patients must be provided with adequate information (education, understanding, and counseling). Management should address the following aspects: psychology support, ovarian hormone replacement for the prevention of long-term complications, and therapy for fertility.

6.1. Psychologic support

The diagnosis of POI is an extremely devastating psychologic disturbance [35]. Some will experience a range of emotions such as high levels of depression and low levels of self-esteem with negative effects on sexuality [82], and providers should offer support regarding infertility, altered self-image, and sexual dysfunction. Patients may benefit from referral to a psychologist and support groups [83].

6.2. Hormone replacement therapy

Hormone replacement therapy (HRT) remains the cornerstone of treatment for relief of menopausal symptoms (including vasomotor instability, sexual dysfunction, mood, fatigue, and skin issues) and prevention of long-term morbidity and earlier mortality related to prolonged estrogen deficiency [84]. The results of Women's Health Initiative (WHI) study should not be applied to young women with POI [85, 86]. In contrast with women older than 50s, POI is a pathologic condition in which young women have low serum E2 levels compared with their peers. For young women with E2 deficiency, hormone therapy is indeed a "replacement," whereas in women with normal menopause, hormone therapy is hormone "extension." Physiological replacement of ovarian steroid hormones until the age of 50 years (the average age of natural menopause) is generally accepted as routine, unless a specific contraindication exists, such as an estrogen-dependent malignancy. At present, very little evidence exists regarding the optimum method of hormone replacement, and options include both the combined oral contraceptive pill (COC) and hormone replacement. Data regarding the optimal estradiol levels in POI are lacking; however, the average serum estradiol level during the menstrual cycle in normal women is approximately 100 pg/ml [87]. Transdermal and transvaginal replacement of 100 μg/day of estradiol achieves physiologic blood levels in this range and provides adequate symptomatic relief. The transdermal route has the advantage of avoidance of first-pass hepatic metabolism and appears to be free of an excess risk of thrombosis compared with oral estrogen [88–90]. To reduce the risk of endometrial hyperplasia, 5–10 mg of medroxyprogesterone acetate should be given for 12 days of the month, provided that the uterus is present and intact [90, 91]. However, the optimum type of progestogen is unclear. With the use of this regimen, most of women will develop monthly withdrawal bleeding, which may be psychologically important to the patient. The COC is also commonly used as hormone replacement in POI. However, they should not be recommended as first-line hormone replacement. Indeed, they result in supraphysiological doses of sex steroid hormones and are associated with an increased risk of thromboembolic events related to the first-pass effect on the liver [27]. Androgen replacement could be carefully considered for women who have persistent fatigue and low libido despite optimized estrogen replacement [92]. Transdermal testosterone administration and dehydroepiandrosterone treatment are two of the options for androgen replacement in these women [93]. Importantly, this should be performed with great caution and for relatively short periods until more data are available. When there has been no spontaneous start to puberty or progression of breast development, many options for HRT are suggested for puberty induction. However, systemic administration of increasing doses of estradiol, preferably by transdermal application, is the only form of therapy to achieve natural levels of estradiol in blood and mimic normal estradiol physiology in adolescence and adulthood [94, 95]. Patients who do not want to get pregnant should be offered contraception due to the 5–10% chance of spontaneous conception. Women with untreated POI are at increased risk of developing long-term comorbidities such as cardiovascular disease [96], metabolic syndrome [97], osteoporosis, dementia, cognitive impairment, Parkinsonism, reduced sexual function, and psychological well-being. Untreated POI can induce specific increase in mortality rate due to complications of the prolonged estrogen deficiency compared to those with a menopause after the age of 50 years [98]. The main reason for shortened life expectancy in women with POI is cardiovascular disease. The Framingham study was one of the first to show a higher incidence of cardiovascular disease among postmenopausal women than age-matched women who were premenopausal [99]. A number of studies have subsequently demonstrated higher rates of coronary artery disease, higher rates of heart failure, and higher rates of mortality in women reaching menopause before 40–45 years of age, and it has been demonstrated that this impairment was reversed by estrogen replacement [100]. Compared with control women, women with premature ovarian insufficiency have reduced bone mineral density. The prevalence of osteoporosis in POI appears to be in the range of 8–14% [101]. Multiple studies have shown that the lower bone mineral density (BMD) seen in women with POI is associated with significantly higher overall fracture risk, and this has been associated with the presence, degree, and duration of estrogen deficiency. Studies on fracture risk in early menopause compared to natural menopause have demonstrated that fracture rates are reduced among women with POI or early menopause who are treated with the use of HRT [101–103]. Early data demonstrate an increased risk of cognitive impairment [104]. Some studies suggest that estrogen is neuroprotective. The Mayo Clinic Cohort Study of Oophorectomy and Aging demonstrated that women who underwent either unilateral or bilateral oophorectomy before the onset of the menopause had an increased risk of cognitive impairment or dementia [105] and Parkinsonism [104] compared to controls and that this risk increased with younger age at oophorectomy. They also demonstrated a protective role for estrogen replacement in women with bilateral oophorectomy when taken until at least 50 years of age. A similar finding was noted in a Danish cohort study, revealing an increased risk of dementia in women undergoing oophorectomy prior to the age of 50 years, with a similar trend of increasing risk with earlier age at oophorectomy [106].

6.3. Fertility

6.3.1. Spontaneous conception and POI

For many women with POI, infertility is the most devastating aspect of the diagnosis.

Fertility of women with POI is severely diminished, but unlike menopause, POI may be accompanied with spontaneous ovarian activity and natural pregnancies in approximately 5–10% [107]. Currently, no fertility treatment has been found to effectively increase fertility in women with POI including estrogens [108–110], 5-dehydroepiandrosterone (DHEA) [111], corticosteroids [112], and azathioprine [113].

6.3.2. Assisted reproductive technology (ART) and POI

6.3.2.1. Oocyte donation

The only proven therapy for obtaining a pregnancy in patients with POI is fertilization of a donor oocyte. At present IVF with donor oocytes confers the highest chance of pregnancy for women with POI with high success rates of around 40–50% per cycle.

The pregnancy rate from oocyte donation is not greatly affected by the recipient's age [114, 115].

6.3.2.2. Fertility management of the Turner syndrome

There are special considerations regarding oocyte donation in women with Turner syndrome. If pregnancy is desired, hormone replacement therapy can be initiated to increase uterine size, followed by assisted reproductive technology, namely, in vitro fertilization with an oocyte donor. However, coexisting cardiac abnormalities associated with Turner syndrome may increase the risk of pregnancy for the mother, and therefore this type of approach to achieve pregnancy is strongly discouraged [116, 117]. Should a Y chromosome be identified with or without an SRY gene mutation, the patient should be counseled about the risk of development of a gonadal tumor, and gonadectomy should be advised [118, 119].

6.3.2.3. Fertility preservation and POI

Fertility preservation may also be considered for women at risk of POI; in young women who require cancer treatments, including chemotherapy, radiotherapy, and surgery; or for those who have a strong family history of POI. Options for fertility preservation include ovarian transposition, oocyte or embryo cryopreservation, and ovarian tissue cryopreservation. Ovarian transposition remains the standard of care for women undergoing pelvic radiation, although it has been suggested that it may be combined with ovarian tissue cryopreservation. Embryo cryopreservation remains the most successful technique, with success rates approaching that of fresh embryo transfer [120, 121]. Live birth rates of approximately 30% per embryo transfer have been reported, depending on the age of the patient [120]. The success of oocyte cryopreservation has also improved significantly in recent years, and birth rates similar to that of fresh oocytes have been reported [122]. Oocyte cryopreservation is a potential option for women without a partner. Since the initial report of successful pregnancy following ovarian tissue cryopreservation and subsequent transplant in 2000 [123], there has been increasing success with the technique [124, 125].

7. Prediction and genetic counseling

Contrary to the induced POI occurring in cancer survivors, the spontaneous POI particularly the idiopathic form is still difficult to be predicted in the general population. Low circulating AMH level is currently thought to be the most reliable measure of reduced ovarian reserve and may play a role in predicting age at menopause [23]. Sowers et al. (2008) have shown that AMH starts declining 5 years before the final menstrual period. All these observations suggest a potential role for AMH in screening women at high risk for POI and in well woman screening programs [24]. Autoantibody screening, for anti-adrenal, anti-ovarian, and antithyroid antibodies, is also recommended [25]. Genetic counseling is nowadays recommended for several reasons, when a genetic form of POI is suspected or identified. The prevalence of familial POI has been reported to be between 4 and 31% of cases in various series [126–129]. The early diagnosis of familial POI will provide the opportunity to predict the likelihood of early menopause and allow other reproductive choices to be made, such as freezing embryos or having children earlier. Karyotyping and screening for the FMR1 gene permutation are especially important in younger patients with or without mental retardation or when a female is born from a family with female members affected with POI. The review of McConkie-Rosell states that approximately 13–24% of women who are fragile X premutation carriers (identified through families with fragile X syndrome) have POI [130].

8. Future

Continued advances in DNA sequencing techniques will facilitate finding additional genes responsible for POI in other portions of the genome. Besides, the future holds the possibility of restoring ovarian function with ovarian or oogonial stem cell (OSC) therapy which may open the door to novel fertility preservation strategies for women with both age-related and POI [131]. More recently, Kawamura et al. (2013) have successfully promoted follicle growth, retrieved mature oocytes, and performed IVF. Following embryo transfer, a healthy baby was delivered [132]. This in vitro activation (IVA) approach has been reproduced by a group in Zhengzhou University, China, with two cases [133]. Up to the summer of 2018, there were more than one dozen of successful cases.

9. Summary

The POI represents a continuum of declining ovarian function with intermittent ovulation in women below the age of 40 years resulting usually in an earlier than average menopause. Its incidence is gradually increasing secondary to the improved survival of young women with cancer. In most cases, the etiology is unknown, but known causes include genetic disorders, particularly involving the X chromosome, associations with autoimmune diseases, cancer therapy, pelvic surgery, and also environmental toxic agents. A timely diagnosis of POI is the main challenge. The typical disorder is characterized by the loss of regular menstrual cycles, and the diagnosis is confirmed by the detection of menopausal-level serum gonadotropins in repeated blood tests. Second-line investigations should be directed by specific clinical indications. Regardless of the etiology, patients with POI are estrogen deficient. The aims of HRT extend beyond simply symptom relief to levels that support cardiovascular, bone, and cognitive health. Only 5–10% of women with POI may conceive spontaneously. Currently, there are no proven treatments to improve ovarian function, and only the use of donor eggs with IVF confers the highest chance of pregnancy. However, in women with Turner syndrome, this approach is strongly discouraged. To date, the prediction of POI is difficult in the general population. However, in women at risk of POI particularly those who have a strong family history of POI, or require cancer treatments, a screening program will provide the opportunity to predict the likelihood of early onset menopause and to consider fertility preservation as well. Further research is needed particularly in idiopathic POI to identify mechanisms and specific molecular defects which may offer a better opportunity for early therapeutic interventions.

Financial support and sponsorship

Nil.

Author details

Abdelhamid Benmachiche[1*] and Amel Dammene Debbih[2]

*Address all correspondence to: benmachiche@gmail.com

1 Center for Reproductive Medicine, Clinique Ibn Rochd, Constantine, Algeria,

2 Faculty of Medicine of Algiers, Bologhine University Hospital Center, Algiers, Algeria

References

[1] Coulam CB, Adamson SC, Annegers JF. Incidence of premature ovarian failure. Obstetrics and Gynecology. 1986;**67**(4):604-606

[2] Webber L, Davies M, Anderson R, et al. ESHRE Guideline: Management of Women With Premature Ovarian Insufficiency. Grimbergen, Belgium: European Society of Human Reproduction and Embryology; 2015

[3] Welt CK. Primary ovarian insufficiency: A more accurate term for premature ovarian failure. Clinical Endocrinology. 2008;**68**:499-509

[4] Kalu E, Panay N. Spontaneous premature ovarian failure: Management challenges. Gynecological Endocrinology. 2008;**24**:273-279

[5] Sowers MF et al. Premature menopause in a multi-ethnic population study of the menopause transition. Human Reproduction. 2003;**18**:199-206

[6] Panay N, Fenton A. Premature ovarian failure: A growing concern. Climacteric. 2008; **11**:1-3

[7] Islam R, Cartwright R. The impact of premature ovarian failure on quality of life: Results from the UK 1958 Birth Cohort. Presented at: 27th Annual Meeting of ESHRE; 3-6 July 2011; Stockholm. Sweden

[8] Luborsky JL, Meyer P, Sowers MF, et al. Premature menopause in a multi-ethnic population study of the menopause transition. Human Reproduction. 2003;**18**:199-206

[9] Chang SH, Kim CS, Lee KS, et al. Premenopausal factors influencing premature ovarian failure and early menopause. Maturitas. 2007;**58**:19-30

[10] Conway GS, Kaltsas G, Patel A, Davies MC, Jacobs HS. Characterization of idiopathic premature ovarian failure. Fertility and Sterility. 1996;**64**:337-341

[11] Cramer DW, Xu H, Harlow BL. Family history as a predictor of early menopause. Fertility and Sterility. 1995;**64**:740-745

[12] Torgerson DJ, Thomas RE, Reid DM. Mothers and daughters menopausal ages: Is there a link? European Journal of Obstetrics, Gynecology, and Reproductive Biology. 1997;**74**:63-66

[13] Morris DH, Jones ME, Schoemaker MJ, Ashworth A, Swerdlow AJ. Familial concordance for age at natural menopause: Results from the breakthrough generations study. Menopause. 2011;**18**:956-961

[14] Alzubaidi NH, Chapin HL, Vanderhoof VH, et al. Meeting the needs of young women with secondary amenorrhea and spontaneous premature ovarian failure. Obstetrics and Gynecology. 2002;**99**:720-725

[15] McKinlay SM, Brambilla DJ, Posner JG. The normal menopause transition. Maturitas. 1992;**14**:103-115

[16] Hoek A, Schoemaker J, Drexhage HA. Premature ovarian failure and ovarian autoimmunity. Endocrine Reviews. 1997;**18**:107-134

[17] Gallagher JC. Effect of early menopause on bone mineral density and fractures. Menopause. 2007;**14**:567-571

[18] Atsma F, Bartelink ML, Grobbee DE, van der Schouw YT. Postmenopausal status and early menopause as independent risk factors for cardiovascular disease: A meta-analysis. Menopause. 2006;**13**:265-279

[19] van der Stege JG, Groen H, van Zadelhoff SJ, Lambalk CB, Braat DD, van Kasteren YM, et al. Decreased androgen concentrations and diminished general and sexual well-being in women with premature ovarian failure. Menopause. 2008;**15**:23-31

[20] Goldenberg RL, Grodin JM, Rodbard D, Ross GT. Gonadotropins in women with amenorrhea. The use of plasma follicle-stimulating hormone to differentiate women with and without ovarian follicles. American Journal of Obstetrics and Gynecology. 1973 Aug 1;**116**(7):1003-1012

[21] La Marca A, Marzotti S, Brozzetti A, Stabile G, Artenisio AC, Bini V, et al. Primary ovarian insufficiency due to steroidogenic cell autoimmunity is associated with a preserved pool of functioning follicles. The Journal of Clinical Endocrinology and Metabolism. 2009 Oct;**94**(10):3816-3823. DOI: 10.1210/jc.2009-0817. Epub 2009 Jul 21

[22] Rebar RW. Premature ovarian failure. Obstetrics and Gynaecology. 2009;**113**:1355-1363. DOI: 10.1097/AOG.0b013e3181a66843

[23] Tehrani A, Shakeri N, Azizi F. Whether age at menopause is predictable using serum anti-Mullerian hormone concentration? Human Reproduction. 2010;**25**:i1-i3

[24] Sowers MR, Eyvazzadeh AD, McConnell D, et al. Antimullerian hormone and inhibin B in the definition of ovarian aging and the menopause transition. The Journal of Clinical Endocrinology and Metabolism. 2008;**93**:3478-3483

[25] Webber L, Davies M, Anderson R, Bartlett J, Braat D, Cartwright B, et al. Vermeulen N ESHRE guideline: Management of women with premature ovarian insufficiency. European Society for Human Reproduction and Embryology (ESHRE) Guideline Group on POI. Human Reproduction. 2016 May;**31**(5):926-937

[26] Persani L, Rossetti R, Cacciatore C. Genes involved in human premature ovarian failure. Journal of Molecular Endocrinology. 2010;**45**:257-279

[27] Nelson LM. Clinical practice. Primary ovarian insufficiency. The New England Journal of Medicine. 2009;**360**:606-614

[28] North American Menopause Society. Menopause Practice: A Clinician's Guide. 3rd ed. Cleveland, OH: North American Menopause Society; 2007

[29] Santoro N. Mechanisms of premature ovarian failure. Annales d'Endocrinologie. 2003; **64**:87-92

[30] Kalantari H, Madani T, Zari Moradi S, Mansouri Z, Almadani N, Gourabi H, Mohseni Meybodi A. Cytogenetic analysis of 179 Iranian women with premature ovarian failure. Gynecological Endocrinology. 2013;**29**:588-591

[31] Jiao X, Qin C, Li J, Qin Y, Gao X, Zhang B, et al. Cytogenetic analysis of 531 Chinese women with premature ovarian failure. Human Reproduction. 2012;**7**:2201-2207

[32] Luisi S, Orlandini C, Regini C, Pizzo A, Vellucci F, Petraglia F. Premature ovarian management. Journal of Endocrinological Investigation. 2015;**38**:597-603

[33] Bianco B, Nunes Lipay MV, Guedes AD, Verreschi IT. Clinical implications of the detection of Y-chromosome mosaicism in Turner's syndrome: Report of 3 cases. Fertility and Sterility. 2008 Oct;**90**(4):1197.e17-1197.e20

[34] Hook EB, Warburton D. Turner syndrome revisited: Review of new data supports the hypothesis that all viable 45, X cases are cryptic mosaics with a rescue cell line, implying an origin by mitotic loss. Human Genetics. 2014;**133**(4):417-424

[35] Goswami R, Goswami D, Kabra M, Gupta N, Dubey S, Dadhwal V. Prevalence of the triple X syndrome in phenotypically normal women with premature ovarian failure and its association with autoimmune thyroid disorders. Fertility and Sterility. 2003;**4**:1052-1054

[36] Villanueva AL, Rebar RW. Triple-X syndrome and premature ovarian failure. Obstetrics and Gynecology. 1983;**62**(3 Suppl):70s-73s

[37] Krauss CM, Turksoy RN, Atkins L, Laughlin C, Brown LG, Page DC. Familial premature ovarian failure due to an inter-stitial deletion of the long arm of the X chromosome. The New England Journal of Medicine. 1987;**317**:125-131

[38] Zhao H, Chen ZJ. Genetic association studies in female reproduction: From candidate-gene approaches to genome-wide mapping. Molecular Human Reproduction. 2013;**19**: 644-654

[39] Cox L, Liu JH. Primary ovarian insufficiency: An update. International Journal of Women's Health. 2014;**6**:235-243

[40] Simpson JL. Gonadal dysgenesis and abnormalities of the human sex chromosomes: Current status of phenotypic-karyotypic correlations. Birth Defects Original Article Series. 1975;**11**:23-59

[41] Willemsen R, Levenga J, Oostra B. CGG repeat in the FMR1 gene: Size matters. Clinical Genetics. 2011;**80**:214-225

[42] Marozzi A, Vegetti W, Manfredini E, et al. Association between premature ovarian failure and fragile x premutation. Human Reproduction. 2000;**15**:197-202

[43] Murray A. Premature ovarian failure and the FMR1 gene. Seminars in Reproductive Medicine. 2000;**18**:59-66

[44] Bussani C, Papi L, Sestini R, et al. Premature ovarian failure and fragile X premutation: A study on 45 women. European Journal of Obstetrics, Gynecology, and Reproductive Biology. 2004;**112**:189-191

[45] Dube JL, Wang P, Elvin J, Lyons KM, Celeste AJ, Matzuk MM. The bone morphogenetic protein 15 gene is X-linked and expressed in oocytes. Molecular Endocrinology. 1998;**12**:1809-1817

[46] Aaltonen J, Laitinen MP, Vuojolainen K, Jaatinen R, Horelli-Kuitunen N, Seppa L, et al. Human growth differentiation factor 9 (GDF-9) and its novel homolog GDF-9B are

expressed in oocytes during early folliculogenesis. The Journal of Clinical Endocrinology and Metabolism. 1999;**84**:2744-2750

[47] Laissue P, Christin-Maitre S, Touraine P, et al. Mutations and sequence variants in GDF9 and BMP15 in patients with premature ovarian failure. European Journal of Endocrinology. 2006;**154**:739-744

[48] Di Pasquale E, Rossetti R, Marozzi A, et al. Identification of new variants of human BMP15 gene in a large cohort of women with premature ovarian failure. The Journal of Clinical Endocrinology and Metabolism. 2006;**91**:1976-1979

[49] Rossetti R, Di Pasquale E, Marozzi A, et al. BMP15 mutations associated with primary ovarian insufficiency cause a defective production of bioactive protein. Human Mutation. 2009;**30**:804-810

[50] Tiotiu D, Alvaro Mercadal B, Imbert R, et al. Variants of the BMP15 gene in a cohort of patients with premature ovarian failure. Human Reproduction. 2010;**25**:1581-1587

[51] Sutherland GR, Baker E. Characterisation of a new rare fragile site easily confused with the fragile X. Human Molecular Genetics. 1992;**1**:111-113

[52] Ellis NA, German J. Molecular genetics of Bloom's syndrome. Human Molecular Genetics. 1996;**5**:1457-1463

[53] Gatti RA, Boder E, Vinters HV, Sparkes RS, Norman A, Lange K. Ataxia-telangiectasia: An interdisciplinary approach to pathogenesis. Medicine. 1991;**2**:99-117

[54] Epstein CJ, Martin GM, Schultz AL, Motulsky AG. Werner's syndrome a review of its symptomatology, natural history, pathologic features, genetics and relationship to the natural aging process. Medicine. 1966;**3**:177-221

[55] Wang LL, Levy ML, Lewis RA, Chintagumpala MM, Lev D, Rogers M, et al. Clinical manifestations in a cohort of 41 Rothmund-Thomson syndrome patients. American Journal of Medical Genetics. 2001;**1**:11-17

[56] Silva CA, Yamakami LY, Aikawa NE, Araujo DB, Carvalho JF, Bonfa E. Autoimmune primary ovarian insufficiency. Autoimmunity Reviews. 2014;**13**:427-430

[57] Bakalov VK, Anasti JN, Calis KA, et al. Autoimmune oophoritis as a mechanism of follicular dysfunction in women with 46, XX spontaneous premature ovarian failure. Fertility and Sterility. 2005;**84**:958-965

[58] Rebar RW, Cedars MI. Hypergonadotrophic forms of amenorrhea in young women. Endocrinology and Metabolism Clinics of North America. 1992;**21**:173-191

[59] Betterle C, Dal Pra C, Mantero F, Zanchetta R. Autoimmune adrenal insufficiency and autoimmune polyendocrine syndromes: Autoantibodies, autoantigens, and their applicability in diagnosis and disease prediction. Endocrine Reviews. 2002;**23**:327-364

[60] Kauffman RP, Castracane VD. Premature ovarian failure associated with autoimmune polyglandular syndrome: Pathophysiological mechanisms and future fertility. Journal of Women's Health (2002). 2003;**12**:513-520

[61] Kaufman FR, Kogut MD, Donnell GN, Goebelsmann U, March C, Koch R. Hypergonadotrophic hypogonadism in female patients with galactosemia. The New England Journal of Medicine. 1981;**304**:994-998

[62] Bjursell C, Stibler H, Wahlström J, et al. Fine mapping of the gene for carbohydrate-deficient glycoprotein syndrome, type 1 (CDG1): Linkage disequilibrium and founder effect in Scandinavian families. Genomics. 1997;**39**:247-253

[63] Yanase T. 17α-hydroxylase/17, 20-lyse defects. The Journal of Steroid Biochemistry and Molecular Biology. 1995;**53**:153-157

[64] Mullis PE, Yoshimura N, Kuhlmann B, Lippuner K, Jaeger P, Harada H. Aromatase deficiency in a female who is compared heterozygote for two new point mutations in the P450arom gene: Impact of estrogens on hypergonadotrophic hypogonadism, multicystic ovaries, and bone densitometry in childhood. The Journal of Clinical Endocrinology and Metabolism. 1997;**82**:1739-1745

[65] Van Dorp W, Mulder RL, Kremer LCM, et al. Recommendations for premature ovarian insufficiency surveillance for female survivors of childhood, adolescent, and young adult cancer: A report from the international Late Effects of Childhood Cancer Guideline Harmonization Group in collaboration with the PanCareSurFupConsortium. Journal of Clinical Oncology. 2016;**34**:3440-3450

[66] Wallace WH. Oncofertility and preservation of reproductive capacity in children and young adults. Cancer. 2011;**117**:2301-2310

[67] Beerendonk CC, Braat DD. Present and future options for the preservation of fertility in female adolescents with cancer. Endocrine Development. 2005;**8**:166-175

[68] Lie Fong S, Laven JS, Hakvoort-Cammel FG, Schipper I, Visser JA, Themmen AP, et al. Assessment of ovarian reserve in adult childhood cancer survivors using anti-Mullerian hormone. Human Reproduction. 2009;**24**:982-990

[69] Wallace WH, Thomson AB, Saran F, Kelsey TW. Predicting age of ovarian failure after radiation to a field that includes the ovaries. International Journal of Radiation Oncology, Biology, Physics. 2005;**62**:738-744

[70] Gracia CR, Sammel MD, Freeman E, Prewitt M, Carlson C, Ray A, et al. Impact of cancer therapies on ovarian reserve. Fertility and Sterility. 2012;**97**:134-140. e131

[71] Siddle N, Sarrel P, Whitehead M. The effect of hysterectomy on the age at ovarian failure: Identification of a subgroup of women with premature loss of ovarian function and literature review. Fertility and Sterility. 1987;**47**:94-100

[72] Visvanathan N, Wyshak G. Tubal ligation, menstrual changes, and menopausal symptoms. Journal of Women's Health & Gender-Based Medicine. 2000;**9**:521-527

[73] Coccia ME, Rizzello F, Mariani G, Bulletti C, Palagiano A, Scarselli G. Ovarian surgery for bilateral endometriomas influences age at menopause. Human Reproduction. 2011;**26**:3000-3007

[74] Fenton A, Panay N. Does routine gynecological surgery contribute to an early menopause? Climacteric. 2012;**15**:1-2

[75] Api M. Is ovarian reserve diminished after laparoscopic ovarian drilling? Gynecological Endocrinology. 2009;**25**:159-165

[76] Koh JM, Kim CH, Hong SK, Lee KU, Kim YT, Kim OJ, et al. Primary ovarian failure caused by a solvent containing 2- bromopropane. European Journal of Endocrinology. 1998;**138**(5):554-556

[77] Kappeler CJ, Hoyer PB. vinylcyclohexene diepoxide: A model chemical for ovotoxicity. Systems Biology in Reproductive Medicine. 2012 Feb;**58**(1):57-62. DOI: 10.3109/19396368.2011.648820. 4

[78] Matkainen T. Aromatic hydrocarbon receptor-driven Bax gene expression. Nature Genetics. 2001;**28**:355-360. DOI: 10.1038/ng575

[79] Kokcu A. Premature ovarian failure from current perspective. Gynecological Endocrinology. 2010;**26**:555-562

[80] Morrison JC, Givens JR, Wiser WL, Fish SA. Mumps oophoritis: A cause of premature menopause. Fertility and Sterility. 1975;**26**:655-659

[81] Imai K, Sutton MY, Mdodo R, Del Rio C. HIV and menopause: A systematic review of the effects of HIV infection of age at menopause and the effects if menopause on response to antiretroviral therapy. Obstetrics and Gynecology International. 2013;**2013**:11. Article ID: 340309. http://dx.doi.org/10.1155/2013/340309

[82] Liao KL, Wood N, Conway GS. Premature menopause and psychological well-being. Journal of Psychosomatic Obstetrics and Gynaecology. 2000;**21**:167-174

[83] International Premature Ovarian Failure Association. Alexandria, VA, USA. Available from: http://www.pofsupport.org [Accessed: August 10, 2013]

[84] Rivera CM, Grossardt B, Rhodes D, et al. Increased cardiovascular mortality after early bilateral oophorectomy. Menopause. 2009;**16**:15-23

[85] Welt CK. Primary ovarian insufficiency: A more accurate term for premature ovarian failure. Clinical Endocrinology. 2009;**68**:449-509. DOI: 10. 1111/j.1365-2265.2007. 03073.x

[86] Rossouw JE, Anderson GL, Prentice RL, LaCroix AZ, Kooperberg C, Stefanick ML, et al. Risks and benefits of estrogen plus progestin in healthy postmenopausal women: Principal results from the women's health initiative randomized controlled trial. JAMA. 2002;**288**:321-333

[87] Mishell DR Jr, Nakamura RM, Crosignani PG, et al. Serum gonadotropin and steroid patterns during the normal menstrual cycle. American Journal of Obstetrics and Gynecology. 1971;**111**(1):60-65

[88] Scarabin PY, Alhenc-Gelas M, Plu-Bureau G, et al. Effects of oral and transdermal estrogen/progesterone regimens on blood coagulation and fibrinolysis in postmenopausal women. A randomized controlled trial. Arteriosclerosis, Thrombosis, and Vascular Biology. 1997;**17**(11):3071-3078

[89] Scarabin PY, Oger E, Plu-Bureau G. Differential association of oral and transdermal oestrogen replacement therapy with venous thromboembolism risk. Lancet. 2003; **362**(9382):428-432

[90] Canonico M, Oger E, Plu-Bureau G, et al. Hormone therapy and venous thromboembolism among postmenopausal women: Impact of the route of estrogen administration and progestogens: The ESTHER study. Circulation. 2007;**115**(7):840-845

[91] Gibbons WE, Moyer DL, Lobo RA, et al. Biochemical and histologic effects of sequential estrogen/progestin therapy on the endometrium of postmenopausal women. American Journal of Obstetrics and Gynecology. 1986;**154**(2):456-461. PubMed: 3004222

[92] Davis SR, Burger HG. The role of androgen therapy. Best Practice & Research. Clinical Endocrinology & Metabolism. 2003;**17**:165-175

[93] Arlt W. Androgen therapy in women. European Journal of Endocrinology. 2006;**154**:1-11

[94] Ankarberg-Lindgren C, Elfving M, Wikland KA, Norjavaara E. Nocturnal application of transdermal estradiol patches produces levels of estradiol that mimic those seen at the onset of spontaneous puberty in girls. The Journal of Clinical Endocrinology and Metabolism. 2001;**86**:3039-3044

[95] Davenport ML. Approach to the patient with Turner syndrome. The Journal of Clinical Endocrinology and Metabolism. 2010;**95**:1487-1495

[96] Schenck-Gustaffson K, Brincat M, Erel T, Gambacciani M, Lamberdounaki I, Tremorrlieres F, et al. EMAS position statement: Managing the menopause in the context of coronary heart disease. Maturitas. 2011;**68**:94-97

[97] Beljic T, Zivkovic T, Vuksanovic M, Andjelic-Jelic M, Stojanovic J, Buric B, et al. Obesity and metabolic syndrome during the menopausal transition. Climacteric. 2011;**14**:643-648

[98] Shuster LT, Rhodes DJ, Gostout BS, Grossardt BR, Rocca WA. Premature menopause or early menopause: Long-term health consequences. Maturitas. 2010;**65**:161-166

[99] Kannel WB, Hjortland MC, McNamara PM, Gordon T. Menopause and risk of cardiovascular disease. The Framingham study. Annals of Internal Medicine. 1976;**85**:447-452

[100] Faubion SS, Kuhle CL, Shuster LT, Rocca WA. Long-term health consequences of premature or early menopause and considerations for management. Climacteric. 2015;**18**:483-491

[101] Popat VB, Calis KA, Vanderhoof VH, Cizza G, Reynolds JC, Sebring N, et al. Bone mineral density in estrogen-deficient young women. The Journal of Clinical Endocrinology and Metabolism. 2009;**94**(7):2277-2283

[102] Vega EM, Egea MA, Mautalen CA. Influence of the menopausal age on the severity of osteoporosis in women with vertebral fractures. Maturitas. 1994;**19**:117-124

[103] Van der Klift M, de Laet CE, McCloskey EV, et al. Risk factors for incident vertebral fractures in men and women: The Rotterdam study. Journal of Bone and Mineral Research. 2004;**19**:1172-1180

[104] Rocca WA, Bower JH, Maraganore DM, et al. Increased risk of parkinsonism in women who underwent oophorectomy before menopause. Neurology. 2009;**70**:200-209

[105] Rocca WA, Bower JH, Maraganore DM, et al. Increased risk of cognitive impairment or dementia in women who underwent oophorectomy before menopause. Neurology. 2007;**69**:1074-1083

[106] Phung TK, Waltoft BL, Laursen TM, et al. Hysterectomy, oophorectomy and risk of dementia: A nationwide historical cohort study. Dementia and Geriatric Cognitive Disorders. 2010;**30**:43-50

[107] Nelson LM, Covington SN, Rebar RW. An update: Spontaneous premature ovarian failure is not an early menopause. Fertility and Sterility. 2005;**83**:1327-1332

[108] Nelson LM, Anasti JN, Kimzey LM, et al. Development of luteinized graafian follicles in patients with karyotypically normal spontaneous premature ovarian failure. The Journal of Clinical Endocrinology and Metabolism. 1994 Nov;**79**(5):1470-1475

[109] Taylor AE, Adams JM, Mulder JE, Martin KA, Sluss PM, Crowley WF,J. A randomized, controlled trial of estradiol replacement therapy in women with hypergonadotrophic amenorrhea. The Journal of Clinical Endocrinology and Metabolism. 1996;**81**:3615-3621

[110] Tartagni M, Cicinelli E, De Pergola G, et al. Effects of pretreatment with estrogens on ovarian stimulation with gonadotropins in women with premature ovarian failure: A randomized, placebo-controlled trial. Fertility and Sterility. 2007;**87**:858-861

[111] Mamas L, Mamas E. Premature ovarian failure and dehydroepiandrosterone. Fertility and Sterility. 2009;**91**:644-646

[112] Badawy A, Goda H, Ragab A. Induction of ovulation in idiopathic premature ovarian failure: A randomized double-blind trial. Reproductive Biomedicine Online. 2007;**15**:215-219

[113] Ferrau F, Gangemi S, Vita G, Trimarchi F, Cannavo S. Pregnancy after azathioprine therapy for ulcerative colitis in a woman with autoimmune premature ovarian failure and Addison's disease: HLA haplotype characterization. Fertility and Sterility. 2011;**95**:2430 e2415-2430 e2437

[114] Sauer MV, Paulson RJ, Ary BA, Lobo RA. Three hundred cycles of oocyte donation at the University of Southern California: Assessing the effect of age and infertility diagnosis on pregnancy and implantation rates. Journal of Assisted Reproduction and Genetics. 1994;**11**:92-96

[115] Templeton A, Morris JK, Parslow W. Factors that affect outcome of in-vitro fertilisation treatment. Lancet. 1996;**348**:1402-1406

[116] Foudila T, Soderstrom-Antilla V, Hovatta O. Turner's syndrome and pregnancies after oocyte donation. Human Reproduction. 1999;**14**:532-535

[117] Practice Committee of the American Society for Reproductive Medicine. Increased maternal cardiovascular mortality associated with pregnancy in women with Turner syndrome. Fertility and Sterility. 2012 Feb;**97**(2):0015-0282. DOI: 10.1016/j.fertnstert.2011.11.049

[118] Michala L, Goswami D, Creighton SM, Conway GS. Swyer syndrome: Presentation and outcomes. BJOG. 2008;**115**:737-741

[119] Rocha VB, Guerra-Júnior G, Marques-de-Faria AP, de Mello MP, Maciel-Guerra AT. Complete gonadal dysgenesis in clinical practice: The 46, XY karyotype accounts for more than one third of cases. Fertility and Sterility. 2011 Dec;**96**(6):1431-1434. DOI: 10.1016/j.fertnstert.2011.09.009. Epub 2011 Oct 6

[120] Wong KM, Mastenbroek S, Repping S. Cryopreservation of human embryos and it contribution to *in vitro* fertilization success rates. Fertility and Sterility. 2014;**102**:19-26

[121] Evans J, Hannan NJ, Edgell TA, et al. Fresh versus frozen embryo transfer: Backing clinical decisions with scientific and clinical evidence. Human Reproduction Update. 2014;**20**:808-821

[122] Grifo JA, Noyes N. Delivery rate using cryopreserved oocytes is comparable to conventional *in vitro* fertilization using fresh oocytes: Potential fertility preservation for female cancer patients. Fertility and Sterility. 2010;**93**:391-396

[123] Oktay K, Karlikaya G. Ovarian function after transplantation of frozen, banked autologous ovarian tissue. The New England Journal of Medicine. 2000;**342**:1919

[124] Donnez J, Silber S, Andersen CY. Children born after autotransplantation of cryopreserved ovarian tissue: A review of 13 live births. Annals of Medicine. 2011;**43**:437-450

[125] Schmidt KT, Resendahl M, Ernst E. Autotransplantation of cryopreserved ovarian tissue in 12 women with chemotherapy-induced premature ovarian failure: The Danish experience. Fertility and Sterility. 2011;**95**:695-701

[126] Conway GS, Payne NN, Webb J, Murray A, Jacobs PA. Fragile X premutation screening in women with premature ovarian failure. Human Reproduction. 1998;**13**:1184-1187

[127] Vegetti W, Grazia Tibiletti M, Testa G, de Lauretis Y, Alagna F, Castoldi E, et al. Inheritance in idiopathic premature ovarian failure: Analysis of 71 cases. Human Reproduction. 1998;**13**:1796-1800

[128] van Kasteren YM, Hundscheid RD, Smits AP, Cremers FP, van Zonneveld P, Braat DD. Familial idiopathic premature ovarian failure: An overrated and underestimated genetic disease? Human Reproduction. 1999;**14**:2455-2459

[129] Janse F, Knauff EA, Niermeijer MF, Eijkemans MJ, Laven JS, Lambalk CB, et al. Dutch Premature Ovarian Failure C. Similar phenotype characteristics comparing familial and sporadic premature ovarian failure. Menopause. 2010;**17**:758-765

[130] McConkie-Rosell A, Finucane B, Cronister A, Abrams L, Bennett RL, Pettersen BJ. Genetic counseling for fragile x syndrome: Updated recommendations of the national society of genetic counselors. Journal of Genetic Counseling. 2005;**14**:249-270

[131] Dunlop CE, Telfer EE, Anderson RA. Ovarian stem cells--potential roles in infertility treatment and fertility preservation. Maturitas. 2013 Nov;**76**(3):279-283. DOI: 10.1016/j.maturitas.2013.04.017. Epub 2013 May 18

[132] Kawamura K, Cheng Y, Suzuki N, Deguchi M, Sato Y, Takae S, et al. Hippo signaling disruption and Akt stimulation of ovarian follicles for infertility treatment. Proceedings of the National Academy of Sciences of the United States of America. 2013 Oct 22;**110**(43):17474-17479. DOI: 10.1073/pnas.1312830110

[133] Zhai J, Yao G, Dong F, Bu Z, Cheng Y, Sato Y, et al. In vitro activation of follicles and fresh tissue auto-transplantation in primary ovarian insufficiency patients. The Journal of Clinical Endocrinology & Metabolism. 2016 Nov 1;**101**(11):4405-4412. DOI: 10.1210/jc.2016-158

2

Menopause in Nonhuman Primates: A Comparative Study with Humans

María de Jesús Rovirosa-Hernández,
Marisela Hernández González,
Miguel Ángel Guevara-Pérez,
Francisco García-Orduña,
Abril de los Ángeles Aguilar-Tirado,
Abraham Puga-Olguín and
Brisa Patricia Vásquez-Domínguez

Abstract

Although menopause is a phenomenon predominantly studied in humans or laboratory animals, this chapter discussed the case of nonhuman primates (NHPs), not only with the objective of employing them as study models but also to better understand phylogenetic divergence among species. Those taxonomic differences are reflected in reproductive processes that may be similar to those of human beings, with the presence of a defined cycle or periods of estrus, but perhaps at different ages as well, where menopause plays a crucial role. First, it is important to delimit the concept of menopause by considering its anatomical, physiological, and biochemical parameters, including the cessation of menstrual bleeding or perineal swelling—when present—or follicular depletion and hormonal changes. Thus, the aim of this chapter is to discuss some of the similarities between NHPs and human females, during the menopause period. Studying these phenomena should help us achieve a better understanding of the social, physiological, and environmental factors without adopting any particular cultural view of menopause.

Keywords: nonhuman primate, ovarian cycle, reproductive cessation, new world monkeys, old world monkeys

1. Introduction

Menopause is a process of the reproductive aging [1] manifested in the depletion of ovarian follicles, the reduction of ovarian hormones to castration levels, and the increase in the concentration of serum gonadotropins [2]. In human beings, this process occurs in midlife, heralded by the gradual disappearance of menstrual cycles accompanied by the end of reproductive capacity, which correlates with functional and structural changes in the hypothalamic-pituitary-ovarian axis [3].

This process is not exclusive to humans, for it also occurs in all iteroparous organisms that exhibit declining fertility as a function of general senescence [4]. However, in contrast to human beings, nonhuman primates (NHPs) and even longer lived species like tortoises, elephants, and whales retain their capacity to reproduce until relatively advanced age [5]. Studies in NHPs, such as monkeys and apes, both in the wild and in conditions of captivity, have reported menopause as a physiological phenomena [6–8], but they clearly show that the reproductive changes observed in NHPs differ from those of human menopause, at least from a perspective of comparative life history [6]. This is because most of the oldest individuals in all wild species studied showed no signs of ovarian failure, while studies of captive primate species have observed that 67% of old females continued reproducing throughout their lives [7].

It has been suggested that the differences between the human fertility pattern and those of other NHPs are evident in the maximum age of reproduction and mean life expectancy at maturity of both. This refers to the fact that human beings have an early fertility peak that begins to decrease when they are in their mid-1920s, followed by a general decline and then a steep drop that normally begins around age 35; being this age the specific moment fertility functions of NHPs as macaques remain relatively constant over a long period, terminating abruptly only a few years before age death [9].

NHPs are used in medical and scientific research due to their similarities in physiology, neuroanatomy, reproduction, development, cognition, and social complexity to humans, which reflect their close phylogenetic relationship between NHPs and human beings. Primates are divided phylogenetically into strepsirrhines (galagos, lorises, and Malagasy lemurs) and haplorhines (tarsiers and anthropoids). There are three major branches of extant anthropoids or higher primates: the Platyrrhini or New World monkeys (South and Central America) and two groups of Catarrhini (the Cercopithecoids or Old World monkeys (Africa, Europe, and Asia) and Hominoids (Apes and human beings)) (**Figure 1**) [10].

The aim of the present chapter is to discuss and analyze some similarities between female NHPs and human females during natural or surgically induced menopause, since expanding our knowledge of this phenomenon in mammals with such a close phylogenetic relationship so to human beings should lead to a more comprehensive understanding of this biological process.

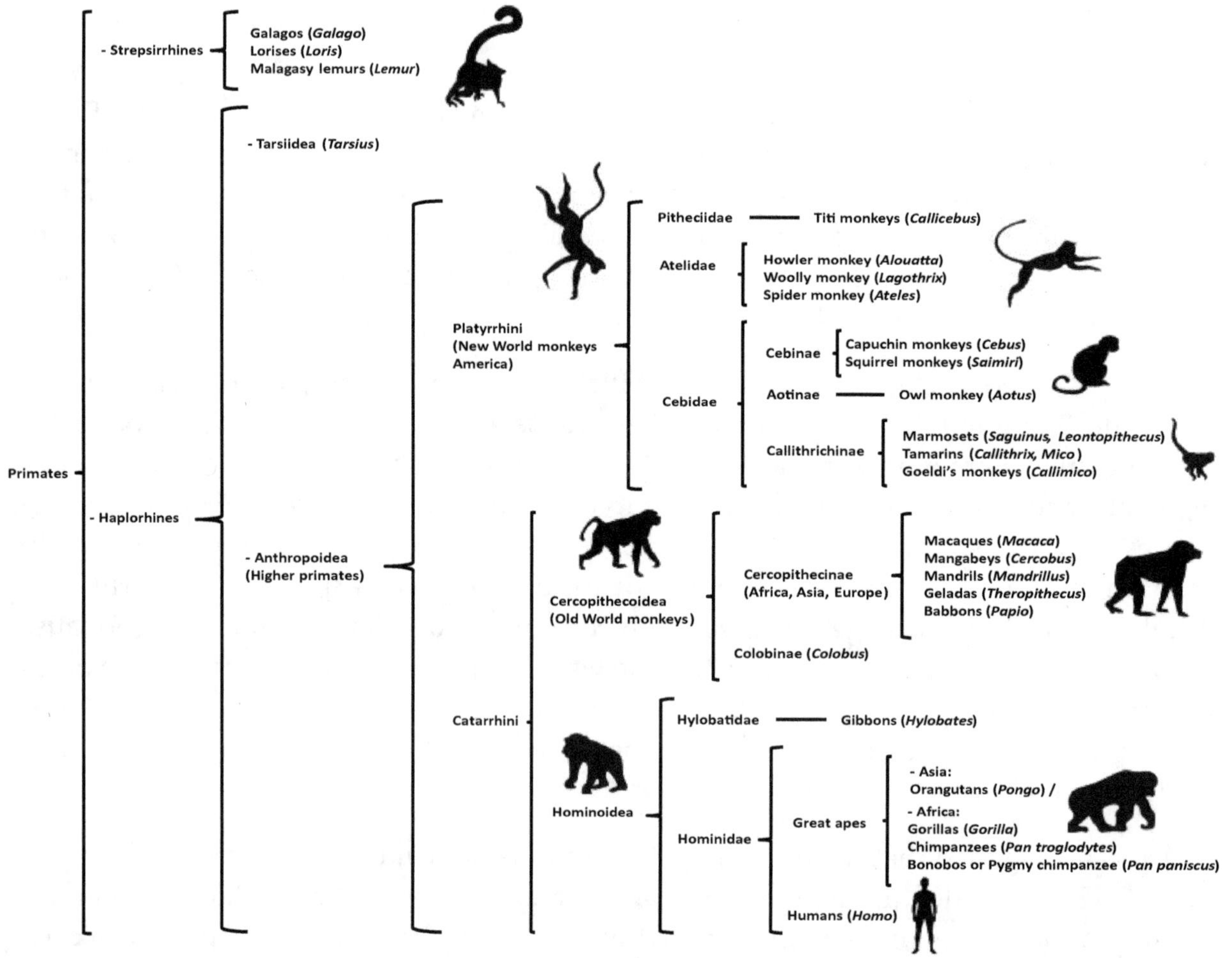

Figure 1. Taxonomic classification of extant primates with branch lengths in millions of years. Representative genus is shown in brackets (modified from Ref. [10]).

2. Reproductive cycles in nonhuman primate females and their relation with cycles in human beings

For many mammals, estrus is not only confined to a brief portion of the reproductive cycle that is characterized by an increase in attractivity and in the proceptive and receptive behaviors of females but is also strictly seasonal. In NHPs the reproductive cycles occur for only a few weeks of the year, as occurs among Madagascar prosimians, such as the sifakas. In some New World primates, such as squirrel monkeys, sexual cycles occur only during 3 months of the year [11], but many catarrhine primates do not follow this strict pattern circumscribed by the estrous period [12]. The literature mentioned that apes, human beings, and many monkeys have reproductive cycles that differ in two ways: first, the cycles include menstruation, a cyclical sloughing of the uterine lining. Second, there is greater flexibility in the time of proceptive and receptive behaviors with a longer duration of estrus [13]. Apes and Old World monkeys, meanwhile, exhibit menstrual cycles that range from 25 to 35 days similar to those human females. Also in NHPs, mating activity is not restricted to the periovulatory period as occurs in other mammals since female receptivity is not under strict control of ovarian hormones, but is more closely related to the social context, also as in human beings [14]. Finally, circulating steroid hormones reflect the process of ovulation and ovarian cycling [15].

2.1. Ovarian cycle in nonhuman primates

Ovarian cycles in primates begin with a follicular phase during which the follicle matures, follicular secretion of estrogen increases, and the circulating concentration of progesterone (P_4) decreases [16]. In most primates, only one follicle ovulates in each cycle. It emerges during the mid-follicular phase and inhibits maturation of other follicles by secreting large amounts of estrogen that, in turn, reduce concentrations of the follicle-stimulating hormone (FSH) below the threshold level required for maturation of early antral follicle [17]. Second, ovulation occurs immediately after the follicular phase, and this maintains high circulating concentrations of estrogens from the mature follicle while exerting positive feedback on the hypothalamus and pituitary that triggers secretion of the gonadotropin-releasing hormone (GnRH), as well as FSH and luteinizing hormone (LH). The increased LH reaches the ovaries where it causes the follicle to rupture [18]. Third, during the luteal phase, the concentration of P_4 rises, but that of estrogens declines. Fertilization can take place during the early luteal phase of the cycle only during the first 24 h after ovulation. This is because the oocyte has a short life span. If the ovum is fertilized, then the corpus luteum does not degrade and continues to secrete P_4 until the placenta develops [19].

Some of these processes are similar to the ovarian cycles in the human beings [20]; however, studies have found that in all primate species studied, follicular development, ovulation, and corpus luteum formation occur spontaneously and independent of mating-induced stimuli [21]. Also, NHPs have been shown to have extended ovarian cycles, especially prolonged luteal phases, compared to those of other mammals [22]. Also, the duration of the follicular and luteal phases differs among NHPs. Cycle lengths vary among different primate groups: in prosimians, from 30 to 50 day; in New World monkeys, from 16 to 30 days; in Old World monkeys, from 24 to 35 days; in lesser apes, from 20 to 30 days; and in great apes—including humans—from 25 to 50 days [14, 15, 21, 23]. In contrast, squirrel monkeys have a mean cycle length of just 7–12 days, with a follicular phase of about 5 days [24].

Menstruation appears to be absent in all prosimians and possibly in tarsiers, presumably associated with the noninvasive form of placentation characteristic of these primates [21]. However, menstruation does occur in most Old World monkeys and apes, as well as in several New World monkeys [25], and prosimians may be considered to have an estrous cycle, because they exhibit distinct cyclical changes in relation to sexual receptivity, with a peak during the periovulatory period. Finally, many New World monkeys do not exhibit either menstruation or strict estrous cyclicity [20].

2.2. Ovarian cycle in humans

In human beings menstrual bleeding is the visible sign of cyclicity; it has a length of 3–6 days and occurs at the end of the luteal phase and the beginning of the follicular. While fertile phase has a length of 5 days and is associated with the end of follicular phase and an increase of estradiol (E_2) before ovulation, during this period conception can occur. Recent studies have found that human females possess dual sexuality, which consists of a fertile phase where they are more sexually attractive to men and a phase extended (non-fertile), which presents a motivation or interest in sex with the aim of obtaining some benefits, without conception occurring [26].

2.3. Reproductive aging

Female reproductive output differs markedly in relation to species and time. As females of many species age, a period of reproductive instability with perimenopausal-like hormonal changes has been observed. Like many other mammals, NHP females show fertility parameters that are related to age [7]. Anovulation, insufficient luteolysis, and impairment of gestation and lactation processes all become more common toward the end of reproductive life [27]. Female reproductive senescence differs among mammalian taxonomic groups. For example, in NHPs, the end of reproductive life is characterized by the loss of the follicular pool, whereas in rodents, variations are seen in the size of the follicular pool that remains at the end of reproductive life. In humans, experiencing follicular depletion early in the maximum life span is not usual; rather, it is the result of an extended period of altered hormonal environments. These alterations may be caused by reduced circulating estrogens, P_4, and inhibin, resulting in elevated gonadotropin concentrations (GTHs) for a time, followed by their decline [28]. Monkeys and apes also experience follicular depletion and associated hormonal alterations [8, 29], but the stage of life at which these occur is generally later than in humans. Some reports on lemurs and callitrichids indicate an age-related decline in reproduction in many species that is reflected in diminished reproductive success [30]. Older female sifakas (*Propithecus edwardsi*), a Madagascar lemur, show decreased rates of infant survival, and studies have affirmed that this effect can be attributed to the females' deteriorating dentition resulting in inability to support lactation [31]. This indicates that reduced fertility in old age does not, in and of itself, reflect impaired neuroendocrine or gonadal function [20].

Considering the taxonomic scale of primates, we can observe the variability in physiological characteristics, like it is reflected in aging process. As much NHPs get closer to human beings, more similarities are found, going through estrous cycles for strepsirrhines (galagos, lorises, and lemurs), to ovarian cycles, and hormonal profiles similar to human being females, in great apes (orangutans, gorillas, and chimpanzees), and Old World monkeys (macacos and baboons). Also in both cases, at the end of their reproductive life, different physiological and hormonal changes occur, which are associated with the loss of ovarian function that are characteristic of aging, where this gives us the opportunity to study in a comparative way different alterations that could be related to the absence of ovarian hormones.

3. Menopause in *Homo sapiens* females and nonhuman primates

Menopause has been defined as a series of changes in the termination of reproductive viability, of which the discontinuation of menstruation is but one component. Menstrual bleeding is a marker of the ovarian and neuroendocrine phenomena of reproductive viability in humans [32], but not all NHPs exhibit this [24]. Consequently, menopause must encompass hormonal, physiological, and biochemical changes that play essential roles in the cessation of ovarian cyclicity, regardless of whether menstrual bleeding is present. However, Walker and Herndon [1] have defined menopause in NHPs as the permanent, non-pathological, age-associated cessation of ovulation, so to infer this event would require considering such biological parameters as menstrual bleeding, perineal swelling, follicular depletion, and hormonal changes.

Some species of NHPs seem to present processes that are quite similar to what human females experience during menopause, but differences also exist, such as the shorter postmenopausal life span and differences in the timing of hormonal changes during the menopausal transition [33]. It is important to consider the time of menopause relative to the average and maximum life span of individuals. For example, humans may be unique among primates in that they have a long post-reproductive survival potential [34]. In human females, the reproductive function does not begin with puberty nor does it end with menopause at a certain chronological age. Instead, both of these are dynamic periods for the reproductive axis, during which development or senescence occurs relatively rapidly. In fact, the reproductive axis ages to a nonfunctional state (menopause) much earlier than other organs, while the reproductive system reaches the point of failure at a relatively young average age of 51 + 8 years [35]; considering that the maximum span for humans is around 80 years, they spend nearly 35% of her life in a post-reproductive state and in very special cases to 60% (122 years). Also, there are significant differences between species of NHPs and humans in terms of life span. For example, the life span of animals after menopause is short compared to humans, as they usually die not long after menopause [1].

Human females are born with a finite number of oocytes; thus, reproductive aging entails the steady loss of these oocytes through atresia and ovulation, processes that do not necessarily occur at constant rates [36]. Peak fertility in humans occurs in the mid-20s, after which it declines steadily until a steep decrease begins after age 35 [37]. This decline in fertility occurs despite normal hormone secretion by the ovaries of "older" reproductive-age humans, which continues until 3–4 years prior to menopause [38].

In spite of the wide age range at which ovarian dysfunction and reproductive failure occur in these species, the sequence of terminal events is fairly predictable. At the beginning of the process, the menstrual cycle length is shortened due to early follicular development and ovulation [39], which reduces fertility (premenopause). This is followed by disruption of regular menstrual cyclicity (perimenopause) and, finally, complete ovarian failure (menopause). Studies have observed that perimenopause is an indication that the number of remaining ungrown ovarian follicles has dropped below a critical threshold [40]. The period of transition from the reproductive phase to the nonreproductive state is called climacteric. Finally, postmenopause is the period following climacteric and occurs when the hormonal instability that characterizes perimenopause is replaced by the relative stability of the post-reproductive life stage when the reproductive function has ceased [41].

Declining fertility with age is manifested more commonly in monkeys and apes, to the point that some females cease to reproduce altogether before they die. Some reports on Old World monkeys in the wild mention that old toque macaque (*Macaca sinica*) and gray-cheeked mangabey (*Lophocebus albigena*) females no longer breed, perhaps due to increasingly long birth intervals that terminate with death or the cessation of ovulation [42]. In contrast, NHP females living in captivity may show life cycles marked by irregular and lengthened menstrual cycles, reduced estrogen levels, very long birth spacing and, in a few cases—such as chimpanzees—total cessation of ovulation [8, 43]. In captive rhesus monkeys (*Macaca mulatta*), menstruation ends at approximately 25 years of age [44], and their maximum life span is around 30 years [45]; thus, this species may have a maximum post-reproductive life span of approximately 20%, similar to what happens in chimpanzees (*Pan troglodytes*). There are also differences in life span among species of NHPs and humans. For example, the life span of other animals after menopause is short compared to humans, since they usually die after only a short time, while humans have an extended postmenopausal life expectancy [1].

The perimenopause period is also highly variable in human beings, as age at the onset of this period ranges from the mid-1930s to the early 1950s [46]. This wide range impedes gaining a better understanding of the mechanisms that control the onset of menopause in humans. In NHPs, this is even more difficult, since reproductive cessation occurs so late in their life span that relatively few individuals actually live to those ages. However, there are data that support the existence of a perimenopausal in NHPs [33, 47–49], a condition that indicates a transitional stage between fertility and age-associated infertility. Also, it has been reported that patterns of vaginal bleeding and serum hormone profiles of macaques in the third decade of life are similar to those described for peri- and postmenopausal human [29].

Although originally the term menopause was coined in human being context, there are some approaches toward NHPs, which let us build it, considering not only the cessation of menstrual bleeding but also other changes, such as the cessation of perineal swelling, follicular depletion, and hormonal-associated changes. So this term has been adapted focusing in the physiological characteristics of each species. By other hand the life span between species should be considered, because unlike human beings, some species usually transit immediately from the reproductive end to death. Therefore, it is of great importance to know what are the differences between species that could help us identify the age of onset of menopause according to the species of the study, and, since this information, it will depend on whether or not our data can be extrapolated to the human.

4. Menopause in nonhuman primates in wild versus captive conditions

Specific studies over physiological mechanisms that govern the timing of menopause in wild NHPs are scarce [42, 50], because many factors could mask the accuracy of these results, including the ages of subjects—which often must be estimated [51]—predation pressures [52], limited survivability [23], infant mortality [53], food availability and nutrition [54], and social dynamics [55]. Therefore, this information is taken as complementary to data derived from captive animals [1].

4.1. Macaques (*Macaca* spp.)

Hodgen et al. [29] reported that female rhesus monkeys (*Macaca mulatta*), in captivity and at least 22 years of age, showed true menopause, confirmed by circulating levels of pituitary and ovarian hormones and the pattern of vaginal bleeding. Female rhesus monkeys older than 22 years are considered aged, as the maximum average life span for this species is estimated at 30 years [44, 45]. Hence, these females are close to the end of their life span, compared to humans, who arc considered as "aged" at around 75 years.

Graham et al. [8] examined the reproductive history and histology of pigtail macaques (*Macaca nemestrina*) by observing females divided into three age classes (4, 10, and 20 years). They reported that one female over 20 years of age showed functional, hormonal, and morphological characteristics of human menopause (i.e., complete follicular depletion, absence of luteal tissue, amenorrhea, increased LH levels, atrophic uterus, and vagina). Miller et al. [56], meanwhile, reported an age-associated decline in fertility in pigtail macaques, similar to the findings for *Macaca sylvanus* reported by Paul et al. [57].

Walker's study [47], of 15 female *Macaca mulatta* aged 8–34 years, was designed to characterize the endocrine and menstrual changes associated with menopause in this species. Findings indicate that females aged 24–26 years were in transition to menopause, evidenced by elevated LH concentrations consistent with a low E_2 concentration and no indication of bleeding menstrual. Also, the histological analysis of their ovaries showed little or no evidence of follicular activity. Finally, the females aged 27–34 years clearly showed a postmenopausal process, marked by high LH concentrations and uniformly low E_2 concentrations. This finding was corroborated by Gilardi et al. [48], who suggest that in female rhesus monkeys menopause does not occur until the second half of the third decade of life. Recent studies have also reported that postmenopausal females show low E_2 and P_4 levels, high indexes of FSH and LH, and a significant decline in the anti-Mullerian hormone and inhibin B. All these findings indicate that these endocrine parameters may be associated with menopause [49]. On the other hand, Johnson and Kapsalis [58] reported a median age >27 years for menopause in free-ranging rhesus monkeys.

Recent studies have concluded that reproductive senescence correlates with overall health [23]. Gore et al. [59], for example, reported that neuroendocrine changes in senescent rhesus monkeys are consistent with those reported in humans [60] and that ovarian changes are related to menopause [61], thus suggesting that these NHPs undergo ovarian changes as a function of aging, similar to humans [40] and chimpanzee [62]. A study of Japanese macaques (*Macaca fuscata*) reported that in free-ranging individuals, fertility rates diminish at around 25 years of age [63], but those normal menstrual cycles continue when they are in captivity, despite a loss of fertility [64]. Finally, recent studies of cynomolgus monkeys (*Macaca fascicularis*) have shown an endocrine pattern similar to that of humans during the postmenopause period [65].

4.2. Great apes

The menstrual cycles, pregnancy, and genital pathology of common chimpanzees (*Pan troglodytes*) were analyzed to determine the extent of perimenopausal changes in females with aged approximately 35–48 years. However, those analyses showed no clear evidence of menopause, because several females continued cycling until death [8]. But the authors did observe a reduced likelihood of conception in those female chimpanzees, even though they did not "run out" of oocytes before the end of the maximum life span. They concluded that female chimpanzees aged 35 years of age or more show increased reproductive senescence that is quite comparable to what is seen during human climacteric.

Other studies of common chimpanzees aged approximately 48–50 years and of bonobos—pygmy chimpanzees (*Pan paniscus*)—aged approximately 40 years reported that even though the former were extremely aged, they continued to have menstrual cycles and perineal swelling but with increased cycle length. Also, these aged females continue to secrete GnRH in a pulsatile fashion, although the levels of this hormone are higher than younger females [43]. Recent studies by Lacreuse et al. [66] found that many aged chimpanzees continued to menstruate at age 50 or more, but the length of their cycles increased after age 20. Similar results were reported by Videan et al. [67], who concluded that menopause in *Pan troglodytes* occurs at approximately 35–40 years of age. These data concur with the report on wild chimpanzee by Nishida et al. [50]. These authors reported that the females ceased cycling after 30 years of age. On the other hand, Thompson et al. [68] observed that healthy free-ranging chimpanzees remained reproductively viable well past 40 years. They suggested that in *Pan troglodytes,* menopause occurs as a by-product of ill health, interpreting that the onset of menopause may be delayed in relatively healthy, long-lived animals. Studies of female chimpanzees have shown that reproductive aging is similar to that seen in human females, including higher fetal loss as a function of advancing age [69] and the age-related depletion of ovarian follicles [62]. Thus, these studies showed that *Pan troglodyte* females continued cycling into extreme old age, which distinguishes them from human females in terms of menopause.

Other studies in *Pan paniscus* females, aged at least 40 years, showed no external evidence of menstrual cycling preceding death, and hormone levels consistent with clinically observed amenorrhea, but an exaggerated response to the exogenous GnRH challenge. Histological examination of ovaries showed similar characteristics to those described for senile ovarian tissue in humans [43].

Studies of captive orangutan (*Pongo* ssp.) females have reported the endocrine characteristics of their menstrual cycle and similarities to the human cycle [70]. These reports considered births and inter-birth intervals across the life span and demonstrated an age-specific decline in the fertility of captive female orangutans (*Pongo pygmaeus*; [7]). Other studies with wild female Sumatran orangutans (*Pongo abelii*) failed to document menopause, inferred from increased inter-birth intervals in females of estimated age [51]. Interpreting data from wild animals is difficult because of such countervailing factors as female rank, uncertain age, infant mortality, and food availability [1].

An earlier study that described the reproductive physiology of female gorillas (*Gorilla gorilla*) mentioned a correlation of perineal tumescence with circulating hormones and reported a pattern of cyclic hormone secretion similar to that of humans [71]. Recently, fecal hormone determination in two captive female gorillas aged approximately 40 years showed evidence of the protracted luteal phases that are typical of aging human females [72].

Information related to the occurrence of menopause in baboons (*Papio* ssp.) was based on menstrual cycle length, total cessation of cycling that occurs at 26 years of age in captivity [73]. Similar results were reported by Lapin et al. [74], and other studies of wild baboons have reported increased cyclic variability with age and a complete loss of fertility by the age of 25 years. This suggests that baboons undergo age-linked alterations in reproductive function similar to those of humans.

The living conditions of primates have an impact over the animal life span, so the observations in captivity are not always the same as in wild conditions. Although there are some reports about NHP aging process and menopause, they are scarce. Most of the studies report animal physiology and behavior in captivity, because to follow animals in wild by a long period is a very difficult process due to the NHP living conditions.

5. Nonhuman primates as a model to study human being menopause

Due to the biological similarities between human beings and NHPs, the latter have been studied in the search for an adequate model of menopause. However, it is necessary to clearly delimit the similarities and differences among reproductive characteristics, perimenopausal and menopausal changes, and the average life span of different species [1]. Establishing similarities with humans during this search requires considering the characteristics of menopausal processes when animals are in captivity versus those who are free-ranging, in order to avoid the confusions that have led to the assertion that menopause is a uniquely human event [1]. Walker and Herndon [1] suggested that a comparative analysis of female reproductive senescence should focus on the anatomical, physiological, and biochemical changes that are essential to the cessation of ovarian cyclicity, regardless of the presence of menstrual bleeding. There are few reports on menopause in New World primates compared to Old World monkeys, but studies of the latter have observed declines in sexual activity and decreased birth rates. Also, reports on captive apes suggest a long post-reproductive life span, though this has not been confirmed in the wild [30].

Among the different primate taxa, menopause is manifested along an evolutionary continuum: in some species—such as cercopithecines and apes—it is followed by an extended post-reproductive life span, while in others it may presage death. In terms of NHPs as models for menopause, the species that have most often been employed are baboons and chimpanzees. Studies of these primates have attempted to simulate all the consequences that characterize menopause, namely, hormonal and cognitive changes, cardiovascular alterations, and osteoporosis.

Until recently, the occurrence of reproductive termination in NHPs was widely questioned. However, numerous studies have reported that this does indeed occur in several species of Old World monkeys and great apes. Most of this research has been conducted with *Macaca mulatta* [29, 33, 47–49, 59, 61], but other species also experience menopause, including *Pan troglodytes* [43, 62, 67] and *Gorilla gorilla* [27]. For example, the hormonal profiles of peri- and postmenopausal macaques, chimpanzees, and gorillas [1, 61, 67], as well as the age-related decline in the number of primordial follicle in macaques [61] and chimpanzees [62], share many similarities and occur in a pattern like to that of aging women [40]. On the basis of data from various studies, Fedigan et al. [75] affirmed that "from an endocrinological perspective, reproductive decline may well follow a similar pattern in all primates, and we could use cases of individual post-reproductive monkeys and apes as clinical models of the physiological basis for menopause in human being. However, from an evolutionary perspective, these studies fail to demonstrate similarity between reproductive senescence in NHPs and menopause in the human female. Instead, they highlight the critical differences: female macaques and chimpanzees that cease to cycle very close to age at death, whereas human females cease to cycle in middle age; female macaques and chimpanzees cease to cycle on an idiosyncratic basis, whereas human females universally cease to cycle at the average age of approximately 50 years."

In light of these data, it is clear that regardless of the age at the onset of menopause, there are numerous physiological similarities between the females of NHPs and human females with respect to the gradual decline and eventual cessation of reproductive capacity. For this reason, several authors of excellent reviews [1, 29, 30] have proposed that NHPs provide the most appropriate animal models available for analyzing menopause in human females and the processes associated with it.

Although NHPs present a rich opportunity to study the process of reproductive senescence or menopause (i.e., the permanent, non-pathological, age-associated cessation of ovulation, [1]) and play a unique role in translational science by bridging the gap between basic and clinical research [76], their use as experimental subjects is limited by the lack of available NHPs that are undergoing the perimenopausal transition and natural menopause, their short menopausal compared to that of human being, high costs, and the strict ethical guidelines that researchers must follow when studying them (see Ref. [33, 76]).

Despite these difficulties, the use of NHPs as study models has several advantages. Macaques (*Macaca* spp.), including *Macaca mulatta* and *Macaca fascicularis* monkeys, for example, have been particularly useful due to their availability, moderate size, and ability to adapt to laboratory conditions. Also, approximately 95% of the overall genetic coding sequence of macaques is identical to that of humans [77], and many of their physiological systems are comparable. Finally, because they are relatively long lived, they are effective models for studying a number of diseases and conditions that increase in frequency with aging. These factors explain why female macaques have been the preferred model for examining critical health concerns of human beings, including luteal phase deficiencies and hypothalamic amenorrhea [78], obesity and diabetes [79], cardiovascular diseases [80], osteopenia, osteoporosis [81], osteoarthritis [82], cognitive deficits associated with age [76], and—at least potentially—decreased interest in mating [83].

If a single conclusion can be gleaned from this brief summary, it is that a large number of physiological conditions and pathologies that human beings experience during their lifetime appear to be broadly manifested in primate taxa, though information is lacking in other regards, such as the interaction between deficits in cognitive processes and their effect on the modulation of social and sexual interaction.

Primates are mammals distinguished by their large brains, advanced cognitive abilities, flexible behavior, and sophisticated social systems [84]. For example, chimpanzees have the ability to recognize themselves in a mirror [85] and perform tasks involving concept formation [86]. Moreover, the structure and function of human and NHP brains are very similar. In this regard, we can mention nuclear organization, projection pathways, and innervation patterns [87], as well as similar cortical development and organization [88], including visual cortical functional divisions and prefrontal cortex subdivisions [89] that are critical for cognitive processes [90].

In human beings and NHPs, cognitive and reproductive functions decline gradually with advancing age and more precipitously with the loss of circulating estrogen that occurs during menopause. Cognitive deficits in NHPs can be quantified over their life span using a battery of cognitive tests that are similar to, if not the same as, those used with humans [91]. These include the monkey version of the Wisconsin Card Sorting Test (WCST) [92], which is the gold standard for assessing cognitive flexibility in humans. Using a version of WCST (without the numerosity category), executive function deficits have been reported in both middle-aged and older rhesus monkeys [93], as well as in middle-aged menopausal rhesus monkeys [91]. However, the limited availability of animals of adequate age [33] means that studies with monkeys typically involve only a few animals and use premenopausal ovariectomized subjects rather than naturally menopausal females.

Given the dramatic effects of sex steroids on neuronal morphology and brain activity in regions involved in cognition, one might expect that age-related changes in the endocrine milieu will have important consequences for cognitive functions. In effect, data on aged, naturally or surgically menopausal monkeys indicate that estrogen does indeed modulate a broad range of cognitive domains, such as learning and memory. These effects observed appear to be task specific and sensitive to the time that passed without estrogen prior to estrogen replacement. For example, on the delayed response (DR) task—a test of prefrontal functioning—it was noted that performance was impaired in postmenopausal individuals compared to age-matched premenopausal rhesus monkeys [94]. This result suggests that the absence of estrogen, associated with menopause, could be detrimental to prefrontal functioning.

Although the effects of the menstrual cycle, estrogen withdrawal, and estrogen replacement in young monkeys appear limited to non-mnemonic functions, such as attention or aspects of face processing [95], a broad range of cognitive functions, including memory, are sensitive to estrogen deprivation and replacement in older monkeys [92]. Neurobiological data are consistent with such cognitive findings and demonstrate an array of morphological and physiological changes following ovariectomy and/or estrogen replacement in brain areas that are important for cognition.

Although the specific mechanisms through which estrogens may affect cognition remain to be elucidated, it is clear that these hormones have broad effects on areas of the brain that play key roles in cognitive functions [96]. Estrogen receptors are found in the cerebral cortex, hippocampus, and amygdala in both monkeys [97] and human beings [98]. Estrogens alter the neuronal morphology and physiology of some of these areas [99].

NHPs provide valuable animal models that have significantly advanced our understanding of numerous behavioral and biological phenomena in humans and other primates. Their value as models for studying menopause in humans derives from their common ancestry, as well as a series of hormonal, cognitive, and social influences that are similar to those experienced by human beings. The aging process or menopause has been also explored focusing through the neural basis of cognitive functioning, revealing not only alterations over specific neural systems but also differences in the affectation level among brain regions and neurobiological parameters. Therefore, further research into the interactions among hormones and various neurotransmitter systems could potentially produce improved knowledge of the neural and hormonal bases that comprehend the gamma of alterations that human beings suffer before, during, and after menopause.

5.1. Anxiety and depression during natural or surgical menopause of nonhuman primates

The decrease in ovarian hormones during natural and surgical menopause is associated with a higher incidence of psychiatric disorders, such as anxiety and depression in vulnerable women, where the decrease of hormones—principally E_2 and P_4—can induce neural changes that exert affects on both the emotional and affective levels [100]. In this regard, ovariectomies in NHPs have been used as a model of surgical menopause at the experimental level, given that the absence of certain hormones induced by ovariectomy can reproduce the physiological, emotional, and affective change characteristic of menopause.

At the behavioral level, ovariectomized primates may exhibit anxiety and depression-related behaviors. For example, long-term ovariectomy may increase anxiety in Japanese macaques (*Macaca fuscata*), associated with decreases in such behaviors as positive social contact, dominance, and the time spent receiving grooming. Similarly, temperament tests performed on these individuals show an increase in anxiogenic behavior [101]. Furthermore, ovariectomized pigtail macaques (*Macaca nemestrina*) present higher scratching rates [102], a well-established indicator of anxiety in NHPs, while in Japanese macaques, a reduction in locomotion has been observed after ovariectomy [101], in association with depressive behavior. Therefore, these behavioral alterations are probably due to the absence of ovarian hormones, given that after ovariectomy in rhesus (*Macaca mulatta*) and pigtail macaques a reduction in E_2 and P_4 concentrations is detected, in relation to increased anxiety [102].

The absence of ovarian hormones in NHPs may also generate neural changes in the brain (**Table 1**). Studies of ovariectomized Japanese monkeys have detected downregulation of estrogen receptor beta (ER-β) in the subiculum of hippocampal formation, while postmenopausal monkeys of the same species have shown upregulation of ER-β [103]. On the other hand, in ovariectomized African green monkeys (*Cercopithecus aethiops sabaeus*), a reduction of synaptic plasticity of the hippocampus was detected [104]. Given that the reduced density of dendritic spines and ER-β in the hippocampus is related to an increase in indicators of anxiety and depression in ovariectomized rodents [105], this is probably occurring as well in nonhuman primates that experience surgical menopause. In addition, the long-term absence of ovarian hormones may impact serotonergic activity. For example, it has been demonstrated that ovariectomy in rhesus macaques reduces expression of the mRNA of the tryptophan

Species	Natural menopause/ ovariectomy	Neural changes	Related behavior	References
African green monkeys (*Cercopithecus aethiops sabaeus*)	Ovariectomy	Reduced density of dendritic spines in the CA1 layer of the hippocampus	Not reported	[104]
Pigtail macaques (*Macaca nemestrina*)	Ovariectomy	Not reported	Anxiety	[102]
Rhesus macaques (*Macaca mulatta*)	Ovariectomy	Increased expression of MAO-A protein and decreased expression of TPH and SERT proteins in the dorsal raphe nucleus	Not reported	[107]
Rhesus macaques (*Macaca mulatta*)	Ovariectomy	Decreased expression of TPH2 mRNA in the dorsal raphe nucleus	Not reported	[108]
Rhesus macaques (*Macaca mulatta*)	Ovariectomy	Increased DNA fragmentation of serotonin neurons in the dorsal raphe nucleus	Not reported	[106]
Japanese macaques (*Macaca fuscata*)	Ovariectomy	Not reported	Anxiety and depression	[101]
Japanese macaques (*Macaca fuscata*)	Ovariectomy	Reduced Fev, TPH-2, SERT, and $5HT_{1A}$ gene expression in the dorsal raphe nucleus	Not reported	[109]
Japanese macaques (*Macaca fuscata*)	Natural menopause	Upregulation in the ER-β immunoreactivity in the subiculum of the hippocampal formation	Not reported	[103]
Japanese macaques (*Macaca fuscata*)	Ovariectomy	Downregulation in the ER-β immunoreactivity in the subiculum of the hippocampal formation	Not reported	[103]

Table 1. Neural changes related to anxiety and depressive-like behaviors in nonhuman primates with natural or surgical menopause.

hydroxylase-2 (TPH-2) enzyme, increases the expression of MAO-A, and increases DNA fragmentation of serotonin neurons in the dorsal raphe nucleus [106]. These events could lead, on the one hand, to greater serotonin degradation and, on the other, neuronal death and, finally, a malfunction of the serotonergic system.

Furthermore, long-term ovariectomy in Japanese macaques reduces the expression of serotonergic neurons and gene expression of TPH-2, the serotonin reuptake transporter (SERT), and $5HT_{1A}$ autoreceptors in the dorsal raphe nucleus [109]. This agrees with data showing that in depressed female of *Macaca fascicularis* the binding potential of $5HT_{1A}$ receptors is reduced in the hippocampus, amygdala, and cingulate cortex [110], three of the structures involved in the pathophysiology of anxiety and depression. In contrast, stress-sensitive female monkeys of the same species decrease levels of Fev (transcription factor that determines whether a neuron is serotonergic),

TPH-2, SERT, and $5HT_{1A}$ mRNAs in the dorsal raphe nucleus [111]. Thus, in the long term, the reduction of TPH-2, which is important for serotonin synthesis, together with determinant markers for serotonergic function, could generate a higher incidence of anxious and depressive behaviors in NHPs with menopause, as occurred in human beings.

On the other hand, exogenous administration of E_2 or P_4 in ovariectomized primates has the capacity to restore serotonergic neurotransmission [106]. Further, serotonin neurons can express the ER-β protein and ER-β mRNA [112]. And, therefore, estrogens could increase the availability of serotonin in the brain by interacting with its receptor. Thus, the absence of ovarian hormones, such as E_2 and P_4, has the ability to induce changes at the level of the the central nervous system in primates [103]. This evidence suggests that neural changes could be related to anxiety and depression behaviors, which could indicate some vulnerability in NHPs that experience natural or surgical menopause or suffer changes in different neurotransmission systems in which ovarian hormones participate, all of which could affect the emotional and affective state of these individuals.

6. Conclusion

Menopause is a natural process that entails the permanent cessation of ovulation. It is associated with physiological and structural changes in aging females. Although it has long been assumed that menopause occurs only in human beings, the search for medical/clinical models to aid in research on this process has revealed that some species of NHPs also exhibit menopause. However, certain differences between human females and NHPs are clear: shorter postmenopausal life spans and variations in the timing of hormonal changes during the menopausal transition. But NHP models allow us to better understand not only several of the processes that occur during human aging—such as cognitive changes, cardiovascular alterations, and osteoporosis—but also similarities among species along the taxonomic scale.

On the other hand, increases in anxiety and depression behaviors may be observed in NHPs that undergo natural or surgical menopause. In a comparative perspective, these findings could improve our understanding of the neurobiological mechanisms that underlie emotional and affective disorders associated with the absence of ovarian hormones, given that experiments have demonstrated that long-term hormonal absence has the ability to affect numerous neurotransmission systems involved in mood disorders. In addition to reproducing various neural changes that can be correlated with depressive and anxious behaviors in NHPs, this might help understand the neurobiological substrate of emotional and affective disorders that can appear in women who experience natural or surgical menopause.

Acknowledgements

The authors of the present chapter received support from the following institutions: Sistema Nacional de Investigadores, SNI 60372-0 (AAA-T); Consejo Nacional de Ciencia y Tecnología (CONACyT), 297410 (AP-O); and Universidad Veracruzana, 46392 (BPV-D).

Author details

María de Jesús Rovirosa-Hernández[1*], Marisela Hernández González[2], Miguel Ángel Guevara-Pérez[2], Francisco García-Orduña[1], Abril de los Ángeles Aguilar-Tirado[1], Abraham Puga-Olguín[3] and Brisa Patricia Vásquez-Domínguez[4]

*Address all correspondence to: jrovirosa@uv.mx

1 Instituto de Neuroetología, Universidad Veracruzana, Xalapa, Veracruz, México

2 Instituto de Neurociencias, Universidad de Guadalajara, Jalisco, México

3 Posgrado en Neuroetología, Universidad Veracruzana, Xalapa, Veracruz, México

4 Facultad de Medicina, Universidad Veracruzana, Zona-Xalapa, Veracruz, México

References

[1] Walker ML, Herndon JG. Menopause in nonhuman primates?. Biology of Reproduction. 2008;**79**:398-406. DOI: 10.1095/biolreprod.108.068536

[2] Rance N. Menopause and the human hypothalamus: Evidence for the role of kisspeptin/neurokinin B neurons in the regulation of estrogen. Peptides. 2009;**30**:111-122. DOI: 10.1016/j.peptides.2008.05.016

[3] Hall J. Neuroendocrine changes with reproductive aging in women. Seminars in Reproductive Medicine. 2007;**25**:344-351. DOI: 10.1055/s-2007-984740

[4] Wilson EO. The Relevant Principles of Population Biology: Sociobiology. Cambridge: The Belknap Press; 1975. pp. 32-47

[5] Hill K, Hurtado A. Ache life history: The ecology and demography of a foraging people. American Ethonologist. 1996;**26**:531-532. DOI: 10.1525/ae.1999.26.2.531

[6] Pavelka M, Fedigan L. Reproductive termination in female Japanese monkeys: A comparative life history perspective. American Journal of Physical Anthropology. 1999;**109**: 455-464

[7] Caro TM, Sellen DW, Parish A, Frank R, Brown DM, Voland E, Borgerhoff Mulder M. Termination of reproduction in nonhuman and human primate females. International Journal of Primatology. 1995;**16**:205-220. DOI: 10.1007/BF02735478

[8] Graham CE, Kling OR, Steiner RA. Reproductive senescence in female nonhuman primates. In: Bowden DM, editor. Aging in Nonhuman Primates. New York: Van Nostrand Reinhold; 1979. 183-202

[9] Scott P. Menopause: Adaptation or epiphenomenon?. Evolutionary Anthropology. 2001; **10**:43-57. DOI: 10.1002/evan.1013

[10] Fleagle J. Apes and humans. In: Fleagle J, editor. Primate Adaptation and Evolution. 3rd ed. New York, Elsevier; 2013. Pp. 151-168. DOI: 10.1016/B978-0-12-378632-6.0007-0

[11] DuMond FV. The Squirrel Monkey in a Seminatural Environment. New York: Academic Press; 1968

[12] Keverne E. Do Old World primates have oestrus. Malaysian Applied Biology. 1981;**10**: 119-126

[13] Hrdy SB, Whitten P. Patterning of sexual activity. In: Smuts BB, Cheney DL, Seyfarth RM, Wrangham RW, Struhsaker TT, editors. Primates Societies. Chicago and London, University of Chicago Press; 1986; **30**:359-370

[14] Dixson AF. Primate Sexuality: Comparative Studies of the Prosimians, Monkeys, Apes, and Human Beings. Trends in Ecology and Evolution. Inglaterra: Oxford University Press; 1998

[15] Ziegler T, Strier K, Van S. The reproductive ecology of South American primates: Ecological adaptations in ovulation and conception. In: Garber PA, Estrada A, Bicca-Marques JC, Heymann EW, Strier KB, editors. South American Primates: Comparative Perspectives in the Study of Behavior, Ecology, and Conservation. New York: Springer; 2009. pp. 191-210 . DOI: 10.1007/978-0-387-78705-3_8

[16] Yen SC, Jaffe RB. Reproductive Endocrinology: Physiology, Pathophysiology and Clinical Management. Philadelphia: Saunders Company; 1986

[17] Zeleznik AJ, Pohl CR. Control of Follicular development, Corpus Luteum function, the maternal recognition of pregnancy, and the Neuroendocrine regulation of the menstrual cycle in higher primates. Academic Press. 2006; **45**:2449-2510. DOI: 10.1016/b978-012515400-0/50050-6

[18] Bonello N, Jasper MJ, Norman RJ. Periovulatory expression of intercellular adhesion molecule-1 in the rat ovary. Biology Reproduction. 2004;**71**:1384-1390. DOI: 10.1095/biolreprod.104.030650

[19] Hodgen GD, Itskovitz J. Recognition and maintenance of pregnancy. In: Knobil E, Neill J, editors. The Physiology of Reproduction. New York: Raven Press; 1988

[20] Saltzman W, Tardif S, Rutherford J. Hormones and reproductive cycles in primates. In: Hormones and Reproduction of Vertebrates. United States of America, Elsevier Inc. 2011;**5**:291-327. DOI: 10.1016/B978-0-12-374928-4.10013-6

[21] Martin RD. The evolution of human reproduction: A primatological perspective. American Journal of Physical Anthropology. 2007;**50**:59-84. DOI: 10.1002/ajpa.20734

[22] Johnson MH. Everitt B. Essential Reproduction. Oxford, OXF, Inglaterra: Blackwell Science; 2000

[23] Thompson ME. The endocrinology of intersexual relationships in the apes. In Thorpe P, Grey P, editors. The Endocrinology of Social Relationships. Cambridge: Harvard University Press; 2009. pp. 196-222

[24] Dukelow W. Reproductive cyclicity and breeding in the squirrel monkey. In: Rosenblum LA, Coe CL, editors. Handbook of Squirrel Monkey Research. NY: Plenum Press; 1985. pp. 169-190 . DOI: 10.1007/978-1-4757-0812-7_7

[25] Strassmann BI The evolution of endometrial cycles and menstruation. The Quarterly Reviex of Biology. 1996;**71**:181-220. DOI: 10.1086/419369

[26] Gangestad SW, Thornhill R. Human oestrus. Proceeding of the Royal Society B. 2008;**275**:991-1000. DOI: 10.1098/rspb.2007.1425

[27] Atsalis S, Margulis SW. Perimenopause and menopause: Documenting life changes in aging female gorillas. In: Atsalis S, Margulis SW, Hof PR, editors. Primate Reproductive Aging. Switzerland: Kargel AC; 2008. pp. 119-146 . DOI: 10.1159/000137704

[28] Wise PM. Aging of the female reproductive system. In: Masoro EJ, Austad SN, editors. Handbook of the Biology of Aging. London: Elsevier; 2006. pp. 570-590 . DOI: 10.1016/B978-012088387-5/50024-8

[29] Hodgen G, Goodman A, O'Connor A, Johnson D. Menopause in rhesus monkeys: Model for study of disorders in the human climacteric. American Journal of Obstetrics Gynecology. 1977;**127**:581-584. DOI: 10.1016/0002-9378(77)90352-0

[30] Atsalis S, Margulis SW. Primate reproductive aging: From lemurs to humans. In: Atsalis S, Marguli S, Hof P, editors. Primate Reproductive Aging. Switzerland: Kargel AC. 2008. pp. 186-194 . DOI: 10.1159/000137710

[31] Wright P, King S, Baden A, Jernvall J. Aging in wild female lemurs: Sustained fertility with increased infant mortality. In: Primate Reproductive Aging. Vol. **36**. Chicago, New York, Karger Publishers; 2008. pp. 17-28 . DOI: 10.1159/000137677

[32] Vom Saal FS, Finch CE. Reproductive senescence: Phenomena and mechanisms in mammals and selected vertebrates. In: Knobil E, Neill J, editors. The Physiology of Reproduction. New York: Raven Press; 1988. pp. 2351-2413

[33] Bellino FL, Wise PM. Nonhuman primate models of menopause workshop. Biology of Reproduction. 2003;**68**:10-18. DOI: 10.1095/biolreprod.102.005215

[34] Hawkes K, O'Connell JF, Blurton Jones NG, Alvarez H, Charnov EL. Grandmothering, menopause, and the evolution of human life histories. Proceedings of the National Academy of Sciences. 1998:**95**:1336-1339

[35] Hansen K, Knowlton N, Thyer A, Charleston J, Soules M, Klein N. A new model of reproductive aging: The decline in ovarian non-growing follicle number from birth to menopause. Human Reproduction. 2008;**23**:599-708. DOI: 10.1093/humrep/dem408

[36] Soules M, Sherman S, Parrot E, Rebar R, Santoro N, Utian W, Woods N. Executive summary: Stages of Reproductive Aging Workshop (STRAW). Climacteric. 2001;**4**:267-272. DOI: 10.1080/cmt.4.4.267.272

[37] Van Noord-Zaadstra B, Looman C, Alsbach H, Habbema J, te Velde E, Karbaat J. Delayed childbearing: Effect of age on fecundity and outcome of pregnancy. British Medical Journal. 1991;**302**:1361-1365

[38] Hansen K, Thyer A, Sluss P, Bremner W, Soules M, Klein N. Reproductive ageing and ovarian function: Is the early follicular phase FSH rise necessary to maintain adequate secretory function in older ovulatory women? Human Reproduction. 2005;**20**:89-95. DOI: 10.1093/humrep/deh54

[39] Klein NA, Harper AJ, Houmard BS, Sluss P, Soules M. Is the short follicular phase in older women secondary to advanced or accelerated dominant follicle development? The Journal of Clinical Endocrinology and Metabolism. 2002;**87**:5746-5750. DOI: 10.1210/jc.2002-020622

[40] Richardson SJ, Senikas V, Nelson JF. Follicular depletion during the menopausal transition: Evidence for accelerated loss and ultimate exhaustion. The Journal of Clinical Endocrinology & Metabolism. 1987;**65**:1231-1237. DOI: 10.1210/jcem-65-6-1231

[41] Gosden RG. Biology of Menopause: The Cause and Consequence of Ovarian Ageing. London: Academic Press; 1985

[42] Waser P. Postreproductive survival and behavior in a free-ranging female mangabey. Folia Primatologica. 1978;**29**:142-160. DOI: 10.1159/000155836

[43] Gould K, Flint M, Graham C. Chimpanzee reproductive senescence: A possible model for evolution of the menopause. Maturitas. 1981;**3**:157-166. DOI: 10.1016/0378-5122(81)90007-4

[44] Van Wagenen G. Menopause in subhuman primate. The Anatomical Record. 1970;**166**:392.

[45] Tigges J, Gordon TP, McClure HM, Hall EC, Peters A. Survival rate and life span of rhesus monkeys at the Yerkes Regional Primate Center. American Journal Primatology. 1988;**15**:263-273 DOI: 10.1002/ajp.1350150308

[46] Zapantis G, Santoro N. The menopausal transition: Characteristics and management. Best Practice and Research: Clinical Endocrinology and Metabolism. 2003;17:33-52 DOI: 10.1016/S1521-690X(02)00081-7

[47] Walker ML. Menopause in female rhesus monkeys. American Journal of Primatology. 1995;**35**:59-71. DOI: 10.1002/ajp.1350350106

[48] Gilardi KVK, Shideler SE, Valverde CR, Roberts JA, Lasley BL. Characterization of the onset of menopause in the rhesus macaque. Biology of Reproduction. 1997;**57**:335-340. DOI: 10.1095/biolreprod57.2.335

[49] Downs JL, Urbanski HF. Neuroendocrine changes in the aging reproductive axis of female rhesus macaques (*Macaca mulatta*). Biology of Reproduction. 2006:**75**:539-546. DOI: 10.1095/biolreprod.106.051839

[50] Nishida T, Corp N, Hamai M, Hasegawa Y, Hiraiwa-Hasegawa M, Hosaka K, et al. Demography, female life history, and reproductive profiles among the chimpanzees of Mahale. American Journal Primatology. 2003;**59**:99-121. DOI: 10.1002/ajp.10068

[51] Wich SA, Utami-Atmoko SS, Setia TM, Rijksen HD, Schürmann C, van Hooff JA, et al. Life history of wild Sumatran orangutans (*Pongo abelii*). Journal Human Evolution. 2004;**47**:385-398. DOI: 10.1016/j.jhevol.2004.08.006

[52] Hamilton WD III, Busse C, Smith KS. Adoption of infant orphan chacma baboons. Animal Behavior. 1982;**30**:29-34. DOI: 10.1016/S0003-3472(82)80233-9

[53] Teleki G, Hunt EE, Pfifferling JH. Demographic observations (1963-1973) on the chimpanzees of Gombe National Park, Tanzania. Journal of Human Evolution. 1976;**5**:559-598. DOI: 10.1016/0047-2484(76)90004-X

[54] Van Noordwijk MA, Van Schaik CP. Development of ecological competence in *Sumatran orangutans*. American Journal Physical Anthropology. 2005;**127**:79-94. DOI: 10.1002/ajpa.10426

[55] Machatschke IH, Wallner B, Dittami J. Impact of social environment on female chimpanzee reproductive cycles. Hormones and Behavior. 2006;**50**:126-131. DOI: 10.1016/j.yhbeh.2006.02.003

[56] Miller PB, Charleston JS, Battaglia DE, Klein NA, Soules MR. Morphometric analysis of primordial follicle number in pigtailed monkey ovaries: Symmetry and relationship with age. Biology of Reproduction. 1999;**61**:553-556

[57] Paul A, Kuester J, Podzuweit D. Reproductive senescence and terminal investment in female Barbary macaques (*Macaca sylvanus*) at Salem. International Journal of Primatology. 1993;**14**:105-124. DOI: 10.1007/BF02196506

[58] Johnson R, Kapsalis E. Menopause in free-ranging rhesus macaques: Estimated incidence, relation to body condition and adaptive significance. International Journal of Primatology. 1998;**19**:751-765. DOI: 10.1023/A:1020333110918.

[59] Gore AC, Windsor-Engnell BM, Terasawa E. Menopausal increases in pulsatile gonadotropin-releasing hormone release in a nonhuman primate (*Macaca mulatta*). Endocrinology. 2004;**145**:4653-4659. DOI: 10.1210/en.2004-0379

[60] Gill S, Sharpless JL, Rado K, Hall JE. Evidence that GnRH decreases with gonadal steroid feedback but increases with age in postmenopausal women. Journal of Clinical Endocrinology and Metabolins. 2002;**87**:2290-2296. DOI: 10.1210/jcem.87.5.8508

[61] Nichols SM, Bavister BD, Brenner CA, Didier, PJ, Harrison R, Kubisch, HM. Ovarian senescence in the rhesus monkey (*Macaca mulatta*). Human Reproduction. 2005;**20**:79-83. DOI: 10.1093/humrep/deh576

[62] Jones KP, Walker LC, Anderson D, Lacreuse A, Robson SL, Hawkes K. Depletion of ovarian follicles with age in chimpanzees: Similarities to humans. Biology of Reproduction. 2007;**77**:247-251. DOI: 10.1095/biolreprod.106.059634

[63] Itogawa N, Tanaka T, Ukai N, Fujii H, Kurokawa T, Ando A, Watanabe Y, Imakawa S. Demography and reproductive parameters of a free-ranging group of Japanese macaques (*Macaca fuscata*) at Katsuyama. Primates. 1992;**33**:49-68. DOI: 10.1007/BF02382762

[64] Nozaki M, Mitsunaga F, Shimizu K. Reproductive senescence in female Japanese monkeys (*Macaca fuscata*): Age- and season-related changes in hypothalamic-pituitary-ovarian functions and fecundity rates. Biology of Reproduction. 1995;**52**:1250-1257

[65] Kavanagh K, Koudy Williams J, Wagner JD. Naturally occurring menopause in cynomolgus monkeys: Changes in hormone, lipid, and carbohydrate measures with hormonal status. Journal of Medical Primatology. 2005;**34**:171-177. DOI: 10.1111/j.1600-0684.2005.00114.x

[66] Lacreuse A, Chennareddi L, Johnson J, Gould KG, Hawkes K, Wijayawardana S, et al. Menstrual cycles continue into advanced old age in the common chimpanzee (*Pan troglodytes*). Biology of Reproduction. 2008;**79**:407-412. DOI: 10.1095/biolreprod.108.068494.

[67] Videan E, Fritz J, Heward C, Murphy J. The effects of aging on hormone and reproductive cycles in female chimpanzees (*Pan troglodytes*). Comparative Medicine. 2006;**56**:291-299.

[68] Thompson ME, Jones JH, Pusey AE, Brewer-Marsden S, Goodall J, Marsden D, et al. Aging and fertility patterns in wild chimpanzees provide insights into the evolution of menopause. Current Biology. 2007;**17**(24):2150-2156. DOI: 10.1016/j.cub.2007.11.033

[69] Holman DJ, Wood JW. Pregnancy loss and fecundity in women. In: Ellison PT, editor. Reproduction, Ecology, and Human Evolution. New York: Aldine de Gruyter; 2001. pp. 15-38

[70] Collins DC, Graham CE, Preedy JR. Identification and measurement of urinary estrone, estradiol-17-beta, estriol, pregnanediol and androsterone during the menstrual cycle of the orangutan. Endocrinology. 1975;**96**:93-101. DOI: 10.1210/endo-96-1-93

[71] Nadler RD. Reproductive physiology and behavior of gorillas. Journal of Reproduction and Fertility. 1980;(Suppl 28):79-89

[72] Margulis SW, Atsalis S, Bellem A, Wielebnowski N. Assessment of reproductive behavior and hormonal cycles in geriatric western Lowland gorillas. Zoo Biology. 2007;**26**:117-139. DOI: 10.1002/zoo.20124

[73] Martin LJ, Carey KD, Comuzzie AG. Variations in menstrual cycle length and cessation of menstruation in captive raised baboons. Mechanisms of Ageing and Development. 2003;**124**:865-871. DOI: 10.1016/S0047-6374(03)00134-9

[74] Lapin BA, Krilova RI, Cherkovich GM, Asanov NS. Observations from Sukhumi. In: Bowden DB, editor, Aging in Nonhuman Primates. New York: Van Nostrand Reinhold; 1979. pp. 14-37

[75] Fedigan LM, Pavelka MSM Campbell C, Fuentes A, MacKinnon KC, Panger M, et al. Reproductive cessation in female primates comparisons of Japanese macaques and humans. In: Campbell C, Fuentes A, MacKinnon K, Panger M, Bearder S, editors. Primates in Perspective. United Kingdom, Oxford University Press; 2006. pp. 437-447

[76] Shively CA, Clarkson TB. The unique value of primate models in translational research. American Journal of Primatology. 2009;**71**:715-721. DOI: 10.1002/ajp.20720

[77] Magness CL, Fellin PC, Thomas M, Korth M, Agy M, Proll, S, et al. Analysis of the *Macaca mulatta* transcriptome and the sequence divergence between *Macaca* and human. Genome Biology. 2005;**6**:60. DOI: 10.1186/gb-2005-6-7-r60

[78] Kaplan JR, Manuck SB. Ovarian dysfunction, stress, and disease: A primate continuum. ILAR Journal. 2004; **45**:89-115. DOI: 10.1093/ilar.45.2.89

[79] Wagner JD, Kavanagh K, Ward GM, Auerbach BJ, Harwood H, Kaplan JR. Old world nonhuman primate models of type 2 diabetes mellitus. ILAR Journal. 2006;**47**:259-271. DOI: 10.1093/ilar.47.3.259

[80] Shively CA, Kaplan JR, Clarkson T. Carotid artery atherosclerosis in cholesterol-fed cynomolgus monkeys: The effects of oral contraceptive treatments, social factors and regional adiposity. Arteriosclerosis Thrombosis and Vascular Biology. 1990;**10**:358-366. DOI: 10.1161/01.ATV.10.3.358

[81] Jerome CP, Peterson PE. Nonhuman primate models in skeletal research. Bone. 2001;**29**:1-6. DOI: 10.1016/S8756-3282(01)00477-X

[82] Carlson CS, Loeser RF, Purser CB, Gardin JF, Jerome CP. Osteoarthritis in cynomolgus macaques. III: Effects of age, gender, and subchondral bone thickness on the severity of disease. Journal of Bone and Mineral Research. 1996;**11**:1209-1217. DOI: 10.1002/jbmr.5650110904

[83] Wallen K. Sex and context: Hormones and primate sexual motivation. Hormones and Behavior. 2001;**40**:339-357. DOI: 10.1006/hbeh.2001.1696

[84] Hartwig W. Primate evolution and Taxonomy. In: Campbell C, Fuentes A, MacKinnon, K, Bearder S Stumpf R, editors. Primates in Perspective. 2nd ed. New York: Oxford University Press. 2007. pp. 11-22

[85] Povinelli DJ, Rulf AB, Landau KR, Bierschwale DT. Self-recognition in chimpanzees (*Pan troglodytes*): Distribution, ontogeny, and patterns of emergence. Journal of Comparative Psychology. 1993;**107**(4):347

[86] Thompson R, Oden DL. Categorical perception and conceptual judgements by non-human primates: The paleological monkey and the analogical ape. Cognitive Science. 2000;**24**:363-396. DOI: 10.1016/S0364-0213(00)00029-X

[87] Amaral D, Lavenex P. Hippocampal neuroanatomy. In: Anderson P, Morris R, Amaral D, Bliss T, O'Keefe J, editors. The Hippocampus Book. New York: Oxford University Press; 2009. DOI: 10.1093/acprof:oso/9780195100273.003.0003.

[88] Hutchison RM, Everling S. Monkey in the middle: Why non-human primates are needed to bridge the gap in resting-state investigations. Frontiers in Neuroanatomy. 2012;**6**:1-19. DOI: 10.3389/fnana.2012.00029

[89] Uylings HBM, Groenewegen HJ, Kolb B. Do rats have a prefrontal cortex?. Behavioural Brain Research. 2003;**146**:3-17. DOI: 10.1016/j.bbr.2003.09.028

[90] Phillips K, Bales K, Capitanio J, Conley A, Czoty P, t Hart B, et al. Why primate models matter. American Journal of Primatology. 2014;**76**:801-827. DOI: 10.1002/ajp.22281

[91] Voytko M, Tinkler G. Cognitive function and its neural mechanisms in nonhuman primate models of aging, Alzheimer disease, and menopause. Frontiers in Bioscience. 2004;**9**:1899-1914. DOI: 10.2741/1370

[92] Lacreuse A, Chhabra R, Hall M, Herndon J. Executive function is less sensitive to estradiol than spatial memory: Performance on an analog of the card sorting test in ovariectomized aged rhesus monkeys. Behavioural Processes. 2004;**67**:313-319. DOI: 10.1016/j.beproc.2004.05.004

[93] Moore TL, Killiany RJ, Herndon JG, Rosene DL. Moss M. Executive system dysfunction occurs as early as middle-age in the rhesus monkey. Neurobiology of Aging. 2006;**27**:1484-1493. DOI: 10.1016/j.neurobiolaging.2006.08.004

[94] Roberts JA, Gilardi K, Lasley B, Rapp PR. Reproductive senescence predicts cognitive decline in aged female monkeys. Neuroreport. 1997;**8**:2047-2051

[95] Landauer N, Kohama SG, Voytko ML, Neuringer M. Effects of menstrual cycle status on visuospatial attention in aged rhesus monkeys. Society for Neuroscience Abstract. 2004;**34**:779-782

[96] McEwen BS, Alves SE. Estrogen actions in the central nervous system 1. Endocrine Reviews. 1999;**20**:279-307. DOI: 10.1210/edrv.20.3.0365

[97] Gundlah C, Kohama SG, Mirkes SJ, Garyfallou VT, Urbanski HF, Bethea C. Distribution of estrogen receptor beta (ERbeta) mRNA in hypothalamus, midbrain and temporal lobe of spayed macaque: Continued expression with hormone replacement. Molecular Brain Research. 2000;**76**:191-204. DOI: 10.1016/S0006-8993(99)02475-0

[98] Osterlund M, Gustafsson JA, Keller E, Hurd YL. Estrogen receptor beta (ERbeta) messenger ribonucleic acid (mRNA) expression within the human forebrain: Distinct distribution pattern to ERalpha mRNA. The Journal of Clinical Endocrinology & Metabolism. 2000;**85**:3840-3846. DOI: 10.1210/jcem.85.10.6913

[99] Tang Y, Janssen WGM, Hao J, Roberts JA, McKay H, Lasley B, et al. Estrogen replacement increases spinophilin-immunoreactive spine number in the prefrontal cortex of female rhesus monkeys. Cerebral Cortex. 2004;**14**:215-223. DOI: 10.1093/cercor/bhg121

[100] Rodríguez-Landa JF, Puga-Olguín A, Germán-Ponciano LJ, García-Ríos RI, Soria-Fregozo C. Anxiety in natural and surgical menopause—Physiologic and therapeutic bases. In: Durbano F, editor. A Fresh Look at Anxiety Disorders. Rijeka: InTech; 2015. pp. 173-198 . DOI: 10.5772/60621

[101] Coleman K, Robertson ND, Bethea CL. Long-term ovariectomy alters social and anxious behaviors in semi-free ranging Japanese Macaques. Behavioural Brain Research. 2011;**225**:317-327. DOI: 10.1016/j.bbr.2011.07.046

[102] Pazol K, Wilson ME, Wallen K. Medroxyprogesterone acetate antagonizes the effects of estrogen treatment on social and sexual behavior in female macaques. Journal of Clinical Endocrinology & Metabolism. 2004;**89**:2998-3006. DOI: 10.1210/jc.2003-032086

[103] Higaki S, Takumi K, Itoh M, Watanabe G, Taya K, Shimizu K, Hayashi M, Oishi T. Response of ERβ and aromatase expression in the monkey hippocampal formation to ovariectomy and menopause. Neuroscience Research. 2012;**72**:148-154. DOI: 10.1016/j.neures.2011.10.007

[104] Leranth C, Shanabrough M, Redmond D. Gonadal hormones are responsible for maintaining the integrity of spine synapses in the CA1 hippocampal subfield of female nonhuman primates. Journal of Comparative Neurology. 2002;**447**:34-42. DOI: 10.1002/cne.10230

[105] Velázquez-Zamora DA, González-Tapia D, González-Ramírez MM, Flores-Soto ME, Vázquez-Valls E, Cervantes M, González-Burgos I. Plastic changes in dendritic spines of hippocampal CA1 pyramidal neurons from ovariectomized rats after estradiol treatment. Brain Research. 2012;**1470**:1-10. DOI: 10.1016/j.brainres.2012.06.012

[106] Lima FB, Bethea CL. Ovarian steroids decrease DNA fragmentation in the serotonin neurons of non-injured rhesus macaques. Molecular Psychiatry. 2010;**15**:657-668. DOI: 10.1038/mp.2009.97

[107] Smith LJ, Henderson JA, Abell CW, Bethea CL. Effects of ovarian steroids and raloxifene on proteins that synthesize, transport, and degrade serotonin in the raphe region of Macaques. Neuropsychopharmacology. 2004;**29**:2035-2045. DOI: 10.1038/sj.npp.1300510

[108] Sanchez RL, Reddy AP, Centeno ML, Henderson JA, Bethea CL. A second tryptophan hydroxylase isoform, TPH-2 mRNA, is increased by ovarian steroids in the raphe region of macaques. Molecular Brain Research. 2005;**135**:194-203. DOI: 10.1016/j.molbrainres.2004.12.011

[109] Bethea CL, Smith AW, Centeno ML, Reddy AP. Long-term ovariectomy decreases serotonin neuron number and gene expression in free ranging macaques. Neuroscience. 2011;**192**:675-688. DOI: 10.1016/j.neuroscience.2011.06.003

[110] Shively CA, Friedman DP, Gage HD, Bounds MC, Brown-Proctor C, Blair JB, Henderson JA, Smith MA, Buchheimer N. Behavioral depression and positron emission tomography-determined serotonin 1A receptor binding potential in cynomolgus monkeys. Archives of General Psychiatry. 2006;**63**:396-403. DOI: 10.1001/archpsyc.63.4.396

[111] Lima FB, Centeno ML, Costa ME, Reddy AP, Cameron JL, Bethea CL. Stress sensitive female macaques have decreased fifth Ewing variant (Fev) and serotonin-related gene expression that is not reversed by citalopram. Neuroscience. 2009;**164**:676-691. DOI: 10.1016/j.neuroscience.2009.08.010

[112] Gundlah C, Lu NZ, Mirkes SJ, Bethea CL. Estrogen receptor beta (ERβ) mRNA and protein in serotonin neurons of macaques. Molecular Brain Research. 2001;**91**:14-22. DOI: 10.1016/s0169-328x(01)00108-5

3

The Benefits of Physical Activity on Climacteric Women

Simoni T. Bittar, José O.R. de Macêdo,
Elisio A. Pereira Neto, Hidayane G. da Silva,
Patrick A.S. Pfeiffer, Janine A. Padilha,
Wagner V. dos Santos and Maria do S. Cirilo-Sousa

Abstract

As the population ages, there is a need of developing ways to prevent or revert the deleterious effects of aging, especially in climacteric women who suffer with the problems caused by hormonal changes. Exercise is a nonmedicated intervention that can be applied on that population. The benefits of physical activity can positively change body composition, increase levels of muscular strength, balance, and functional capacity. Strength training, aerobic exercise, whole body vibration, and aquatic exercises are some of the modalities that health professionals can prescript to these individuals. Although there are many studies about these exercises, a technique called blood flow restriction is emerging as an alternative to high load exercises but with the same benefits.

Keywords: climacteric women, exercise, body composition, strength, blood flow restriction

1. Introduction

The aging process, also called senescence, is characterized by gradual and irreversible changes in an organism's structure and operation as a result of the time passing. The World Health Organization (WHO), in the end of the 1990s, adopted the term "active aging" to describe the process of the health, participation, and security opportunities. The aim of the active aging is to increase the expectation and quality of life to all the people who are aging, including the fragile, physically impaired, and the ones that require special care [1]. Data from the WHO indicate that in 2025, the life expectation in the developed countries will be 81 years; and 78 years in the ones that are in the development process [2].

The word "health," according to the WHO, refers to the physical, mental, and social well-being where the organism works optimally without any disease. Therefore, in an active aging project, the politics and programs that promote mental health and social living are just as important as the ones that improve the physical health conditions. Furthermore, the individual will be able to stay physically active and able to work [2].

During the adult life, the physiological functions of our organism decline, which is part of the senescence. The capacity of protein synthesis reduces significantly, there is a decrease of the immunological functions and changes in the body composition. Also, in elderly, the motor performance falls down expressively as a result of physiological degeneration and extrinsic factors such as environment conditions, task requirements, state of the disease, life style, or the combination of these elements. More than just biological and physiological changes, the aging process brings loss of psychological and social character, as well as elderly isolation, with the understanding that they are no longer active, or the fact that they think that are an obstacle to their families what causes sadness, low self-steam, even causing emotional diseases like depression [3].

In the middle-age, about 45 years old, the non-transmissible diseases are responsible for most part of the health complications and deaths. The researches show the risk of chronic diseases as the age advances, such as diabetes, cardiopathy, osteoarthritis, osteoporosis, and sarcopenia. However, what raises the risk of development of chronic diseases at older ages is smoking, sedentarism, inadequate diet, and hormonal alterations [1]. On the other hand, the enrolment in adequate physical activities, healthy diet, nonsmoking, not drinking alcohol, and the right use of the medicaments prescribed by the doctor may prevent diseases and the functional fall, increase the longevity and the individual's quality of life. Regarding specifically the indication of physical activity for the population over 65 years, the American College of Sports Medicine (ACSM) [4] recommends that along with aerobic exercises (moderate or intense), 8–10 strength exercises must be performed, with 8–12 repetitions for each exercise, two time a week.

The reduction of the lean mass close to 50 years is more expressive in women than men. The peak of this reduction happens on the postmenopause period, when occurs the loss of skeletal muscle, which is related to the fall on the production of ovarian hormones (especially, estrogen). The sarcopenia is a syndrome characterized by progressive and generalized reduction of the skeletal muscle mass associated with the loss of muscular strength, having as a consequence the physical impairment (reduction of muscular function and speed), fall in the quality of life and greater mortality. The European Study Group in Sarcopenia on the Elderly recommends that for the sarcopenia diagnostic the individual must have, necessarily, low lean mass associated with one of these two factors: low muscular function or strength. The preservation of the skeletal muscle mass is connected to the well-being and the disease prevention in the elderly [5].

Among the events that happen during the aging process, the reduction on the mineral bone density has a particular important role for the possible development of osteoporosis in both the genders but mostly in the female. After 40 years, the annual bone loss average is from 2 to 3% and elevates to more than 5% in the early years of climacteric [6]. The WHO defines osteoporosis as the reduction of bone mass associated with the disarrangement of the bone microarchitecture resulting in increased fragility of the bone and an elevated fracture risk [2].

Women in the postmenopause, when submitted to an exercise program based on stretching, balance, strength exercises, and impact exercises associated with hormone therapy (HT), show greater bone mineral density on the femoral neck when compared to the women that only do hormone therapy [7]. The muscle strength reduces fracture risks caused by osteoporosis because it increases the bone mineral content, the strength supported by the noncontractile tissues (tendons and ligaments), improvement in the postural function, and decrease in the risk of fall. Some studies suggest that the growth of muscle mass leads to a rise on the muscular strength, stimulating the bone remodeling through the piezoelectric effect, which is the capacity of the bone to transform mechanic signals into electrical signals [8].

2. Body composition

2.1. Lean and fat mass

The role of physical activity on body and fat mass control is extremely important. Studies demonstrated that there is a negative correlation between regular physical activities and body mass index (BMI). Since the exercise enhances energy expenditure, it plays an important part on reaching the ideal weight and body composition related to the health of elderly people. Therefore, the morbi-mortality, associated with non-transmissible chronic diseases, could be reduced with prevention, including physical activity as a change on the lifestyle to improve the aspects of body composition. Also, a reduction on the muscle mass on climacteric women results in a decrease of the basal metabolic rate, strength, and level of physical activity. However, it is already established that the reduction of these energetic needs is not followed by a decrease on the caloric ingestion, which causes a rise in the body fat mass with aging [9].

The aerobic exercise is a modality that has the power of promoting positive changes in the body composition. However, there is a need of controlling the intensity of the exercise because literature shows that when realized with a very small load, it will not modify the aspects of body composition [10]. A group of postmenopause women performed a 1-hour walking protocol three times a week for 6 months at 60% of the maximum oxygen volume (VO_{2max}) intake, whereas the other group performed walking 5 days a week for the same period but without controlling the intensity. Despite both the groups had shown reduction in fat mass and percentage, only the controlled one had decrease in the body mass.

Still regarding the effects of exercise on body composition, eight postmenopause women and seven men, aged between 61 and 77 years, caucasian, healthy and sedentary, with body mass index (BMI) with normal levels (24.8 kg/m^2) performed a 26-week resistance training protocol to upper and lower limbs and lumbar extensors, three times a week, two series of 10 repetitions for each exercise at 65–80% of one maximum repetition (1RM), totaling 45 min [11]. There were no changes on body mass; however, there was a reduction on fat percent (3.4%) and fat mass (3.1 kg) and an increase of the free-fat mass (2.0 kg), strength (14.9–49.0 kg), total energy expenditure, and basal metabolic rate.

Another aspect that can interfere on the results of exercise on the body composition is the presence or absence of a certified supervisor for the physical activity. Recently, the effects of an exercise program composed of stretching, weight bearing, resistance training for upper and lower limbs, and leisure activities in postmenopause women were evaluated where one group had the supervision of a physiotherapist and the other did not have; the exercises were performed at home. The upper and lower limbs and total body lean mass of the supervised group was increased. On the other hand, that did not happen on the other group, showing that supervision is important to obtain the desired results and also to prevent injuries [12].

The effects of a 16-week variable load resistance exercise protocol on body composition, associated with diet or not, were evaluated in 15 postmenopause women (50–69 years) who performed strength training three times a week with a load of 90% of 1RM [13]. The sample was divided according to the BMI: G1 ($n = 7$; IMC > 27 kg/m^2) and G2 ($n = 8$; IMC < 27 kg/m^2). Group 1 was submitted to the exercise protocol plus diet, whereas the other group did not have the diet controlled. The exercise-only group did not show significant changes on body composition. In comparison, the on-the-exercise + diet group showed a reduction on weight, fat mass, and fat percentage. In that perspective, although the exercise can promote a lot of benefits to climacteric women, if other aspects such as the diet are not well controlled, these benefits may not appear.

2.2. Bone mass

Positive effects of the exercise on the increase or maintenance of bone mineral density (BMD) were already observed in post menopause women with osteopenia or osteoporosis. However, the benefits depend on the type of exercise, intensity, frequency, and duration of the session [14].

Strength training can increase the mechanical stress on bone throughout the tendon promoting an osteogenic response and the piezoelectric effect, justifying the maintenance or increase of BMD. Because of that mechanism, forces of compression, tension, or torsion can generate electric signals that stimulate bone activity and deposition of minerals in stress points caused by muscle contraction. The muscle contraction can increase the BMD and, possibly, block the bone reabsorption [8, 15].

A positive linear relation between BMD and the increase of load during 1 year of strength training in postmenopause women was observed [16]. Exercise programs from low to moderate impact (running, walking, steps up-and-down) are more effective for the preservation of BMD on the lumbar area and femoral neck when combined with strength training than high-impact exercises such as jumping [17].

Many meta-analyses point out that high-intensity aerobic and resistance exercises tend to be more effective for the increase of lumbar spine BMD than low-intensity walking. Nevertheless, when there is an association between low-intensity walking and a high-calcium diet is also effective on elevating BMD. Furthermore, these exercises can promote a 2% elevation on the BMD of postmenopause women, which is a very important improvement in their bone health [18, 19].

Moderate aerobic exercise (50% of the maximum VO_2) seems to be safe and easy to execute in osteoporotic women and effectively increase BMD of the lumbar spine after 12 months of intervention [20]. A well-regulated bone metabolism is extremely important for the prevention and maintenance of the bone system properties. Likewise, a training program can help on the reduction of reabsorption bone biomarkers, reducing the risk of vertebral fracture up to 25%, even if the BMD does not increase significantly [21].

Besides the discrete effect of walking on the lumbar vertebrae BMD, there are other benefits related to that exercise. A 4-hour walking per week showed to be associated to a 41% less hip fracture risk compared to less than 1-hour per week [22]. In the same perspective, 40-minute brisk walking, three times a week, promoted a clinical improvement on the femoral neck BMD and a 35% reduction on the risk of fall on the elderly after 2 years of exercise [23]. **Table 1** sums up a few studies that investigated the benefits of exercise on body composition of climacteric women.

Year	Sample			Exercise protocol	Main results
	n	Age (years)	Stage		
1995 [10]	15	50–69	Postmenopause women	G1: strength training + diet G2: strength training 16 weeks	G1: ↓weight, ↓Percentage fat mass, ↓fat mass, ↑lean mass
1996 [11]	36	X	Postmenopause women	G1: walking, three times a week G2: walking five times a week 24 weeks	G1: ↓Weight, ↓fat mass, ↓ Percentage fat mass G2: ↓Fat mass, ↓ Percentage fat mass
2000 [24]	Eight men and seven women	61–77	Postmenopause	65–80% 1RM strength training, three times a week, 45 minutes' session 26 weeks	↓3, 4% fat mass, ↓fat mass, ↑lean mass
2016 [13]	34	60–74	Postmenopause women	G1: stretching, walking or step, upper and lower limbs strength training, leisure activities, all with supervision G2: same protocol, but without supervision Two times a week 12 months	G1: ↑arms, legs and total lean mass
1997 [23]	97	59–75	Postmenopause women with upper limb fractures	G1: walking, 40 min, three times/week G2: upper limb exercises, guided to perform exercises that improve wrists and arms function, visited each 3 month. Reassessed after 1 and 2 years.	G1: a tendency on the increase of the BMD of the femoral neck; increase on the lumbar BMD in both groups, however not statistically significant

Year	Sample			Exercise protocol	Main results
	n	Age (years)	Stage		
2001 [14]	35	53–77	Osteoporotic postmenopause women	G1: daily walking + 2 series of 15 repetitions per day of exercises for trunk and lower limb muscles and ingestion of calcium and D vitamin G2: detraining group G3: control group	No difference on the BMD of the lumbar vertebral in none of the groups; ↑ Percentage average BMD of the G1 when comparing the baseline to the 1st and 2nd year of training
2003 [7]	140	X	Osteoporotic postmenopause women	G1: hormone therapy + strength training G2: hormone therapy only	There was a positive association between the amount of weight lifted and the BMD of the femur independent from factors such as age, weight, and hormone therapy
2004 [20]	50	X	Osteoporotic postmenopause women	G1: outside walking (50% VO_{2max}, 1 h per day, 4 days a week, for 12 months G2: control group	There was no significant difference on the BMD of both groups The bone marker NTX showed a reduction on the G1

Table 1. Studies related to exercise and body composition in climacteric women.

3. Neuromuscular variables

As an important consequence caused by the many endocrine, neuroendocrine, behavioral, and metabolic changes that occur on the climacteric period, the decline of neuromuscular variables is one of the most frequent that brings important alterations to the life of this population [24]. During this chapter, the term "neuromuscular variables" will be used to make reference to all capacities that are related to neural stimulus and muscle health such as strength, agility, speed, flexibility, balance, and others.

There is a direct relation between muscle mass loss and strength decrease in women with more than 40 years. It is estimated that the muscle strength has a 15% fall on the period between 60 and 79 years, and 30% from the eighth life decade, with the lower limbs being more affected than the upper limbs [25, 26].

The diminution of muscle strength as a result of changes in the composition of the subtypes of muscle fiber, oxidative stress, variations of the growing hormone (GH), IGF-1, insulin, among others, also leads to a reduction in other important physical capacities that depends on the strength [27]. Body balance, walking speed, stepping up-and-down, recovery after a stability loss and standing up from the chair are some examples of variables that, with the fall in strength, end up being negatively affected.

The Brazilian Society of Sports Medicine [28] published an official statement regarding physical activity and women's health pointing that there is an inverse relation between exercising regularly and the main causes of death in menopause women. Thus, performing physical exercises regularly is the most effective way of avoiding strength loss, or try to regain part of the strength that was lost, similarly all the other capacities that depends on strength [26].

There are many types of exercise that promote benefits for the neuromuscular variables of climacteric women. Strength training, in general, is the most well-studied and used to achieve that goal. To prescribe correctly the most adequate training, few factors are to be taken into consideration such as the number of repetitions, load, series, resting interval, seminal frequency and others. The American College of Sports Medicine [4] states that to have effective results with the strength training, the load should be bigger than 65% of one maximum repetition (1RM), three series with 8–12 repetitions for the main muscle groups of the upper and lower limbs should be performed, at least three times a week. Nonetheless, those training variables can be manipulated in many ways, allowing the creation of a lot of training programs.

It is also well-known that training with higher intensities promote bigger changes. When comparing a training protocol that followed all the statements of the ACSM, which means exercises that involved the main muscle groups from upper and lower body where one group trained at 40% and the other at 80% of 1RM, it was observed that despite the fact that both showed increase of strength and transverse muscle section, the high intensity group had significantly more gains. In addition, it is important to highlight that in this specific study, emphasis was given to exercises that activated muscles that had origin or insertion on the spine and femur aiming to ally the strength gain with the piezoelectric effect and, consequently, improve the bone mass, which can be an interesting way to potentialize the benefit of the resistance exercise [29].

Although muscle strength happens to be a variable relatively easy to increase or, at least, maintain, it must be highlighted that if the individual stops practicing the physical activity, the detraining also happens fast. To illustrate that 15 postmenopause women practiced strength exercises for upper and lower limbs for 8 weeks with a load of 80% of 1RM and that was effective to increase strength of the trained muscle groups. To analyze the detraining process, those women stopped training and re-evaluated after 8 weeks. The average of strength loss was 4.5% after detraining. Yet, it is important to say that there was no difference between the strength before the training and after detraining [30]. Hence, the strength training is effective to climacteric women, but its benefits are easily lost in cases of abandoning the exercise program, pointing out the importance of developing strategies that increase the adherence of these women to the training.

A group of researchers from the Idaho State University, United States, developed a training program called POWIR (Prevent Osteoporosis with Impact + Resistance) with the initial goal of bone improvement but was modified to improve strength and function also. The basis of this program is composed of a progressive training that uses dumbbells, barbells, and weighted vests as ways of applying resistance focusing on exercises for the lower limbs, hips, chest, and back [31]. This protocol was initially created to healthy climacteric women; however, it was also applied in postmenopause women who had breast cancer.

In this specific population, 106 women who went through breast cancer treatment were separated in two groups where one performed the POWIR protocol and the other an exercise program consisted only of stretching and flexibility, called FLEX. The intervention lasted for 1 year and in addition to the exercises already pointed, both groups performed home exercises one time per week. The POWIR was able to improve aspects such as muscle strength, walking speed, stand up from the chair, among others, showing to be an efficient and safe option for climacteric women, including the ones who had diseases like cancer [31].

Water exercises are another type of physical activity that can improve neuromuscular variables of climacteric women and the changes may be similar to other exercises that are commonly used on the daily practice of physiotherapists and personal trainers, such as elastic bands. A water exercises protocol with the same number of repetitions, rest interval, series, week frequency, duration (35–60 min) and for the same muscle groups of an elastic band protocol promote the similar benefits for climacteric women [32].

Nevertheless, even with the same exercises, some differences still appear when comparing water exercises and elastic bands. The water exercises were more efficient on improving the performance on the 60-second squats (65%) and abdominal crunch (28%), whereas the elastic bands were better to increase flexibility (44.19%) and performance on the knee push-up (29.13%). Still, it is important to highlight that both protocols promoted benefits in all neuromuscular variables [32]. When the protocol is well designed with heating, stretching, strength exercises, and cool down, there is no doubt that the benefits will appear, and both water exercises and strength training with elastic bands are effective to climacteric women.

In fact, to promote a muscle strength gain, it is necessary that the muscle contracts and so activate mechanisms that promote protein synthesis. In more intense exercises such as strength training or water exercises, it is very easy to observe how the contraction needed to win a load stimulates muscle hypertrophy and strength gains. On the other hand, lighter activities such as whole body vibration training (WBVT) sessions also stimulate muscle contraction [33]. The most important mechanism activated is that the vibration has the capacity of stimulating sensorial receptors that lead to a reflect activation of the motor units, similar to what happens on the tonic reflex [34].

Hormone therapy (HT) on climacteric women is an important treatment indicated to reduce the symptoms (such as, heat waves, night sweats, vaginal dryness, changes in sleep, among others) caused by decrease of hormones, mainly estrogen [35, 36]. Studies confirmed the positive effects of this therapy on the quality of life and strength in postmenopausal women [37, 38]. Associated with HT, physical exercise can bring benefits to women's health after menopause, reduce fat mass and the risk of coronary diseases; increase strength, resistance, and flexibility [39–41]. Besides that, weight-bearing, strength, and balance exercises associated with HT are able to help in osteoporosis prevention and treatment in a 1-year period, aiming to increase BMD and, consequently, reducing the number of lumbar and femur neck fractures [16].

It is undeniable that the strength training is the type of exercise mostly used to promote strength gains. In this perspective, to see if the WBVT is also capable of promoting those gains, the results of both types of exercise must be compared. Three times a week WBVT and strength training, for 6 months, were able to increase significantly the isometric (15.10% and 16.49%, respectively) and isotonic (16.47% and 10.59%) strength, those differences being nonsignificant when comparing both types of training [34]. Thus, WBVT can promote a strength increase similar to the strength training. Some studies that analyzed the effects of many types of exercise on the neuromuscular variables are listed on **Table 2**.

Year	Sample			Exercise protocol	Main results
	n	Age (years)	Stage		
2000 [29]	25	41–60	Postmenopause women	G1: strength training at 80% of 1RM G2: strength training at 40% of 1RM G3: control group	G1 and G2: ↑muscle strength, ↑transverse muscle section G1: showed significant greater increases
2002 [30]	15	49–62	Postmenopause women	G1: strength training at 80% of 1RM G2: control group	G1: increased strength after 8 weeks, but that improvement was lost after 8 weeks of detraining
2012 [31]	106	≥50	Postmenopause women survivors of breast cancer G2: FLEX Both interventions lasted 1 year	G1: POWIR	G1: ↑ muscle strength, ↑walking speed, ↑stand up from the chair
2009 [32]	46	54.7 ± 2.0	Postmenopause women	G1: water exercises G2: strength training with elastic bands	Both groups: ↑60-second squats, ↑abdominal crunch, ↑flexibility, ↑knee push-up
2004 [34]	70	58–74	Postmenopause women	G1: whole body vibration (24 weeks) G2: strength training (24 weeks) G3: control group	G1 and G2: ↑isometric and isotonic strength

Table 2. Studies related to exercise and neuromuscular variables in climacteric women.

4. Blood flow restriction—an alternative to high loads

As previously said, to obtain maximum benefits from exercise, for example the strength training, it is indicated that higher loads must be used, which will promote a bigger response of the organism and, consequently, greater benefits [42]. Nevertheless, loads bigger than 65% of 1RM as stated by the ACSM [4] many times are not tolerated by the elderly, individuals with some disease that turns harder performing exercises, such as chronic obstructive pulmonary disease and osteoporosis, among other populations. In this perspective, a Japanese scientist called Yoshaki Sato thought about a method that consisted of low-load exercises associated with some device that could reduce the blood flow, for example pneumatic cuffs, elastic bands, and sphygmomanometers (**Figure 1**), to the muscle that is being used [43]. Initially, the method was called "vascular occlusion", but nowadays, the terms "Kaatsu training" and "blood flow restriction" (BFR) are the most widely used.

There are still many unanswered questions regarding how the BFR is capable of promoting benefits on strength, functionality, muscle activation, and others, similar to the traditional high

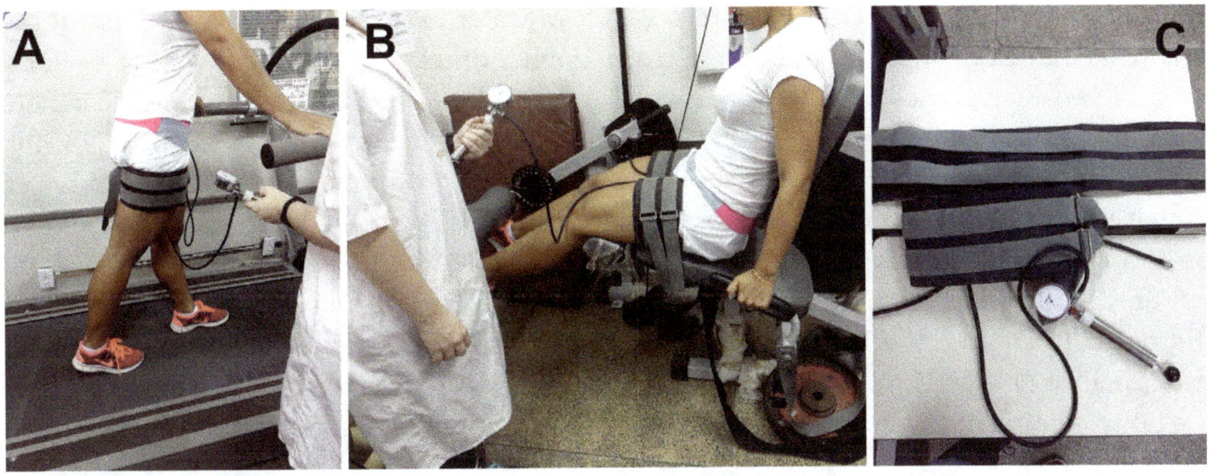

Figure 1. (A) Walking with blood flow restriction, (B) strength training with blood flow restriction, and (C) pneumatic cuff used to promote the blood flow restriction.

load exercise, even being performed with very low loads. However, studies that investigated the BFR mechanisms affirm that the explanation lies on a bigger metabolite concentration, stimulation of anaerobic growth factors, greater fast twitch fibers recruitment, increase on GH secretion, VGF1, fall on miostatine and rise on mTOR levels, greater nitric oxide synthesis, along with other factors that were not yet discovered [44–46].

Most part of the studies with BFR combine this technique with the strength training and in apparently healthy individuals; however, some researchers already have been investigating how the BFR can be used in special populations and associated with other types of exercise [47–52]. In the next session, some studies that used this technique in climacteric women and/or with non-transmissible chronic diseases will be presented.

4.1. Applying the blood flow restriction

The osteoporosis, which is a bone-metabolic disorder characterized by a reduction of the bone mineral density (BMD) with deterioration of the bone micro architecture, leading to an increase of the bone fragility and fracture risk [53], affects climacteric women, and this is a population that needs to practice exercises to improve not only the bone, but also the neuromuscular aspects. Because of that, strength training with blood flow restriction is being used in osteoporotic women due to the fact that it can promote benefits without the need of elevated loads [47].

A low load (30% of 1RM) with BFR and a high load (80% of 1RM) strength training program were applied for 3 months and two times a week in women with osteoporosis (62.60 ± 4.33 years) to compare the alterations on strength levels [47]. Both protocols consisted of four series until concentric failure, but while the BFR group had a 30 seconds' rest between series, the high load group had 2 minutes. The two types of exercises were capable of increasing strength comparing the pre-test in the 6 and 12 weeks, and the gains were similar for both groups, showing that even with low load, the BFR promotes strength gains on the same magnitude of high loads.

There is few literature regarding the use of BFR in water exercises probably because of the problems that can appear on building a restriction equipment that could be easily used on water. Even with those difficulties, two studies were developed by a group of researchers from the Federal University of Paraíba, Brazil, associating water exercises for BFR [48, 49]. Menopaused women (n = 28) were separated in control group, water exercises and water exercises with BFR. For 8 weeks, the experimental groups performed a 45 minutes' exercise protocol for lower limbs in a pool with controlled temperature, being on with and without BFR. The exercise combined with BFR increased lower limbs maximum strength, which did not happen on the other experimental group. Also, both groups improved functional performance [48]. In contrast, neither of the protocols were capable of changing aspects of the body composition, probably because the exercise volume was too low to promote such changes [49].

Elastic band exercises are another type of exercise whose effects associated with BFR were investigated. Similar to the traditional strength training, low-load elastic band exercises with BFR for upper limbs for 2 months, three times a week, showed an increase on the strength similar to the high intensity group. In addition, a tendency for improving the total bone mass was also found [50].

Even though the mechanisms of BFR on the improvement of the muscle health are not completely well known, some studies were already able to partially explain that [44, 45]. Regarding the bone mass, few are the studies explaining the physiological mechanisms caused by BFR. However, since it is a low-load exercise, the improvements do not come from mechanical stimulus or piezoelectric effect but from metabolic and hormonal factors [51, 52]. The low-load strength training with BFR was capable of increasing the bone alkaline phosphatase levels in elderly men after 6 weeks of exercise, correspondingly to the high load group (21% and 23%, respectively) [51]. Besides that, there is the hypothesis that an increase on the intramedullary pressure and interstitial fluid flow within the bone promoted by the BFR leads to favorable responses for bone formation and remodulation [52].

5. Conclusions

With the aging of the world's population, it turns even more necessary that new studies be developed with the goal of finding exercise types that benefits this population group, aiming not only the treatment of non-transmissible chronic disease but also its prevention. The positive effects of exercise in climacteric women were already proved in a lot of studies, and it is essential that the health professionals responsible for the prescription of such exercises (physiotherapists, personal trainers, occupational therapists) have the necessary knowledge to prescribe correctly in a way that brings maximum improvements on body composition, functional performance, strength, balance, and others. On the other hand, new ways of exercise, just like blood flow restriction, are promissory exercise modalities for that the public still needs more studies regarding the ideal prescription to apply this technique on climacteric women.

Author details

Simoni T. Bittar[1*], José O.R. de Macêdo[2], Elisio A. Pereira Neto[3], Hidayane G. da Silva[3], Patrick A.S. Pfeiffer[3], Janine A. Padilha[3], Wagner V. dos Santos[4] and Maria do S. Cirilo-Sousa[3]

*Address all correspondence to: simonibittar@hotmail.com

1 Federal University of Paraíba, João Pessoa, Brazil

2 Patos Integrated Faculties, Patos, Brazil

3 Federal University of Paraíba, João Pessoa, Brazil

4 Faculty of Medical Sciences, João Pessoa, Brazil

References

[1] World Health Organization (WHO). Active Aging: A Health Politics. Brasilia; 2005

[2] World Health Organization (WHO). Global Forum for Health Research: The 10/90 Report on Health Research. Genebra; 2000

[3] Mazo GA, Lopes MA, Bertoldo BT. Atividade física e o idoso: concepção gerontológica. 2nd ed. São Paulo: Sulina; 2004. p. 236

[4] American College of Sports Medicine (ACSM). Position stand: Progression models in resistance training for healthy adults. Medicine and Science in Sports and Exercise. 2009;**3**:687-708

[5] Cruz-Jentoft AJ, Baeyens JP, Bauer JM, Boirie Y, Cederholm T, Landi F, et al. Sarcopenia: European consensus on definition and diagnosis. Age Ageing. 2010;**39**:412-423

[6] Silverman SL, Piziak VK, Chen P, Misurski DA, Wagman RB. Relationship of health related quality of life to prevalent and new or worsening back pain in postmenopausal women with osteoporosis. Journal of Rheumatology. 2005;**32**:2405-2409

[7] Teixeira PJ, Going SB, Houtkooper LB, Metcalfe LL, Blew RM, Flint-Wagner HG, et al. Resistance training in postmenopausal women with and without hormone therapy. Medicine and Science in Sports and Exercise. 2003;**35**:555-562

[8] Fukada E, Yasuda I. On the piezoelectric effect of bone. Journal of the Physical Society of Japan. 1957;**12**:1158-1162

[9] Melby C, Commerford S, Hill J. Perspectives in exercise science and sports medicine vol. 11: Exercise, nutrition, and weight control. In: Lamb D, Murray R, editors. Exercise, Macronutrient Balance, and Weight Control. Carmel: Cooper Publishing Group; 1998. pp. 1-60

[10] Ready AE, Naimark B, Ducas J, Sawatzky J-AV, Boreskie SL, Drinkwater DT, et al. Influence of walking volume on health benefits in women post-menopause. Medicine and Science in Sports and Exercise. 1996;**28**:1097-105

[11] Hunter GR, Wetzstein CJ, Fields DA, Brown A, Bamman MM. Resistance training increases total energy expenditure and free-living physical activity in older adults. Journal of Applied Physiology. 2000;**89**:977-984

[12] Bittar ST, Maeda SS, Marone MMS, Santili C. Physical exercises with free weights and elastic bands can improve body composition parameters in postmenopausal women: WEB protocol with a randomized controlled trial. Menopause. 2016;**23**:383-389

[13] Ryan AS, Pratley RE, Elahi D, Goldberg AP. Resistive training increases fat-free mass and maintains RMR despite weight loss in postmenopausal women. Journal of Applied Physiology. 1995;**79**:818-823

[14] Iwamoto J, Takeda T, Ichimura S. Effect of exercise training and detraining on bone mineral density in postmenopausal women with osteoporosis. Journal of Orthopaedic Science. 2001;**6**:128-132

[15] Bonewald LF, Johnson ML. Osteocytes, mechanosensing and Wnt signaling. Bone. 2017;**42**:606-615

[16] Cussler EC, Lohman TG, Going SB, Houtkooper LB, Metcalfe LL, Flint-Wagner HG, et al. Weight lifted in strength training predicts bone change in postmenopausal women. Medicine and Science in Sports and Exercise. 2003;**35**:10-17

[17] Martyn-St James M, Carroll S. A meta-analysis of impact exercise on postmenopausal bone loss: The case for mixed loading exercise programmes. British Journal of Sports Medicine. 2009;**43**:898-908

[18] Specker BL. Evidence for an interaction between calcium intake and physical activity on changes in bone mineral density. Journal of Bone and Mineral Research. 1996;**11**:1539-1544

[19] Kelley GA, Kelley KS, Tran ZV. Exercise and lumbar spine bone mineral density in postmenopausal women: A meta-analysis of individual patient data. Medical Sciences. 2002;**57**:599-604

[20] Yamazaki S, Ichimura S, Iwamoto J, Takeda T, Toyama Y. Effect of walking exercise on bone metabolism in postmenopausal women with osteopenia/osteoporosis. Journal of Bone and Mineral Metabolism. 2004;**22**:500-508

[21] Cummings SR, Karpf DB, Harris F, Genant HK, Ensrud K, LaCroix AZ, et al. Improvement in spine bone density and reduction in risk of vertebral fractures during treatment with antiresorptive drugs. American Journal of Medicine. 2017;**112**:281-289

[22] Feskanich D, Willett W, Colditz G. Walking and leisure-time activity and risk of hip fracture in postmenopausal women. Journal of the American Medical Association. 2002;**288**:2300-2306

[23] Ebrahim S, Thompson PW, Baskaran V, Evans K. Randomized placebo-controlled trial of brisk walking in the prevention of postmenopausal osteoporosis. Age Ageing. 1997;**26**:253-260

[24] De Villiers TJ, Gass MLS, Haines CJ, Hall JE, Lobo RA, Pierroz DD, et al. Global Consensus Statement on menopausal hormone therapy. Climacteric. 2013;**16**:203-204

[25] Orsatti FL, Dalanesi RC, Maestá N, Náhas EAP, Burini RC. Redução da força muscular está relacionada à perda muscular em mulheres acima de 40 anos. Rev Bras Cineantropometria e Desempenho Hum. 2011;**13**:36-42

[26] Macaluso A, De Vito G. Muscle strength, power and adaptations to resistance training in older people. European Journal of Applied Physiology. 2004;**91**:450-472

[27] Maltais ML, Desroches J, Dionne IJ. Changes in muscle mass and strength after menopause. Journal of Musculoskeletal and Neuronal Interactions. 2009;**9**:186-197

[28] Leitão M, Lazzoli J, Oliveira M, Nóbrega A, Silveira G, Carvalho T, et al. Posicionamento oficial da Sociedade Brasileira de Medicina do Esporte: Atividade física e saúde na mulher. Revista Brasileira de Medicina do Esporte. 2000;**6**:215-220

[29] Bemben DA, Fetters NL, Bemben MG, Nabavi N, Koh ET. Musculoskeletal responses to high- and low-intensity resistance training in early postmenopausal women. Medicine and Science in Sports and Exercise. 2000;**32**:1949-1957

[30] Elliott KJ, Sale C, Cable NT. Effects of resistance training and detraining on muscle strength and blood lipid profiles in postmenopausal women. British Journal of Sports Medicine. 2002;**36**:340-344

[31] Winters-Stone KM, Dobek J, Bennett JA, Nail LM, Leo MC, Schwartz A. The effect of resistance training on muscle strength and physical function in older, postmenopausal breast cancer survivors: A randomized controlled trial. Journal of Cancer Survivorship. 2012;**6**:189-199

[32] Colado JC, Triplett NT, Tella V, Saucedo P, Abellán J. Effects of aquatic resistance training on health and fitness in postmenopausal women. European Journal of Applied Physiology. 2009;**106**:113-122

[33] Moreira L, Oliveira M, Galvão A, Marin-Mio R, Santos R, Castro M. Physical exercise and osteoporosis: Effects of different types of exercises on bone and physical function of postmenopausal women. Arquivos Brasileiros de Endocrinologia & Metabologia. 2014;**58**:514-522

[34] Verschueren SMP, Roelants M, Delecluse C, Swinnen S, Vanderschueren D, Boonen S. Effect of 6-month whole body vibration training on hip density, muscle strength, and postural control in postmenopausal women: A randomized controlled pilot study. Journal of Bone and Mineral Research. 2004;**19**:352-359

[35] Rebar R, Trabal J, Mortola J. Low-dose esterified estrogens (0.3 mg/day): Long term and short-effects on menopausal symptoms and quality of life in postmenopausal women. Climacteric. 2000;**3**:176-182

[36] Dennerstein L, Lehert P, Guthrie J, Burger H. Modeling women's health during the menopausal transition: A longitudinal analysis. Menopause. 2007;**14**:53-62

[37] Genazzani A, Niccolucci A, Campagnoli P, Crosigani P, Nappi C, Serra G. Assessment of the QoL in Italian menopausal women: Comparison between HRT users and non users. Maturitas. 2002;**42**:267-280

[38] Skelton D, Philips S, Bruce S, Naylor C, Woledge R. Hormone replacement therapy increases isometric muscle strength of adductor pollicis in postmenopausal women. Clinical Science (London). 1999;**4**:357-364

[39] Reubinoff B, Wurtman J, Rojansky N, Adler D, Stein P, Schenker J, et al. Effects of hormone replacement therapy on weight, body composition, fat distribution, and food intake in early postmenopausal women: A prospective study. Fertility and Sterility. 1995;**64**:963-968

[40] Schmitz K, Jacobs DJ, Leon A, Schreiner P, Sternfeld B. Physical activity and body weight: Associations over ten years in the CARDIA study. Coronary Artery Risk Development in Young Adult. International Journal of Obesity and Related Metabolic Disorders. 2000;**24**:1475-1487

[41] Teoman N, Ozcan A, Acar B. The effect of exercise on physical fitness and quality of life in postmenopausal women. Maturitas. 2004;**47**:71-77

[42] Laurentino G, Ugrinowitsch C, Aihara AY, Fernandes AR, Parcell AC, Ricard M, et al. Effects of strength training and vascular occlusion. International Journal of Sports Medicine. 2008;**29**:664-667

[43] Sato Y. The history and future of KAATSU Training. International Journal of KAATSU Training and Research. 2005;**1**:1-5

[44] Kawada S. What phenomena do occur in blood flow-restricted muscle? International Journal of KAATSU Training and Research. 2005;**1**:37-44

[45] Loenneke JP, Wilson GJ, Wilson JM. A mechanistic approach to blood flow occlusion. International Journal of Sports Medicine. 2010;**31**:1-4

[46] Pearson SJ, Hussain SR. A review on the mechanisms of blood-flow restriction resistance training-induced muscle hypertrophy. Sport Medicine. 2015;**45**:187-200

[47] Silva J, Neto G, Freitas E, Pereira Neto E, Batista G, Torres M, et al. Chronic effect of strength training with blood flow restriction on muscular strength among women with osteoporosis. Journal of Exercise Physiology. 2015;**18**:33-41

[48] Araújo JP, Neto GR, Loenneke JP, Bemben MG, Laurentino GC, Batista G, et al. The effects of water-based exercise in combination with blood flow restriction on strength and functional capacity in post-menopausal women. Age (Omaha). 2015;**37**:110-118. DOI 10.1007/s11357-015-9851-4

[49] Araújo J, Rodrigues Neto G, Silva J, Silva H, Pereira Neto E, Batista G, et al. Does water aerobics with blood flow restriction change the body composition? Journal of Exercise Physiology. 2015;**18**:25-31

[50] Thiebaud RS, Loenneke JP, Fahs CA, Rossow LM, Kim D, Abe T, et al. The effects of elastic band resistance training combined with blood flow restriction on strength, total bone-free lean body mass and muscle thickness in postmenopausal women. Clinical Physiology and Functional Imaging. 2013;**33**:344-352

[51] Karabulut M, Bemben DA, Sherk VD, Anderson MA, Abe T, Bemben MG. Effects of high-intensity resistance training and low-intensity resistance training with vascular restriction on bone markers in older men. European Journal of Applied Physiology. 2011;**111**:1659-1667

[52] Loenneke JP, Young KC, Fahs CA, Rossow LM, Bemben DA, Bemben MG. Blood flow restriction: Rationale for improving bone. Medical Hypotheses. 2012;**78**:523-527

[53] Pinto Neto AM, Soares A, Urbanetz AA, Souza ACDAE, Ferrari AEM, Amaral B, et al. Brazilian consensus on osteoporosis 2002. Revista Brasileira De Reumatologia. 2002;**42**:343-354

4

Menstrual Cycle and Physical Effort

Magdalena Wiecek

Abstract

In addition to affecting the sexual organs in women, ovarian hormones have a wide impact on processes related to metabolism, water and electrolyte balance, thermoregulation, and redox balance. Differences in the estradiol and progesterone concentrations during the follicular and luteal phases, as well as the increase in the concentration of these hormones under the influence of physical exercise, may cause a different course of exercise response in women depending on the phase of menstrual cycle. Estrogens affect the metabolism of women by reducing the rate of gluconeogenesis and glycogenolysis and, at the same time, by increasing the share of lipids in covering energy requirements. Progesterone affects respiratory system parameters causing, among others, an increase in pulmonary ventilation. The resultant antagonistic action of progesterone and estradiol is the effect on thermoregulatory mechanisms. Increased estradiol concentration at the low progesterone concentration level causes water and electrolyte retention. In turn, an increased level of progesterone leads to loss of water and sodium, causing a decrease in the volume of plasma during the postovulatory phase of the menstrual cycle. The processes described above are related to metabolic changes affecting the ability to perform physical efforts.

Keywords: menstrual cycle, aerobic efforts, anaerobic efforts, acid-base balance, redox balance

1. Introduction

Knowledge about the physiology of physical efforts is mostly based on research results in which only men participated. However, the increasing participation of women in many sports disciplines encourages observation of the physiological reactions and effects regarding intense physical efforts on the body of women associated with the process of sports training [1, 2].

A decrease in the level of sex hormones during rest, as a result of heavy and long-term training, can lead to disorders in the menstrual cycle of a woman [2, 3]. These disorders most have the characteristics of rare menstrual periods (oligomenorrhea) or secondary amenorrhea (amenorrhoea secundaria). In women with regular menstruation, burdened by sports training, anovulatory cycles or shortened luteal phases often occur. It is also possible to exclude the impact of physical exercise related to training on the later menarche age [2, 4]. The factors conducive to hormonal abnormalities are large decreases in body mass and the amount of adipose tissue, resulting not only from significant training loads but also frequent disorders in the way of eating [5]. Long-lasting estrogen deficiency leads to a decrease in bone density, causing deterioration of its structure, which may contribute to osteoporosis in the future [6]. Abnormalities in the way of eating, menstrual disorders, and disturbances in bone metabolism observed in women practicing various sports were called the "triad syndrome" [2, 7, 8]. Therefore, one should look for an answer to the question on how to program women's training in order to achieve high sports results without negative consequences for their health [1].

Assessing physiological responses induced by physical exercise in women, cyclic changes in the level of sex hormones that occur during the reproductive period in every normal menstrual cycle cannot be overlooked. The menstrual cycle is the result of complex interaction of the hypothalamus, pituitary gland, and ovarian hormones, which, apart from acting on the sexual organs, exhibit a broad, nonspecific effect on various processes related to metabolism, water, and electrolyte balance or thermoregulation in women [2, 9–13]. As shown in studies on animals, differences related to estradiol levels are a factor influencing the diversified use of energy substrates [14, 15]. Distinct differences in estradiol and progesterone levels between the follicular and luteal phases, as well as an increase in the concentration of these hormones under the influence of physical exercise, may cause a different course of exercise response in women depending on the phase of the menstrual cycle [2, 10, 16].

Research suggests that estrogens affect the metabolism of women by reducing the rate of gluconeogenesis and glycogenolysis and, at the same time, increase the share of lipids in covering energy demand [17–22]. The increased use of lipids as a source of energy occurs due to the increase in the amount of free fatty acids, which results from the increased synthesis of triglycerides and in the rate of lipolysis [23]. The effect of estradiol on metabolic processes in the liver, muscles, and adipose tissue can be achieved by changing the activity of key enzymes, changing membrane permeability or indirectly through changes in hormone levels: insulin, glucagon, cortisol, hGH, or catecholamines [24, 25].

Progesterone affects the parameters of the respiratory system, causing, inter alia, an increase in pulmonary ventilation per minute (V_E) [26]. In the postovulatory phase, a higher resting level of oxygen uptake (VO_2) is also observed [27].

The resultant antagonistic effect of progesterone and estradiol is the effect on thermoregulatory mechanisms, which leads to an increase in the body's core temperature during the luteal phase of the menstrual cycle [12, 28–30].

In the woman's body, we also observe changes in the total water content associated with the menstrual cycle phase. Observations of some authors indicate that elevated estradiol concentration at low concentration of progesterone causes the retention of water and electrolytes in the body [31]. In turn, the increased level of progesterone, by blocking the action of aldosterone in the kidneys, leads to loss of water and sodium [32], causing a decrease in plasma volume during the postovulatory phase of the menstrual cycle [33].

All processes described above are directly related to metabolic changes affecting the ability to perform physical efforts. Differences in the use of substrates and in the intensity of individual energy changes during muscle work of different intensities, resulting from hormonal changes in the course of the menstrual cycle, may affect, e.g., the activity of the adrenergic system, the amount of lactic acid formed in muscle tissue and its level in the blood, and changes in the level of acid-base balance parameters or indicators of oxidative stress [2, 10, 16, 34]. Therefore, it can be expected that cyclical fluctuations in the level of endogenous ovarian hormones in women will affect the extent and size of exercise responses. However, the test results are not unequivocal.

2. Methods

Original and review scientific publications regarding the level of cardiopulmonary reactions, thermoregulation processes, and oxidative stress as a result of aerobic and anaerobic efforts during various phases of the menstrual cycle were reviewed. Conclusions were formulated on the basis of tests in which hormonal evaluation of the menstrual cycle was conducted.

3. Exercise responses during the menstrual cycle

3.1. Aerobic exercise

It is generally accepted that the maximal oxygen uptake index (VO_{2max}) is the indicator of aerobic efficiency, the level of which is directly determined during gradual physical exercise, performed up to the individual maximum intensity ("until exhaustion"). Such effort leads to the maximum involvement of the oxidative phosphorylation process while activating the processes of anaerobic adenosine triphosphate (ATP) resynthesis (phosphocreatine, anaerobic glycolysis). VE, cardiac output, and blood oxygen capacity are important factors determining the level of VO_{2max} [35].

3.1.1. Cardiorespiratory effect

One of the first studies comparing the physiological and biochemical stress response of women at the time of the menstrual cycle, during which laboratory testing days were determined based on sex hormone levels, was carried out by Jurkowski et al. [36]. In these studies, immediately after two 20-minute physical efforts at an intensity of 40 and 70% VO_{2max}, respectively, the woman performed a physical effort at an intensity of 90% VO_{2max} "until exhaustion." The time of extreme exercise was almost twice as long in the luteal phase. In the luteal phase, higher values of the maximum minute pulmonary ventilation (VE_{max}) were also noted. The maximum heart rate (HR_{max}) and VO_{2max} did not differ between the menstrual cycle phases [36].

However, these data are not fully confirmed in the results of research conducted by other authors. The time of continuing the effort of gradually increasing work intensity did not differ significantly between the follicular and luteal phases of the menstrual cycle [37]. Similar in both phases of the menstrual cycle, Nicklas et al. [17] found that the time of continuing work "until exhaustion " was for the intensity of 70% VO_{2max}, and McCracken et al. [38] noted it for the intensity of 90% VO_{2max}.

The results of some studies indicate a significantly higher level of resting oxygen uptake during the postovulatory phase [27, 39]. However, most authors agree that the menstrual cycle phases do not significantly affect VO_2, neither at rest nor during submaximal and maximal intensity efforts [37, 40–45].

The conclusions from laboratory tests differ regarding the assessment of the influence of the menstrual cycle phases on the level of pulmonary ventilation. Schoene et al. [46] and Das [47] reported higher resting V_E values in the luteal phase of the menstrual cycle. During stress tests, Jurkowski et al. [36], as well as Hessemer and Bruck [39], obtained higher values in the postovulatory phase. However, differences between phases in the exercise level of this parameter are not statistically significant in many studies [37, 43, 45, 48].

Significant inter-phase differences concerning the maximal heart rate were noted by Pivarnik et al. [41]. In this research, HR_{max} was higher in the luteal phase by 10 beats per minute. Higher resting and exercise heart rate in the luteal phase were also noted by other researchers [39, 46, 49]. Some authors, however, did not find significant differences in the values of HR_{max} [37, 40, 43, 45, 48].

De Souza et al. [48], comparing the physiological responses of women with normal menstrual cycles and women with secondary menstrual irregularities, obtained similar results for both groups. In eumenorrheic women, both during the 40-minute effort at 80% intensity VO_{2max} and during the graded test "until exhaustion," in the luteal phase, slightly higher levels of oxygen uptake, pulmonary ventilation, and heart rate were found. However, the postexercise concentration of lactate in the blood was lower in this phase. Nevertheless, the differences between phases were not statistically significant [48].

3.1.2. Metabolic effect

It is undisputed that a gradual increase in the intensity of effort leads to an increase in anaerobic energy recovery processes. This causes an increase in the concentration of lactic acid in the blood, causing changes in the level of acid-base balance parameters [50–52]. Therefore, it is of great importance in the assessment of endurance capacities to determine the location of metabolic thresholds, using blood lactate measurement or based on the dynamics of changes in ventilation indicators. The first metabolic threshold is defined by the first ventilatory threshold, the aerobic or anaerobic threshold (AT), and means the addition of anaerobic metabolism. The second metabolic threshold is referred to as the second ventilatory threshold, respiratory compensation point (RCP), or the threshold of uncompensated metabolic acidosis [50, 52–55]. The severity of anaerobic transformation after exceeding this threshold causes hyperventilation and leads to the development of fatigue induced by incomplete metabolic acidosis [52, 56].

The results of many studies indicate the lack of clear influence of the menstrual cycle phases on resting and postexercise levels of lactate and acid-base balance parameters in the blood [17, 37, 43, 48, 57, 58].

One of the studies [45], during which women performed a graded test, indicated lower blood lactate and lower respiratory exchange ratio (RER) values for submaximal loads in the luteal phase. Resting levels and maximum values of blood lactate concentration did not significantly differ in both phases of the menstrual cycle [45]. Significantly, higher levels of lactate in the follicular phase were found by Lavoie et al. [59] during a 90-minute effort at intensity of approximately 63% VO_{2max}. Similar results were obtained by Jurkowski et al. [36] during an effort of 90% intensity VO_{2max} and McCracken et al. [38] during a graded test. The authors found a statistically significant, higher level of resting blood lactate concentration in the follicular phase of the menstrual cycle. Also, increases in lactate concentration and decreases in buffering bases, after efforts with higher loads, were significantly greater in the follicular phase than the luteal phase [36]. Differences between phases in the postexercise lactate level were maintained for 30 minutes of restitution [38].

The purpose of the Devries et al.'s study [60] was, among others, to determine the effect of menstrual cycle phase upon glucose turnover and muscle glycogen utilization during moderate-intensity endurance exercise. In these studies, healthy, recreationally active young women underwent a primed constant infusion of glucose with muscle biopsies taken before and after a 90-minute cycling exercise at intensity of 65% VO_{2max}. In the studies, it was demonstrated that women in the luteal phase have lesser reliance on carbohydrate sources to fuel endurance exercise compared with follicular phase. It was evidenced by a lower glucose rate of appearance and disappearance as well as metabolic clearance rate and lower glycogen utilization during and at the end of exercise [60].

Higher oxidation of lipids and lower oxidation of carbohydrates in the luteal phase during submaximal efforts at an intensity higher than 50% VO_{2max} have also been demonstrated in other studies [61–63]. It was also noticed that interphase differences in the use of energy substrates are related to the effort intensity. During a 30-minute treadmill run, healthy, well-menstruating women performed three 10-minute efforts at the following intensities: 30, 60, and 75% VO_{2max}, successively. Higher lipid oxidation in the luteal phase was found during low- and moderate-intensity exercise, while there were no interphase differences during exercise at an intensity of 75% VO_{2max} [20]. Similar results were obtained that in cycling efforts, higher lipid oxidation in the luteal phase was found at the 30% intensity VO_{2max} and 50% VO_{2max}, but not at 70% VO_{2max} [64]. On the other hand, they are not confirmed by this study, in which, on the basis of RER, there were no differences between phases in the proportions of energy substrate consumption (lipids/carbohydrates) during efforts of a wide intensity range, i.e., 45% VO_{2max} [65], 50% VO_{2max} [66], 65% VO_{2max} [65], 70% VO_{2max} [67], as well as 80% VO_{2max} [48].

Later research [68], in which young female rowers (female athletes and women practicing recreationally and taking/not taking oral contraceptive pills) performed a graded test on a rowing ergometer during the follicular and luteal phases of the menstrual cycle, showed that there are no interphase differences in the level of power output, ventilator equivalents of O_2 (V_E/VO_2), HR, and blood lactate concentration at maximal and aerobic-anaerobic transition intensities in all three groups. However, higher values were observed for ventilatory equivalents of CO_2 (V_E/VCO_2) at both intensities in the luteal phase compared with the follicular phase in the group of women taking contraceptive pills [68]. There were no significant interphase differences in the oxidation of carbohydrates and fats during resting (before the exercise) or during the 1-hour rowing exercise at 70% VO_{2max}. Energy expenditure, oxygen uptake, HR, and lactate concentration were similar in the follicular and luteal phases during this exercise [69]. In both phases of the menstrual cycle, the female rowers obtained similar values of VO_{2max} and VO_2 at the threshold of anaerobic transitions [69]. These results are consistent with those previously presented by Smekal et al. [70], who showed that there are no significant intergroup differences in the level of power output, VO_2, RER, HR, and blood lactate concentration at rest, at maximal load, and at different thresholds of aerobic and anaerobic metabolism (lactate thresholds, respiratory thresholds: AT and RCP), which were measured during a cycle test in eumenorrheic women. In this study, minute ventilation and V_E/VO_2 and V_E/VCO_2 indices were higher in the luteal phase at rest, exhaustion, and AT [70].

3.1.3. Oxygen capacity of the blood

Another important factor determining the level of VO_{2max} is the oxygen capacity of the blood depending on the content of hemoglobin in the blood and its affinity for oxygen and on the total volume of blood [35]. The high correlation coefficient between hemoglobin concentration and the VO_{2max} value indicates a significant role of this protein in aerobic capacity [71]. A higher level of hemoglobin in the blood in the luteal phase was confirmed by Jurkowski et al. [36]. Increased oxygen availability in tissues during the luteal phase may also result in a higher core temperature during this phase, as well as an elevated level of 2,3-DPG, causing a decrease in the affinity of hemoglobin to oxygen [12, 72]. However, studies carried out by Dombovy et al. [40] showed a slight decrease in the hemoglobin level during the luteal phase. In this research, the differences between phases in the resting level of hemoglobin did not affect the value of VO_{2max}, which did not differ between phases.

Stephenson and Kolka [33] found that the resting values of hemoglobin and hematocrit (HCT) are slightly elevated in the luteal phase. Interphase differences in the level of these parameters increased during passive heating and remained unchanged during the exercise with an intensity of approximately 80% VO_{2max}. Elevated levels of HCT in the luteal phase were also noted by Stachenfeld et al. [11, 12].

3.1.4. Plasma volume

Based on the results of earlier studies [33], it may be assumed that higher resting HCT in the luteal phase results from the smaller plasma volume during it. Gaebelein and Senay [32] suggest that the reason for this phenomenon may be an increase in the luteal phase of vascular wall permeability to plasma proteins. Other studies do not support these views [13]. The authors performed an experiment involving seven women, in whom administering a gonadoliberin inhibitor (GnRH) reduced the level of endogenous estradiol and progesterone. Then, successively at intervals of a few days, they added extrinsic preparations containing synthetic derivatives of estradiol and progesterone. In this way, they obtained a ratio of sex hormone concentrations corresponding to, according to the concept of Janse de Jonge [16], the early-follicular, late-follicular, and middle-luteal phases. They found that at elevated levels of both hormones, which correspond to the middle of the luteal phase, the volume of plasma is the largest and constitutes about 17% of the total volume of extracellular fluids. At the same time, in this situation we observe the lowest permeability of blood vessel walls for plasma proteins. Slightly smaller plasma volume and greater permeability of blood vessel walls were observed in a situation corresponding to the late-follicular phase. However, the differences were not statistically significant. Due to the much smaller volume of extracellular fluids, plasma was then 21%. In the situation when only the GnRH inhibitor was administered, the plasma volume was the lowest, and the permeability of blood vessel walls was the largest for albumin. At the same time, the total volume of extracellular fluids was the highest, with a plasma volume of approximately 16%. Differences in the volume of extracellular fluids may be reflected in small changes in the body mass of women during the menstrual cycle [37].

Stephenson and Kolka [33] found that a 9-minute effort at an intensity of about 80% VO_{2max} caused a significantly larger loss of plasma volume during the follicular phase. The percentage changes in plasma volume reached −15.8 and −13.3% in the follicular and luteal phases, respectively [33]. Other authors did not find significant interphase differences in plasma volume changes immediately after exercise and during the restitution period [12, 37, 38, 48].

3.2. Anaerobic exercise

In the majority of studies assessing the influence of sex hormones on women's exercise responses, efforts were made of constant submaximal intensity or gradually increasing until reaching maximal oxygen uptake, i.e., "until exhaustion." However, there is little information on the interphase variation in response to typical anaerobic efforts [73–78].

The concept of anaerobic capacity of an organism encompasses a set of factors determining the performance of short-term work, during which large force and maximal generated power are developed. These include skeletal muscle mass, the supply of muscle energy substrates [ATP, phosphocreatine (PCr), glycogen], and enzyme activity of anaerobic processes. The large buffer capacity that allows tolerance of homeostatic disorders and rapid restitution in the pH range is also extremely important [79].

Taking the metabolic effects of estradiol and progesterone into account, it can be assumed that the changing ratio of these hormones during the menstrual cycle effects different physiological responses of women under the influence of anaerobic exercise [80]. The presence of estrogen receptors in the human skeletal muscle [81] and the correlation between strength and high concentrations of 17β-estradiol and progesterone have been found [82]. Furthermore, buffering capacity during the 10-s rowing sprint was greater at a higher concentration of 17β-estradiol [83]. Research suggests that ovarian hormones may influence the rate of PCr resynthesis after eutrophic luteal efforts in eumenorrheic women [84]. Other studies also indicate a faster rate of PCr regeneration after anaerobic efforts in the luteal phase due to the greater work performed in this phase of the menstrual cycle during a series of ten 6-s sprints [85]. This indicates the potential for generating more anaerobic power during the luteal phase of the menstrual cycle (high concentration of 17β-estradiol and progesterone) or just before ovulation (high concentration of 17β-estradiol) compared to the follicular phase. In the literature, however, there is little information on the effect of different levels of hormones on the size of the developed strength or the level of anaerobic power indicators during the menstrual cycle, and their results are not consistent.

While some studies show better results during the luteal phase for single and multiple sprints [85, 86], in others, there were no interphase differences in single or repeated anaerobic cycling tests [87, 88]. Bale and Nelson [89], examining 20 women training swimming, found that they achieved the best results for a distance of 50 m in the follicular phase. Also, Parish and Jakeman [90] found that in comparison with the ovulation period and the luteal phase, the highest maximal and average anaerobic power values were obtained by women in the follicular phase.

However, it should be emphasized that the choice of experiment day in some studies was not hormonally confirmed [86–90]. In many experiments on this subject, the research dates were chosen only by calendar or thermal method. Anovulatory cycles may occur without disturbing the length of the menstrual cycle, while in the case of using the calendar method, this may lead to an erroneous indication of the day of laboratory examination. In turn, a reliable diagnosis of the course of the sexual cycle, based on the measurement of basic body temperature, is possible only after the measurements have been performed in at least three consecutive cycles. The erroneous conclusions concerning the division of the cycle into follicular and luteal phases with the use of the thermal method may additionally be caused by factors such as incorrect method of core temperature measurement, night sleep less than 6 hours, disease states, or the use of hypnotics. Inference based on the results obtained by the authors using the calendar method or thermal method is therefore limited [16].

3.2.1. Research based on hormonal verification of menstrual cycle

The results of research based on hormonal verification of the division of the menstrual cycle into phases indicate lack of significant impact of sex hormones on the values of the developed strength [91] and generated anaerobic power [73]. Nonetheless, other studies [76] show that muscle strength returns to the baseline level faster after strenuous stretch-shortening cycle exercise during the ovulatory phase, when the estrogen level is high, compared with the follicular phase. However, the differences in exercise-induced muscle damage markers (CK, soreness, and low-frequency fatigue) between the two menstrual cycle phases were small.

In the research by Wiecek et al. [75], determining the size of the maximal anaerobic power, a 20-second cycle sprint was used (Wingate test version) [92]. The energy medium of this type of effort regards mainly anaerobic processes consisting in the resynthesis of ATP at the expense of PCr and muscle glycogen. According to the research review, participation of these two processes in ATP synthesis starts from the first seconds of effort, with the participation of the phosphagen energy source in favor of anaerobic glycolysis in subsequent seconds [79]. To obtain fully reliable results, Wiecek et al. [75] performed initial assessment of the correctness and regularity of the menstrual cycle on the basis of the registration of basic body temperature. The correctness of experiment day selection was always verified by hormonal assays. In addition, the studies were repeated in two subsequent menstrual cycles. Each woman performed an anaerobic effort twice in the middle of the follicular phase (days 6–9 of the cycle) and two times in the middle of the luteal phase (5–8 days after ovulation). The first day of menstruation was adopted as the first day of the menstrual cycle. The studies concluded that there are no significant differences in the level of indicators determining anaerobic capacity of women in the follicular and luteal phases of the menstrual cycle. No interphase differences were found in the maximal level or average anaerobic power. The time of obtaining and maintaining maximal power and the rate of decrease in anaerobic power were not different either. The effect of anaerobic metabolism during a 20-second effort at supramaximal intensity is a significant increase in blood lactate concentration, which entails changes in the level of acid-base balance parameters. In both phases of the menstrual cycle, the anaerobic effort caused similar disturbances in the acid-base balance [75].

Also, in the research by Tsampoukos et al. [77], the days for exercise were carefully selected. Eumenorrheic women performed a test comprised of two, 30-s sprints separated by a 2-min break. The test was conducted during the follicular phase, just before ovulation and in the luteal phase. The mutual ovarian hormone system was characterized by adequately low levels of progesterone and 17β-estradiol, low progesterone levels and high levels of 17β-estradiol, and high levels of progesterone and 17β-estradiol. It was found that there are no interphase differences in the maximal level or average anaerobic power. Menstrual cycle hormones also did not affect postexercise changes in metabolic parameters (blood lactate and pH, plasma ammonia) or the rate of regeneration between sprints [77].

Furthermore, during the 6-s cycling sprint, there were no interphase differences in the amount of generated anaerobic power and changes in blood lactate or in the sympatho-adrenergic response tested by the measurement of adrenaline and noradrenaline in the blood [93]. The lack of influence of sex hormones on different exercise responses in the follicular and luteal phases was also demonstrated by studies in which no interphase differences were found in maximal accumulated oxygen deficit and sprint performance in repeated sprint cycling, i.e., three times at 120% VO_{2max} with 20-minute resting periods between consecutive sprints [78]. Also, the 40-yd running time preceded by a 15-minute warm-up (jogging, skipping by moving the legs in various directions, and sprinting alternating with jogging), performed at an ambient temperature of about 32.5°C, did not differ between the early-follicular and middle-luteal phases [94]. Regardless of the menstrual cycle phase, the warm-up triggered an increase in the core temperature of about 1°C, which resulted in a better result during the run [94].

Similar results were also obtained in earlier studies [74]. Domagala et al. [74] obtained results indicating a tendency for smaller increases in lactate concentration and changes in acid-base balance parameters in the luteal phase of the menstrual cycle. In the luteal phase, they also noted a slightly higher rate of lactate concentration restitution after exercise with a supramaximal load; however, the interfacial differences were not statistically significant [74].

However, in the research by Redman and Weatherby [83], in which rowers performed a test of anaerobic power (10-s all-out effort) and capacity (1000-m row), it was found that the peak power output was higher and the 1000-m rowing ergometer time was faster when the concentration of progesterone and estradiol was low (quasi-follicular phase), in contrast to when the levels of both hormones were high (quasi-luteal phase). The concentration of sex hormones was regulated by oral contraceptive pills [83]. Julian et al. [95], by examining female soccer players who performed the Yo-Yo intermittent endurance test, multiple jumps, and 3 × 30 m sprints in the early-follicular phase and in the middle of the luteal phase, showed a reduction in maximal endurance performance during the middle-luteal phase. This effect was not observed for jumping or sprint performance.

3.3. Thermoregulation

An important factor conditioning the possibility of performing physical exercise is the efficient functioning of thermoregulation mechanisms. During rest, in thermoneutral conditions, the heat balance of the body is stabilized by the exchange of heat produced in metabolic processes. Heat is exchanged with the environment through conduction and convection, radiation, and evaporation. By these means, approximately 20, 60, and 20%, respectively, of heat is eliminated from the body [96].

During physical exercise, as a result of the intensification of metabolic processes, the thermal balance of the body and the stimulation of thermoregulation systems are disturbed. We observe an increase in the core temperature of the body, depending on the relative load expressed as % VO_{2max}, which during efforts at constant intensity is stabilized at an elevated level. The main role in the elimination of excess endogenous heat during physical exercise is played by evaporation of perspiration from the body's surface, constituting about 80% of heat loss [96]. The effectiveness of exercise-based thermoregulation depends on the rate of sweat secretion and external conditions affecting the efficiency of its evaporation, as well as the correct functioning of the circulatory system, on which the heat transfer from the muscles to the surface of the skin depends [96]. After core temperature exceeds the so-called vasodilation threshold, blood flow through the cutaneous vessels steadily increases along with the increase of exercise intensity to about 60–70% VO_{2max}, after which it gradually decreases due to the increase in muscular flow [97]. Thermoregulatory reactions also depend on hydration status of the body, the concentration of sodium and calcium ions in body fluids, the degree of acclimation to the conditions under which physical exercise is performed, and the level of physical fitness [96].

The increase in resting body temperature during the luteal phase of the menstrual cycle by about 0.3–0.5°C, as compared to the level during the follicular phase, is the result of the antagonistic effect of progesterone and estradiol on the thermoregulatory system in the hypothalamus [12]. Observations of many authors indicate the relationship between thermoregulatory responses in women and the course of the menstrual cycle [29, 39, 41, 98–100].

3.3.1. Core temperature and sweating

The average temperature measured in the esophagus (T_{es}), in thermoneutral conditions, during a 30-minute exercise at an intensity of 40 and 70% VO_{2max}, was higher in the luteal phase [101]. The increase in T_{es} obtained in these studies was the same in both phases of the menstrual cycle [101]. In other studies [102], the temperature measured in the auditory canal (T_{ty}), at rest and during exercise tests (60-minute 50% VO_{2max} and during the graded test), was significantly higher in the luteal phase of the menstrual cycle, and T_{ty} increases were slightly higher in follicular phase.

The increases in core temperature, similar in both phases, during submaximal efforts performed in thermoneutral conditions and in conditions of elevated temperature, were also observed in the studies presented by other authors [12, 94, 100, 103]. These results are only partially consistent with the results of this study, during which a higher level of rectal temperature (T_{re}) was observed in the luteal phase of the menstrual cycle while performing a 60-minute effort at constant intensity of about 60% VO_{2max} (ambient temperature 22°C) [41]. However, T_{re} increments were comparable in both phases of the menstrual cycle only during the initial minutes of exercise, after which the differences between phases increased due to stabilization of T_{re} in the follicular phase at the level of 38.3°C and its continuous increase to 38.9°C (despite the constant load) in the luteal phase [41].

During a 15-minute exercise at a constant intensity of 70% VO_{2max}, performed in an ambient temperature of 18°C, significantly higher T_{re} increments were observed in the follicular phase of the menstrual cycle [39]. In conditions of passive overheating or physical exertion, activation of sweat secretion and dilation of cutaneous blood vessels were observed at higher temperatures as well as a higher intensity of perspiration secretion in the luteal phase [12, 28, 29, 39, 98–102]. There was also later occurrence of perspiration production during exercise tests in the follicular phase [28].

Despite the different course of T_{re} changes in the follicular and luteal phases, the sweat rate was similar in both phases of the menstrual cycle [41]. The authors suggest that this may be related to lower sensitivity of sweat secretion in the luteal phase (sweating rate—increase of core temperature dependency) [41]. However, these results are not confirmed by other laboratory tests, which indicate a slightly higher value in the luteal phase [28, 39, 98] or a similar sensitivity of the perspiration mechanism in both phases [12, 99, 100, 103]. The results obtained during submaximal physical exercise in thermoneutral conditions showed that the increase in rectal temperature in women was lower during the luteal than follicular phase, while the dynamics of sweating were higher in the luteal phase [104].

Tests during which women performed two different stress tests (graded test "to refusal" and 60-minute with 50% intensity of VO_{2max}) show that the temperature threshold for starting the perspiration release reaction is higher in the luteal phase and does not depend on the type of exercise [102]. In contrast, the sensitivity of the perspiration production reaction is independent of the menstrual cycle and is higher during the graded test [102]. According to other authors, the effectiveness of perspiration is greater in the luteal phase of the menstrual cycle [104, 105].

Lower core temperature during exercise in the follicular phase may be due to interphase differences in the value of dermal flow and skin temperature. Some studies [39, 98] show that in thermoneutral conditions, at rest and during submaximal efforts, blood flow through the forearm reaches significantly higher values in the luteal phase. The temperature level at which the cutaneous blood vessels dilate, determined on the basis of temperature measurements, T_{es},

T_{ty}, and T_{re}, shifted toward higher values in the luteal phase by about 0.5°C [39]. However, in other studies, resting blood flow in the forearm did not differ during the menstrual cycle [29]. The exercise-based (30 minutes 80% VO_{2max}) increase in cutaneous flow coincided with the increase in core temperature (T_{es}) to the level of 37.0°C in the follicular phase and 37.4°C in the luteal phase and stabilized at a significantly higher level during the latter phase [29].

3.3.2. Skin temperature

According to some authors, the average skin temperature (T_{sk}) is significantly higher in the luteal phase at rest and during submaximal efforts in thermoneutral conditions [100] at the time of heat exposure [99, 103] and during passive overheating [99]. The lack of differences between phases in the T_{sk} values measured at rest as well as during the exercise tests (30 minutes 40% VO_{2max} and 30 minutes 70% VO_{2max}) performed in thermoneutral conditions was also demonstrated [101]. Cutaneous flow tended to be higher in the luteal phase, but the resulting interphase differences were not statistically significant [101]. Other studies also showed similar resting values and a comparable course of T_{sk} exercise changes in both phases of the menstrual cycle [12, 41, 106]. Cutaneous flow assumed lower values in the luteal phase [106].

3.4. Oxidative stress

The body maintains homeostasis in the scope of redox reactions (prooxidation and antioxidative balance), which affects the proper course of biochemical intracellular processes and intercellular signaling. The condition of redox homeostasis is to maintain balance between the level of reactive oxygen and nitrogen species (RONS) and antioxidant defense. Antioxidative defense is provided by nonenzymatic low-molecular and macromolecular antioxidants and antioxidant enzymes, which together determine total antioxidant capacity. Physical activity gives health benefits by improving, among others, cardiovascular and respiratory system functioning, and metabolic processes as well as by increasing antioxidant capacity [107–109].

3.4.1. Exercise-based sources of oxygen and nitrogen

Research has shown that physical exercise influences prooxidation and antioxidative balance [110–114]. The mechanism of RONS formation depends on the duration, intensity of effort, and type of muscle work. An increase in ATP consumption during aerobic efforts results in an increase in the rate of oxidative phosphorylation and, consequently, increased electron leakage in the internal mitochondrial membrane. As a result, amounts larger than at rest of the superoxide anion ($O_2^{\bullet -}$), hydrogen peroxide (H_2O_2), and hydroxyl radical ($^{\bullet}OH$), which belong to the reactive oxygen species, are formed [109]. The superoxide anion radical is also formed by the reaction of NADPH oxidase in the sarcoplasmic reticulum and transverse tubules (T-tubules) of the sarcolemma, as well as in the reaction of xanthine oxidase, the activity of which increases after anaerobic efforts [108]. The formation of RONS is promoted by the increase in lactate dehydrogenase activity, lowering the pH value, increasing the concentration of catecholamines, as well as increasing intramuscular temperature [108, 109]. Contractile activity also leads to increased nitric oxide (NO) synthesis by induced nitric oxide synthase (iNOS). The consequence of increased NO synthesis, at a high level of $O_2^{\bullet -}$, is the formation of peroxynitrite ($OONO^-$). Peroxynitrite is a reactive form of nitrogen. Excessive RONS production during exercise can also be the result of myocyte micro-injury associated with activation of the leukocytic system [107, 115].

3.4.2. Markers of oxidative stress

Oxidative stress is determined by changes in the level of many, various markers (**Table 1**). Different oxidation rates and different antioxidants are evaluated in the research, the changes of which are not always unidirectional [107].

3.4.3. The significance of reactive oxygen and nitrogen species

The formation of RONS in low concentrations (intracellular signaling) is necessary for the regulation and integration of biochemical processes. They activate primary signaling pathways depending on redox status. The main transcription factor, sensitive to redox status, is the nuclear factor erythroid 2-related factor (Nrf2). Nrf2 activation affects the strengthening of antioxidative defense and cytoprotection. It has been shown that as a result of regular exercise, upregulation of gene expression for peroxisome proliferator-activated receptor-γ coactivator-1α (PGC-1α) occurs, which upregulates Nrf2 in order to regulate the mitochondrial biogenesis. The upstream signals that regulate PGC-1α expression as mitogen-activated protein kinase (MAPK) and nuclear factor κB (NF-κB) are also redox-sensitive. RONS, through

Markers of oxidative stress	Antioxidants
4-Hydroxynonenal (4-HNE)	Endogenous enzymatic
F2-isoprostane	• Superoxide dismutase (SOD)
Isoprostanes (8-iso-PGF2α)	• Catalase (CAT)
Malondialdehyde (MDA)	• Glutathione peroxidase (GPx)
Oxidized low-density lipoprotein (ox-LDL)	• Glutathione reductase (GR)
Thiobarbituric acid reactive substance (TBARS)	Endogenous nonenzymatic
8-Hydroxy-2′-deoxyguanosine (8-OHdG)	• Albumin
3-Nitrotyrosine (3-NTR)	• Uric acid
Protein carbonyl content (PCC)	• Reduced glutathione (GSH)
Advanced oxidation protein products (AOPP)	Exogenous nonenzymatic
Oxidized glutathione (GSSG)	• β-Carotene, vitamin E, vitamin C
Total oxidative status (TOS)	Total antioxidative capacity (TAC)
Oxidative stress index (OSI = TOS/TAC)	

Table 1. Examples of indicators of oxidative stress and antioxidants.

MAPK, activate the NF-κB signaling pathway and, thus, affect the expression of antioxidant enzyme genes such as superoxide dismutase (SOD), catalase (CAT), or glutathione peroxidase (GPx) or glutathione reductase (GR). Therefore, they are responsible for maintaining an appropriate level of endogenous antioxidant defense [107–109, 115].

At high concentrations (oxidative damage level), RONS exhibits inhibitory and damaging effects [107]. Excessive production of RONS with low antioxidant capacity may be the reason for shifting the prooxidation and antioxidant balance toward oxidation and oxidative stress. The consequence of oxidative stress is increased lipid peroxidation, oxidation of thiol groups of proteins, damage to DNA and carbohydrates. Oxidative damage to macromolecules is the cause of disturbance in enzyme activity and permeability of biological membranes [107].

3.4.4. Antioxidant effect of estradiol activity

In women, the antioxidative role is attributed to estrogen. Animal experiments have shown that the amount of H_2O_2 formed in the mitochondria of females is lower than in the mitochondria of male rats. The positive effect of estradiol on oxidative stress has also been demonstrated in women. It was found that estradiol reduces the level of reactive oxygen species, and in postmenopausal women, it intensifies oxidative stress, which is counteracted by hormone replacement therapy. Estradiol, acting indirectly through the estrogen receptor, increases antioxidant capacity, affecting activation of the NF-κB signaling pathway, which consequently results in an increase in enzymatic antioxidant capacity [116–119].

3.4.5. Redox balance in the menstrual cycle

An interesting research model was carried out by Massafra et al. [120]. Young women (aged 20–27) participated in the study, declaring a regular menstrual cycle, the length of which ranged from 28 to 30 days. The first day of menstruation was accepted as the first day of the menstrual cycle. Changes in ovarian hormones were monitored based on the daily determinations of 17β-estradiol and progesterone. A preovulatory peak of 17β-estradiol concentration was determined for each woman, which was the "0" point. In relation to the "0" point, three tests were determined in the follicular phase (early, from bleeding to −10; middle, from days −8 to −4; late, from days −2 to 0) and in the luteal phase (early, from days 2 to 4; middle, from days 6 to 10; late, from days 12 to 14). Significant changes in the menstrual cycle were found in erythrocyte GPx activity, with higher values in the period from late follicular to early luteal phases compared to early-follicular phase. This coincided with the elevated level of 17β-estradiol, and the correlation coefficient was 0.8. In this study, there was no effect of 17β-estradiol, progesterone, and LH or FSH on the activity of CAT and SOD in erythrocytes, which were similar throughout the menstrual cycle [120].

In turn, in another study [121] involving 259 regularly menstruating women aged 18–44, it was found that the level of antioxidants in blood serum is dependent on ovarian hormones. Similar appointments for assays were determined as in previous studies [120]. Among others, antioxidant fat-soluble vitamins and carotenoid micronutrients (α-tocopherol, γ-tocopherol, β-carotene, retinol, lutein, lycopene) and ascorbic acid were determined. The concentration of F2-isoprostane was determined as an indicator of lipid oxidation. In most women, the assays were conducted during two menstrual cycles. Among others, it was found that the concentrations of fat-soluble vitamins and ascorbic acid are lower during menstruation. The concentration of fat-soluble vitamins positively correlated with the concentration of 17β-estradiol. The concentration of ascorbic acid also correlated positively with the concentration of 17β-estradiol and progesterone, while it was lower when the concentration of LH was higher. Women with higher ascorbic acid concentrations had lower F2-isoprostane concentrations. In this study, the ratio of α- to γ-tocopherol was associated with an increased risk of anovulatory cycles [121].

While regularly maturing young women (cycle length 26–31 days) were divided into two groups, i.e., ovulating and non-ovulating, it was found that plasma TBARS (lipid oxidation index), whole blood GSH concentration, and CAT, GPX, and GR activity in erythrocytes are similar in both groups in the first (7–9 days) and in the second (22–25 days) mid-menstrual cycle [122]. However, the activity of SOD in erythrocytes, in both measurements, was significantly higher in the non-ovulating group. In ovulating women, there was a significant negative correlation between the concentration of 17β-estradiol in the blood plasma and the activity of SOD in erythrocytes. Research has shown that the lack of ovulation in menstruating women does not affect increased lipid peroxidation. In contrast to previous studies [120], there was no effect of GSH-dependent erythrocyte antioxidant defense, while it was found that lower plasma estradiol resulted in attenuated erythrocyte SOD inhibition and elevated enzyme activity [122].

There are also studies in which it was concluded that women are subjected to oxidative stress for most of the menstrual cycle. In these studies, oxidative stress was assessed on the basis of the reactive oxygen metabolites-derived compound test (d-ROMs), the results of which correspond to the hydroxyperoxide level. The measurement in the blood was performed every 3 days, starting from the first day of menstruation up to the last day of the menstrual cycle (the day before the next menstruation). The level of dROMs was significantly elevated between days 9 and 24 of the menstrual cycle, when there was a peak of 17β-estradiol at low progesterone concentration, as well as when the levels of both hormones were elevated. However, there was no correlation between 17β-estradiol concentration and the level of dROMs; thus, it can be assumed that other factors influenced the increased lipid oxidation [123].

Other studies do not confirm the relationship between oxidative stress and the course of the menstrual cycle. There were no differences in the level of 8-OHdG in the urine (oxidative DNA damage index) between follicular phase, ovulation, and the luteal phase of the menstrual cycle [124]. There were also no differences between TBARS [34, 125] and MDA [125, 126], i.e., lipid oxidation indices, as well as H_2O_2 and nitrite/nitrate levels [127], nor in total GSH, GSH, and GSSG concentrations [125]. The effect of hormones during the menstrual cycle on the total activity of SOD and the activity of extracellular superoxide dismutase (EC-SOD) [34] or the total antioxidant capacity were not demonstrated [126]. Also, in older postmenopausal women who did not use hormone replacement therapy, there were no higher levels of dROMs or lower antioxidant capacity compared to premenopausal women of similar age (46–55 years). On the basis of dROM values in both groups of women, the middle oxidative stress level was found, and a slight deficit in antioxidant defense was detected [127]. However, the level of lipid oxidation in older women was higher compared to the young (25–35 years), properly menstruating women who did not use contraceptive pills [127].

It was shown that oral contraception (monophasic pills containing 0.02 mg ethinyl estradiol and 3 mg drospirenone) affects the prooxidative and antioxidant status of young women [128]. Compared to women who do not use oral contraception, they cause a decrease in GSH and glutathione S-transferase (GST), GR, and GPx in the blood while increasing CAT activity and lowering GSSG concentration, resulting in the GSH/GSSG oxidative stress index to not change. These studies show that external modification of the concentration of sex hormones causes catalase to play a main antioxidative role, which confirms the positive correlation between CAT activity and MDA concentration. Increased CAT activity may be the result of accumulation of H_2O_2 and other radicals. Detoxification of reactive oxygen species by the GSH system is weakened in this situation [128].

3.4.6. Exercise-induced changes in redox balance

Studies show that high levels of 17β-estradiol in non-training young women with normal biphasic menstrual cycles favor easier elimination of free radicals formed during exercise [34]. Despite the lack of interphase differences in resting TBARS level and SOD activity, after a 30-minute cycling effort with 60% intensity VO_{2max}, it was found that the TBARS level decreased in the follicular phase when the 17β-estradiol concentration was higher than during menstruation and the luteal phase. In the luteal phase, however, the activity of SOD in the blood decreased after the effort. Although in none of the phases (menstruation, follicular phase, luteal phase), neither at rest nor after exercise, was there any correlation between the concentration of 17β-estradiol and oxidative stress markers, it was nonetheless found that along with the higher concentration of this hormone, the decrease in SOD activity was lower [34].

In another study [125], in which young women also performed a 30-minute moderate-intensity exercise (about 75–80% VO_{2max}) in the follicular and luteal phases of the menstrual cycle, a significant postexercise increase in GSSG concentration was noted during the luteal phase (by 28%), while the concentration of total GSH decreased significantly after exercise only in the follicular phase (by 8%). The concentration of GSH after exercise, regardless of the phase of the menstrual cycle, significantly decreased by about 16–17%. These results show that at higher concentrations of 17β-estradiol (late follicular phase), exercise causes slightly less disturbances of redox homeostasis due to more efficient scavenging free radicals with the participation of glutathione [125].

Amenorrheic and eumenorrheic athletes underwent a 90-minute effort at an intensity of 60% VO_{2max} [129]. The level of 17β-estradiol was significantly lower in amenorrheic women both before and during exercises (30, 60, and 90 minutes) and at 15-minute recovery. In these studies, there was a greater effect of the effort on the oxidative stress markers in amenorrheic women. In this group, at rest and during exercise, GPx activity was higher. Before the effort, GR activity in both groups of women was comparable, but as a result of the effort, it also significantly increased in amenorrheic women. Plasma lipid peroxidation concentration and CAT activity were similar in both groups and did not change in response to physical effort. Contrary to other studies [120], there was a negative correlation between GPx activity and 17β-estradiol concentration, but, simultaneously, GPx activity depended positively on cortisol concentration, which was elevated in the group of amenorrheic women [129].

These results are contrary to those of other researchers [130] who found a positive relationship between GPx activity and estradiol levels both before and after physical exercises. Non-training, young women, during menstruation and the preovulatory phase, performed three isokinetic efforts to exhaustion, consisting of performing maximum alternating concentric and eccentric work of the knee extensor muscles of the dominant lower limb, preceded by a 15-minute submaximal bicycle effort at an intensity of 50% VO_{2max}. The concentration of MDA in the blood plasma did not change after exercise, but the activity of SOD and GPx in erythrocytes decreased significantly. The effort-induced changes were lower when the estradiol concentration was higher, what is more, the α-tocopherol supplementation (antioxidant vitamin) did not affect this [130].

Another study [131] showed that a low carbohydrate diet for 3 days (5% carbohydrate, 52% fat, 43% protein), preceded by exertion of glycogen depletion, supports the antioxidant defense system in healthy eumenorrhoeic women, both at rest and during graded exercises performed "until exhaustion," compared to women using a balanced diet at this time (59% carbohydrate, 27% fat, 14% protein). It seems reasonable to assume that the higher daily intake of heme iron, selenium, and α-tocopherol provided with a low carbohydrate diet contributed to the increase of antioxidative capacity by increasing the activity of CAT and increasing the concentration of selenium and α-tocopherol in the plasma, which gave better protection of the cell membranes against peroxidative damage caused by physical effort. This is reflected in the limited release of creatine kinase into the blood, which is an indicator of sarcolemma damage. Physical effort was repeated twice in the follicular phase (6–8 days), when the concentration of 17β-estradiol was low, and twice during the luteal phase (4–6 days after ovulation), when both the concentrations of 17β-estradiol and progesterone in the blood were high. In this study, the phase of the menstrual cycle had only a small effect on antioxidant defenses of blood [131].

3.4.7. Sex differences in exercise-induced oxidative stress

It can be assumed that due to differences in estradiol concentration, disturbances in prooxidative-oxidative balance of the blood after exercise are higher in men than women. In the research carried out by Wiecek et al. [111] among young individuals, it was found that the changes in the prooxidative-antioxidative balance of the blood induced by maximum intensity exercise (graded test) differ in women and in men. In men, there was a significant shift in prooxidant-antioxidant balance toward oxidation without increasing the total plasma antioxidant capacity (TAC). In women, the postexercise changes in total plasma oxidation status (TOS) were low due to the increase in TAC. Exercise-induced changes in TOS concentration depended on VO_{2max} and simultaneously, on the increase in lactate concentration [111]. The lack of such relationships in women may indicate the influence of other factors on postexercise oxidative stress in this group of subjects, such as damage to muscle fibers. Continuing research with the participation of young individuals, it was found that the result of physical effort at maximum intensity is significant, independent of VO_{2max} and VO_2 as well as the work intensity (% VO_{2max}) at the level of the second ventilatory threshold, increase in concentration of ox-LDL and 3-nitrotyrosin in the blood serum, testifying to similar lipid and protein damage in women and men. The significant increase in TAC after exercise at maximum intensity was the result of micro-damage of muscle fibers that occurred in women [114]. However, when young people performed an anaerobic effort, it was found that with similar disturbances of acid-base balance, changes in TAC, TOS, and oxidative stress index (TOS/TAC) in the blood were the same in both women and men. The changes in concentration of low-molecular nonenzymatic antioxidants induced by this effort were also the same in both sexes. The level of the tested markers was indicative of oxidative stress persisting for at least 24 hours after the end of the work [110]. There was no evidence that anaerobic exercise caused muscle damage [113]. During the first hour after completing anaerobic exercise, there were no changes in the activity of xanthine oxidase (XO) in the blood plasma of men or women. The significant increase in the activity of this enzyme was found 24 hours after the completion of anaerobic exercise. The increase in XO activity in the blood after anaerobic exercise was greater in women than men. At the same time, the postexercise increase in XO activity was negatively correlated with the amount of total work performed during anaerobic exercise and with mean and peak anaerobic power, which were significantly lower in women [113]. In turn, the 45-minute submaximal (50% VO_{2max}) effort ending with a 15-minute eccentric exercise [downhill run (−4.5°)] caused oxidative damage to lipids only in women [112]. An increase in ox-LDL concentration indicated redox balance disturbances. In men, regardless of the type of muscle work (eccentric, concentric), submaximal running efforts did not cause oxidative stress. The probable cause of these gender differences was the higher antioxidant capacity of men's blood dependent on greater physical performance [112]. In the above studies, however, the phase of the menstrual cycle was not taken into account; women performed the exercise either during the follicular phase or in a randomly selected phase. Nonetheless, the results indicate that changes in redox balance among women depend on the intensity of the effort and on the type of muscle work involved.

4. Conclusion

Despite many years of interest in this subject, the current research does not allow to draw unambiguous conclusions about the impact of the changing level of sex hormones during individual phases of the menstrual cycle on the exercise capacity of women. There are indications that in the luteal phase, the capacity to perform efforts based mainly on aerobic energy transformations does increase. For example, in one of recent studies [132], an increase in cardiac and respiratory efficiency in the luteal phase of the menstrual cycle for normal-weight females was found, where as in overweight and obese individuals, there was an overall decrease in fitness capacity along with an increase in body mass index (BMI). However, the differences between groups noted by one researcher in the measured effects of the applied test are not confirmed by observations of other authors [133]. Often, however, differences in the results obtained by women in the pre- and postovulatory phase are small. According to a review of studies on women's exercise capacity, in most experiments, efforts were applied with constant submaximal intensity or gradually increasing until the oxygen uptake was achieved. However, there is little information on intergroup variation in response to typical anaerobic efforts. These studies, as one of the most recent [134], indicate a lack of hormone influence in the menstrual cycle on anaerobic efficiency indices. But these tests also provide divergent results.

The question arises as to why there are still no studies that explicitly determine the exercise capacity of women depending on the phase of the menstrual cycle [135].

Difficulties in undertaking research on exercise-related reactions in women lie, inter alia, in obtaining volunteers for research, especially those non-training ones if the experiment requires the implementation of very high intensity efforts. No physical examinations involve large groups of women. Usually, the research group consists of several to a dozen people. The problem is also obtaining the right motivation of the studied women to fully carry out their potential capabilities during laboratory exercise tests. The reason for the discrepancy of some results may be the determination of test date based on measurements of basic body temperature without hormonal determinations. On the other hand, the source of often conflicting results, given by different authors using sex hormone markers, may be the terminology used to determine the location of the performed laboratory test in the course of the menstrual cycle. Some authors use the division of menstrual cycle into follicular and luteal phases, without specifying the days on which the tests were performed and/or concentrations of estradiol and progesterone determined. Considering the changing ratio of these hormones during the menstrual cycle, the following division seems to be more appropriate: early-follicular (low estradiol and progesterone), late-follicular (elevated estradiol and low progesterone), and middle-luteal (high estradiol and progesterone levels) [16] or to reference the day of testing to the day of ovulation [120]. Difficulties in comparing the results obtained by different authors also result from significant differences in the age and level of physical activity of the surveyed women, or from the variety of applied stress tests and performed assays, which mainly concern markers of oxidative stress. Different methodological approaches and inconsistent presentation of data are a limitation when comparing the results of women obtained by them depending on the changing hormone concentrations of the menstrual cycle. So far, it has not been specified whether it is necessary to take the phase of the menstrual cycle into account in sports diagnostics, e.g., during stress tests that check the physical performance of women training different sports. Also, comparisons between exercise reactions of men and women may be imprecise due to methodological differences. A comprehensive and multi-aspect study of the exercise should be carried out, involving training and non-training women of all ages, in the pre- and postmenopausal period, as well as those using and not using hormonal contraceptives or hormone replacement therapy, which would precisely characterize whether there are differences in biochemical-physiological adaptation to the efforts of varying intensity and type of work and the course of changes in the recovery period, related to the level of hormones in the menstrual cycle.

Acknowledgements

This work was supported by the Faculty of Physical Education and Sports, University of Physical Education in Krakow, (Poland) under Grant 153/BS/INB/2018.

Author details

Magdalena Wiecek

Address all correspondence to: magdalena.wiecek@awf.krakow.pl

Department of Physiology and Biochemistry, Faculty of Physical Education and Sport, University of Physical Education, Krakow, Poland

References

[1] Roupas ND, Georgopoulos NA. Menstrual function in sports. Hormones. 2011;**10**(2): 104-116. DOI: 10.14310/horm.2002.1300

[2] Fischetto G, Sax A. The menstrual cycle and performance. New Studies in Athletics. 2013;**3/4**:57-69

[3] Arena B, Maffulli N, Maffulli F, Morelo MA. Reproductive hormones and menstrual changes with exercise in female athletes. Sports Medicine. 1995;**19**(4):278-287. DOI: 10.2165/00007256-199519040-00005

[4] De Souza MJ. Menstrual disturbances in athletes: A focus on luteal phase defects. Medicine and Science in Sports and Exercise. 2003;**35**(9):1553-1563. DOI: 10.1249/01.MSS.0000084530.31478.DF

[5] Bale P. Body composition and menstrual irregularities of female athletes. Are they precursors of anorexia? Sports Medicine. 1994;**17**(6):347-352. DOI: 10.2165/00007256-199417060-00001

[6] Gibbs JC, Nattiv A, Barrack MT, Williams NI, Rauh MJ, Nichols JF, De Souza MJ. Low bone density risk is higher in exercising women with multiple triad risk factors. Medicine and Science in Sports and Exercise. 2014;**46**(1):167-176. DOI: 10.1249/MSS.0b013e3182a03b8b

[7] De Souza MJ, Koltun KJ, Etter CV, Southmayd EA. Current status of the female athlete triad: Update and future directions. Current Osteoporosis Reports. 2017;**15**(6):577-587. DOI: 10.1007/s11914-017-0412-x

[8] Mehta J, Thompson B, Kling JM. The female athlete triad: It takes a team. Cleveland Clinic Journal of Medicine. **85**(4):313-320. DOI: 10.3949/ccjm.85a.16137

[9] Ashley CD, Kramer ML, Bishop P. Estrogen and substrate metabolism. Sports Medicine. 2000;**29**(4):221-227. DOI: 10.2165/00007256-200029040-00001

[10] Lebrun CM, Rumball JS. Relationship between athletic performance and menstrual cycle. Current Women's Health Reports. 2001;**1**(3):232-240

[11] Stachenfeld NS, DiPietro L, Kokoszka CA, Silva C, Keefe DL, Nadel ER. Physiological variability of fluid-regulation hormones in young women. Journal of Applied Physiology. 1999;**86**:1092-1096. DOI: 10.1152/jappl.1999.86.3.1092

[12] Stachenfeld NS, Celso S, Keefe DL. Estrogen modifies the temperature effects of progesterone. Journal of Applied Physiology. 2000;**88**:1643-1649. DOI: 10.1152/jappl.2000.88.5.1643

[13] Stachenfeld NS, Taylor HS. Effects of estrogen and progesterone administration on extracellular fluid. Journal of Applied Physiology. 2004;**96**(3):101-108. DOI: 10.1152/japplphysiol.01032.2003

[14] Hatta H, Atomi Y, Shinohara S, Yamamoto Y, Yamada S. The effects of ovarian hormones on glucose and fatty acid oxidation during exercise in female ovariectomized rats. Hormone and Metabolic Research. 1988;**20**(10):609-611. DOI: 10.1055/s-2007-1010897

[15] Kendrick ZV, Steffen CA, Rumsey WL, Goldberg DI. Effect of estradiol on tissue glycogen metabolism in exercised oophorectomized rats. Journal of Applied Physiology. 1987;**63**:492-496. DOI: 10.1152/jappl.1987.63.2.492

[16] Janse de Jonge XA. Effects of the menstrual cycle on exercise performance. Sports Medicine. 2003;**33**(11):833-851. DOI: 10.2165/00007256-200333110-00004

[17] Nicklas BJ, Hackney AC, Sharp RL. The menstrual cycle and exercise: Performance, muscle glycogen, and substrate responses. International Journal of Sports Medicine. 1989;**10**(4):264-269. DOI: 10.1055/s-2007-1024913

[18] Bunt JC. Metabolic actions of estradiol: Significance for acute and chronic exercise responses. Medicine and Science in Sports and Exercise. 1990;**22**(3):286-290. DOI: 10.1249/00005768-199006000-00003

[19] Hackney AC. Effects of the menstrual cycle on resting muscle glycogen. Hormone and Metabolic Research. 1991;**22**(12):647. DOI: 10.1055/s-2007-1004994

[20] Hackney AC, McCracken-Compton M, Ainsworth B. Substrate metabolism responses to submaximal exercise in the mid-follicular and mid-luteal phases of the menstrual cycle. International Journal of Sport Nutrition. 1994;**4**(3):299-308

[21] Hornum M, Cooper DM, Brasel JA, Bueno A, Sietsema KE. Exercise-induced changes in circulating growth factors with cyclic variation in plasma estradiol in women. Journal of Applied Physiology. 1997;**82**(6):1946-1951. DOI: 10.1152/jappl.1997.82.6.1946

[22] D'Eon TM, Sharoff C, Chipkin SR, Grow D, Ruby BC, Braun B. Regulation of exercise carbohydrate metabolism by estrogen and progesterone in women. American Journal of Physiology, Endocrinology and Metabolism. 2002;**283**(5):E1046-E1055. DOI: 10.1152/ajpendo.00271.2002

[23] Hansen FM, Fahmy N, Nielsen JH. The influence of sexual hormones on lypogenesis and lipolysis in rat fat cells. Acta Endocrinologica. 1980;**95**:566-570. DOI: 10.1530/acta.0.0950566

[24] Hansen AP, Wecke J. Fasting serum growth hormone levels and GH responses to exercise during normal menstrual cycles and cycles of oral contraceptives. Scandinavian Journal of Clinical and Laboratory Investigation. 1974;**34**:199-205. DOI: 10.3109/00365517409081707

[25] Isacco L, Boisseau N. Sex hormones and substrate metabolism during endurance exercise. In: Hackney AC, editor. Sex Hormones, Exercise and Women. Scientific and Clinical Aspects. 1st ed. Basel: Springer International Publishing; 2017. pp. 35-58. DOI: 10.1007/978-3-319-44558-8

[26] Bayliss DA, Millhorn DE. Central neural mechanisms of progesterone action: Application to the respiratory system. Journal of Applied Physiology. 1992;**73**:393-404. DOI: 10.1152/jappl.1992.73.2.393

[27] Das TK, Jana H. Basal oxygen consumption during different phases of menstrual cycle. Indian Journal of Medical Research. 1991;**94**:16-19

[28] Grucza R, Pekkarinen H, Titov EK, Kononoff A, Hänninen O. Influence of the menstrual cycle and oral contraceptives on thermoregulatory responses to exercise in young women. European Journal of Applied Physiology. 1993;**67**:279-285

[29] Kolka MA, Stephenson LA. Effect of luteal phase elevation in core temperature on forearm blood flow during exercise. Journal of Applied Physiology. 1997;**82**(4):1079-1083. DOI: 10.1152/jappl.1997.82.4.1079

[30] Charkoudian N, Johnson JM. Female reproductive hormones and thermoregulatory control of skin blood flow. Exercise and Sport Sciences Reviews. 2000;**28**(3):108-112

[31] Fortney SM, Beckett WS, Carpenter AJ, Davis J, Drew H, LaFrance ND, Rock JA, Tankersley CG, Vroman NB. Changes in plasma volume during bed rest: Effects of menstrual cycle and estrogen administration. Journal of Applied Physiology. 1988;**65**(2):525-533. DOI: 10.1152/jappl.1988.65.2.525

[32] Gaebelein CJ, Senay L. Vascular volume dynamics during ergometer exercise at different menstrual phases. European Journal of Applied Physiology. 1982;**50**:1-11. DOI: 10.1007/BF00952239

[33] Stephenson LA, Kolka MA. Plasma volume during heat stress and exercise in women. European Journal of Applied Physiology. 1988;**57**:373-381. DOI: 10.1007/BF00417979

[34] Joo MH, Maehata E, Adachi T, Ishida A, Murai F, Mesaki N. The relationship between exercise-induced oxidative stress and the menstrual cycle. European Journal of Applied Physiology. 2004;**93**(1-2):82-86. DOI: 10.1007/s00421-004-1168-4

[35] Bassett DR, Howley ET. Limiting factors for maximum oxygen uptake and determinants of endurance performance. Medicine and Science in Sports and Exercise. 2000;**32**:70-84. DOI: 10.1097/00005768-200001000-00012

[36] Jurkowski JE, Jones NL, Toews CJ, Sutton JR. Effects of the menstrual cycle on blood lactate, O_2 delivery, and performance during exercise. Journal of Applied Physiology. 1981;**51**(6):1493-1499. DOI: 10.1152/jappl.1981.51.6.1493

[37] Bemben DA, Salm PC, Salm AJ. Ventilatory and blood lactate responses to maximal treadmill exercise during the menstrual cycle. Journal of Sports Medicine and Physical Fitness. 1995;**35**(4):257-262

[38] McCracken M, Ainsworth B, Hackney AC. Effects of the menstrual cycle phase on the blood lactate responses to exercise. European Journal of Applied Physiology. 1994;**69**:174-175. DOI: 10.1007/BF00609412

[39] Hessemer V, Bruck K. Influence of menstrual cycle on thermoregulatory, metabolic, and heart rate responses to exercise at night. Journal of Applied Physiology. 1985;**59**(6):1911-1917. DOI: 10.1152/jappl.1985.59.6.1911

[40] Dombovy ML, Bonekat HW, Williams TJ, Staats BA. Exercise performance and ventilatory response in the menstrual cycle. Medicine and Science in Sports and Exercise. 1987;**19**(2):111-117. DOI: 10.1249/00005768-198704000-00008

[41] Pivarnik JM, Marichal CJ, Spillman T, Morrow JR. Menstrual cycle phase affects temperature regulation during endurance exercise. Journal of Applied Physiology. 1992;**72**(2):543-548. DOI: 10.1152/jappl.1992.72.2.543

[42] Galliven EA, Singh A, Michelson D, Bina S, Gold PW, Deuster PA. Hormonal and metabolic responses to exercise across time of day and menstrual cycle phase. Journal of Applied Physiology. 1997;**83**(6):1822-1831. DOI: 10.1152/jappl.1997.83.6.1822

[43] Dean TM, Perreault L, Mazzeo RS, Horton TJ. No effect of menstrual cycle phase on lactate threshold. Journal of Applied Physiology. 2003;**95**:2537-2543. DOI: 10.1152/japplphysiol.00672.2003

[44] Zielinski P, Cempla J, Klimek AT, Domagala M. The effect of menstruation on chosen physiological and biochemical reactions caused by the physical effort with the submaximal intensity. Biology of Sport. 2003;**20**(1):53-67

[45] Redman LM, Scroop GC, Norman RJ. Impact of menstrual cycle phase on the exercise status of young, sedentary women. European Journal of Applied Physiology. 2003;**90**(5-6):505-513. DOI: 10.1007/s00421-003-0889-0

[46] Schoene RB, Robertson HT, Pierson DJ, Peterson AP. Respiratory drives and exercise in menstrual cycles of athletic and nonathletic women. Journal of Applied Physiology. 1981;**50**:1300-1305. DOI: 10.1152/jappl.1981.50.6.1300

[47] Das TK. Effects of the menstrual cycle on timing and depth of breathing at rest. Indian Journal of Physiology and Pharmacology. 1998;**42**(4):498-502

[48] De Souza MJ, Maguire MS, Rubin KR, Maresh CM. Effects of menstrual phase and amenorrhea on exercise performance in runners. Medicine and Science in Sports and Exercise. 1990;**22**(5):575-580. DOI: 10.1249/00005768-199010000-00006

[49] Moran VH, Leathard HL, Coley J. Cardiovascular functioning during the menstrual cycle. Clinical Physiology. 2000;**20**(6):496-504. DOI: 10.1046/j.1365-2281.2000.00285.x

[50] Reinhard U, Muller PH, Schmulling RM. Determination of anaerobic threshold by the ventilation equivalent in normal individuals. Respiration. 1979;**38**(1):36-42. DOI: 10.1159/000194056

[51] Skinner JS, McLellan TH. The transition from aerobic to anaerobic metabolism. Research Quarterly for Exercise and Sport. 1980;**51**(1):234-248. DOI: 10.1080/02701367.1980.10609285

[52] Wasserman K, Beaver WL, Whipp BJ. Mechanisms and patterns of blood lactate increase during exercise in man. Medicine and Science in Sports and Exercise. 1986;**18**(3):344-352. DOI: 10.1249/00005768-198606000-00017

[53] Binder RK, Wonisch M, Corra U, Cohen-Solal A, Vanhees L, Saner H, Schmid J-P. Methodological approach to the first and second lactate threshold in incremental cardiopulmonary exercise testing. European Journal of Cardiovascular Prevention and Rehabilitation. 2008;**15**(6):726-734. DOI: 10.1097/HJR.0b013e328304fed4

[54] Faude O, Kindermann W, Meyer T. Lactate threshold concepts. How valid are they? Sports Medicine. 2009;**39**:469-490. DOI: 0112-1642/09/0006-0469/$49.95/0

[55] Beaver WL, Wasserman K, Whipp BJ. A new method for detecting anaerobic threshold by gas exchange. Journal of Applied Physiology. 1986;**60**:2020-2027. DOI: 10.1152/jappl.1986.60.6.2020

[56] Meyer T, Faude O, Scharhag J, Urhausen A, Kindermann W. Is lactic acidosis a cause of exercise induced hyperventilation at the respiratory compensation point? British Journal of Sports Medicine. 2004;**38**:622-625. DOI: 10.1136/bjsm.2003.007815

[57] Lamont LS. Lack of influence of the menstrual cycle on blood lactate. The Physician and Sports Medicine. 1986;**14**(11):159-163. DOI: 10.1080/00913847.1986.11709230

[58] Preston RJ, Aaron P, Heenan P, Wolfe LA. Physicochemical analysis of phasic menstrual cycle effects on acid-base balance. American Journal of Physiology Regulatory, Integrative and Comparative Physiology. 2001;**80**:R481-R487. DOI: 10.1152/ajpregu.2001.280.2.R481

[59] Lavoie JM, Dionne N, Helie R, Brisson GR. Menstrual cycle phase dissociation of blood glucose homeostasis during exercise. Journal of Applied Physiology. 1987;**62**(3):1084-1089. DOI: 10.1152/jappl.1987.62.3.1084

[60] Devries MC, Hamadeh MJ, Phillips SM, Tarnopolsky MA. Menstrual cycle phase and sex influence muscle glycogen utilization and glucose turnover during moderate-intensity endurance exercise. American Journal of Physiology. Regulatory, Integrative and Comparative Physiology. 2006;**291**(4):R1120-R1128. DOI: 10.1152/ajpregu.00700.2005

[61] Campbell SE, Angus DJ, Febbraio MA. Glucose kinetics and exercise performance during phases of the menstrual cycle: Effect of glucose ingestion. American Journal of Physiology. Endocrinology and Metabolism. 2001;**281**:E817-E825. DOI: 10.1152/ajpendo.2001.281.4.E817

[62] Hackney AC. Influence of oestrogen on muscle glycogen utilization during exercise. Acta Physiologica Scandinavica. 1999;**167**:273-274. DOI: 10.1046/j.1365-201x.1999.00605.x

[63] Zderic TW, Coggan AR, Fuby BC. Glucose kinetics and substrate oxidation during exercise in the follicular and luteal phases. Journal of Applied Physiology. 2001;**90**:447-453. DOI: 10.1097/00005768-199805001-01469

[64] Wenz M, Berend JZ, Lynch NA, Chappell S, Hackney AC. Substrate oxidation at rest and during exercise: Effects of menstrual cycle phase and diet composition. Journal of Physiology and Pharmacology. 1997;**48**:851-860

[65] Suh SH, Casazza GA, Horning MA, Miller BF, Brooks GA. Luteal and follicular glucose fluxes during rest and exercise in 3-h postabsorptive women. Journal of Applied Physiology. 2002;**93**:42-50. DOI: 10.1152/japplphysiol.01080.2001

[66] Horton TJ, Miller EK, Glueck D, Tench K. No effect of menstrual cycle phase on glucose kinetics and fuel oxidation during moderate-intensity exercise. American Journal of Physiology, Endocrinology and Metabolism. 2002;**282**:E752-E762. DOI: 10.1152/ajpendo.00238.2001

[67] Bailey SP, Zacher CM, Mittleman KD. Effect of menstrual cycle phase on carbohydrate supplementation during prolonged exercise to fatigue. Journal of Applied Physiology. 2000;**88**(2):690-697. DOI: 10.1152/jappl.2000.88.2.690

[68] Vaiksaar S, Jurimae J, Maestu J, Purge P, Kalytka S, Shakhlina L, Jurimae T. No effect of menstrual cycle phase and oral contraceptive use on endurance performance in rowers. The Journal of Strength and Conditioning Research. 2011;**25**(6):1571-1578. DOI: 10.1519/JSC.0b013e3181df7fd2

[69] Vaiksaar S, Jurimae J, Maestu J, Purge P, Kalytka S, Shakhlina L, Jurimae T. No effect of menstrual cycle phase on fuel oxidation during exercise in rowers. European Journal of Applied Physiology. 2011;**111**(6):1027-1034. DOI: 10.1007/s00421-010-1730-1

[70] Smekal G, von Duvillard SP, Frigo P, Tegelhofer T, Pokan R, Hofmann P, Tschan H, Baron R, Wonisch M, Renezeder K, Bachl N. Menstrual cycle: No effect on exercise cardiorespiratory variables or blood lactate concentration. Medicine and Science in Sports and Exercise. 2007;**39**(7):1098-1106. DOI: 10.1249/mss.0b013e31805371e7

[71] Green HJ, Carter S, Grant S, Tupling R, Coates G, Ali M. Vascular volumes and hematology in male and female runners and cyclists. European Journal of Applied Physiology. 1999;**79**:244-250. DOI: 10.1007/s004210050502

[72] Denis P, Cazor JL, Feret J, Weisang E. Lefrancois. 2,3-Diphosphoglycerate red cell concentration changes during the menstrual cycle in women. Biomedicine. 1976;**25**(4):144-147

[73] Giacomoni M, Bernard T, Gavarry O, Altare S, Falgairette G. Influence of the menstrual cycle phase and menstrual symptoms on maximal anaerobic performance. Medicine and Science in Sports and Exercise. 2000;**32**(2):486-492. DOI: 10.1097/00005768-200002000-00034

[74] Domagala M, Cempla J, Bawelski M, Zielinski P. Changes in a lactate, H^+ ions and base excess concentrations during exercises of different intensities in relation to the phase of menstrual cycle. Biology of Sport. 2001;**18**(4):311-319

[75] Wiecek M, Szymura J, Maciejczyk M, Cempla J, Szygula Z. Effect of sex and menstrual cycle in women on starting speed, anaerobic endurance and muscle power. Physiology International. 2016;**103**(1):127-132. DOI: 10.1556/036.103.2016.1.13

[76] Sipaviciene S, Daniuseviciute L, Kliziene I, Kamandulis S, Skurvydas A. Effects of estrogen fluctuation during the menstrual cycle on the response to stretch-shortening exercise in females. BioMed Research International. 2013;**2013**:243572. DOI: 10.1155/2013/243572

[77] Tsampoukos A, Peckham EA, James R, Nevill ME. Effect of menstrual cycle phase on sprinting performance. European Journal of Applied Physiology. 2010;**109**(4):659-667. DOI: 10.1007/s00421-010-1384-z

[78] Shaharudin S, Ghosh AK, Ismail AA. Anaerobic capacity of physically active eumenorrheic females at mid-luteal and mid-follicular phases of ovarian cycle. Journal of Sports Medicine and Physical Fitness. 2011;**51**(4):576-582

[79] Morales-Alamo D, Calbet JAL. Free radicals and sprint exercise in humans. Free Radical Research. 2014;**48**(1):30-42. DOI: 10.3109/10715762.2013.825043

[80] Oosthuyse T, Bosch AN. The effect of the menstrual cycle on exercise metabolism. Implications for exercise performance in Eumenorrhoeic women. Sports Medicine. 2010;**40**(3):207-227. DOI: 0112-1642/10/0003-0207/$49.95/0

[81] Lemoine S, Granier P, Tiffoche C, Rannou-Bekono F, Thieulant ML, Delamarche P. Estrogen receptor alpha mRNA in human skeletal muscles. Medicine and Science in Sports and Exercise. 2003;**35**(3):439-443. DOI: 10.1249/01.MSS.0000053654.14410.78

[82] Taaffe DR, Newman AB, Haggerty CL, Colbert LH, de Rekeneire N, Visser M, Goodpaster BH, Nevitt MC, Tylavsky FA, Harris TB. Estrogen replacement, muscle composition, and physical function: The health ABC study. Medicine and Science in Sports and Exercise. 2005;**37**(10):1741-1747. DOI: 10.1249/01.mss.0000181678.28092.31

[83] Redman LM, Weatherby RP. Measuring performance during menstrual cycle: A model using oral contraceptives. Medicine and Science in Sports and Exercise. 2004;**36**(1):130-136. DOI: 10.1249/01.MSS.0000106181.52102.99

[84] Harber VJ, Petersen SR, Chilibeck PD. Thyroid hormone concentrations and muscle metabolism in amenorrheic and eumenorrheic athletes. Canadian Journal of Applied Physiology. 1998;**23**:293-306. DOI: 10.1139/h98-017

[85] Middleton LE, Wenger HA. Effects of menstrual phase on performance and recovery in intense intermittent activity. European Journal of Applied Physiology. 2006;**96**(1):53-58. DOI: 10.1007/s00421-005-0073-9

[86] Masterson G. The impact of menstrual cycle phases on anaerobic power performance in collegiate women. Journal of Strength and Conditioning Research. 1999;**13**:325-329

[87] Bushman B, Masterson G, Nelsen J. Anaerobic power performance and the menstrual cycle: Eumenorrheic and oral contraceptive users. Journal of Sports Medicine and Physical Fitness. 2006;**46**(1):132-137

[88] Miskec CM, Potteiger JA, Nau KL, Zebas CJ. Do varying environment and menstrual cycle conditions affect anaerobic power output in female athletes. Journal of Strength and Conditioning Research. 1997;**11**:219-223. DOI: 10.1519/1533-4287(1997)011<0219:DVEAMC>2.3.CO;2

[89] Bale P, Nelson G. The effects of menstruation on performance of swimmers. Australian Journal of Science and Medicine in Sport. 1985;**3**:19-22

[90] Parish H, Jakeman PM. The effects of menstruation upon repeated maximal sprint performance. Journal of Sports Sciences. 1987;**1**:78

[91] Friden C, Hirschberg AL, Saartok T. Muscle strength and endurance do not significantly vary across 3 phases of the menstrual cycle in moderately active premenopausal women. Clinical Journal of Sport Medicine. 2003;**13**(4):238-241. DOI: 10.1097/00042752-200307000-00007

[92] Inbar O, Bar-Or O, Skinner JS. Characteristics of the Wingate anaerobic test: Relative aerobic and anaerobic contributions. In: Inbar O, Bar-Or O, Skinner JS, editors. The Wingate Anaerobic Test. Champaign: Human Kinetics; 1996. pp. 35-37

[93] Botcazou M, Gratas-Delamarche A, Allain S, Jacob C, Bentué-Ferrer D, Delamarche P, Zouhal H. Influence of menstrual cycle phase on catecholamine response to sprint exercise in the woman. Applied Physiology Nutrition and Metabolism. 2006;**31**(5):604-611. DOI: 10.1139/h06-038

[94] Somboonwong J, Chutimakul L, Sanguanrungsirikul S. Core temperature changes and sprint performance of elite female soccer players after a 15-minute warm-up in hot-humid environment. Journal of Strength and Conditioning Research. 2015;**29**(1):262-269. DOI: 10.1519/JSC.0b013e3182aa5f2f

[95] Julian R, Hecksteden A, Fullagar HH, Meyer T. The effects of menstrual cycle phase on physical performance in female soccer players. PLoS One. 2017;**12**(3):e0173951. DOI: 10.1371/journal.pone.0173951

[96] Kenney WL, Wilmore JH, Costill DL. Exercise in hot and cold environments. In: Kenney WL, Wilmore JH, Costill DL, editors. Physiology of Sport and Exercise. 5th ed. Champaign: Human Kinetics; 2011. pp. 283-307

[97] Smolander J, Kolari P, Korhonen O, Ilmarinen R. Skin blood flow during incremental exercise in thermoneutral and hot dry environment. European Journal of Applied Physiology and Occupational Physiology. 1987;**56**(3):273-280. DOI: 10.1007/BF00690892

[98] Hessemer V, Bruck K. Influence of menstrual cycle on shivering, skin blood flow, and sweating responses measured at night. Journal of Applied Physiology. 1985;**59**(6):1902-1910. DOI: 10.1152/jappl.1985.59.6.1902

[99] Kolka MA, Stephenson LA. Control of sweating during the human menstrual cycle. European Journal of Applied Physiology. 1989;**58**:890-895. DOI: 10.1007/BF02332224

[100] Fukuoka Y, Kaneko Y, Takita C, Hirakawa M, Kagawa H, Nakamura Y. The effects of exercise intensity on thermoregulatory responses to exercise in women. Physiology and Behavior. 2002;**76**:567-574. DOI: 10.1016/S0031-9384(02)00781-3

[101] Hirata K, Nagasaka T, Hirai A, Hirashita M, Takahata T, Nunomura T. Effects of human menstrual cycle on thermoregulatory vasodilation during exercise. European Journal of Applied Physiology. 1986;**54**:559-565. DOI: 10.1007/BF00943341

[102] Pokora I, Grucza R. Thermoregulatory responses to exercise in women during follicular and luteal phase of the menstrual cycle. Biology of Sport. 2000;**17**(1):13-24

[103] Carpenter AJ, Nunneley SA. Endogenous hormones subtly alter women's response to heat stress. Journal of Applied Physiology. 1988;**65**(5):2313-2317. DOI: 10.1152/jappl.1988.65.5.2313

[104] Kaciuba-Uscilko H, Grucza R. Gender differences in thermoregulation. Current Opinion in Clinical Nutrition and Metabolic Care. 2001;**4**:533-536

[105] Garcia AMC, Lacerda MG, Fonseca IAT, Reis FM, Rodrigues LOC, Silami-Garcia E. Luteal phase of the menstrual cycle increases sweating rate during exercise. Brazilian Journal of Medical and Biological Research. 2006;**39**:1255-1261. DOI: 10.1590/S0100-879X2006000900014

[106] Frascarolo P, Schutz Y, Jequier E. Decreased thermal conductance during the luteal phase of the menstrual cycle in women. Journal of Applied Physiology. 1990;**69**:2029-2033

[107] Durackova Z. Some current insights into oxidative stress. Physiological Research. 2010;**59**:459-469

[108] Powers SK, Talbert EE, Adhihetty PJ. Reactive oxygen and nitrogen species as intracellular signals in skeletal muscle. The Journal of Physiology. 2011;**9**:2129-2138. DOI: 10.1113/jphysiol.2010.201327

[109] He F, Li J, Liu Z, Chuang CC, Yang W, Zuo L. Redox mechanism of reactive oxygen species in exercise. Frontiers in Physiology. 2016;**7**:486. DOI: 10.3389/fphys.2016.00486

[110] Wiecek M, Maciejczyk M, Szymura J, Szygula Z, Kantorowicz M. Changes in non-enzymatic antioxidants in the blood following anaerobic exercise in men and women. PLoS One. 2015;**10**(11):e0143499. DOI: 10.1371/journal.pone.0143499

[111] Wiecek M, Maciejczyk M, Szymura J, Szygula Z. Changes in oxidative stress and acid-base balance in men and women following maximal-intensity physical exercise. Physiological Research. 2015;**64**(1):93-102

[112] Wiecek M, Maciejczyk M, Szymura J, Szygula Z. Sex differences in oxidative stress after eccentric and concentric exercise. Redox Report. 2017;**22**(6):478-485. DOI: 10.1080/13510002.2017.1304195

[113] Wiecek M, Maciejczyk M, Szymura J, Kantorowicz M, Szygula Z. Impact of single anaerobic exercise on delayed activation of endothelial xanthine oxidase in men and women. Redox Report. 2017;**22**(6):367-376. DOI: 10.1080/13510002.2016.1238991

[114] Wiecek M, Maciejczyk M, Szymura J, Szygula Z. Effect of maximal-intensity exercise on systemic nitro-oxidative stress in men and women. Redox Report. 2017;**22**(4):176-182. DOI: 10.1080/13510002.2016.1169622

[115] Nikolaidis MG, Kyparos A, Spanou C, Paschalis V, Theodorou AA, Vrabas IS. Redox biology of exercise: An integrative and comparative consideration of some overlooked issues. The Journal of Experimental Biology. 2012;**215**:1615-1625. DOI: 10.1242/jeb.067470

[116] Ayers S, Abplanalp W, Liu JH, Subbiah TR. Mechanism involved in the protective effect of estradiol-17β on lipid peroxidation and DNA damage. American Journal of Physiology. 1998;**274**:E1002-E1008. DOI: 10.1152/ajpendo.1998.274.6.E1002

[117] Tiidus PM. Estrogen and gender effects on muscle damage, inflammation, and oxidative stress. Canadian Journal of Applied Physiology. 2000;**25**(4):274-287. DOI: 10.1139/h00-022

[118] Vina J, Gambini J, Lopez-Grueso R, Abdelaziz KM, Jove M, Borras C. Females live longer than males: Role of oxidative stress. Current Pharmaceutical Design. 2011;**17**:3959-3965. DOI: 10.2174/138161211798764942

[119] Sanchez-Rodriguez MA, Zacarias-Flores M, Castrejon-Delgado L, Ruiz-Rodríguez AK, Mendoza-Nunez VM. Effects of hormone therapy on oxidative stress in postmenopausal women with metabolic syndrome. International Journal of Molecular Sciences. 2016;**17**:1388. DOI: 10.3390/ijms17091388

[120] Massafra C, Gioia D, De Felice C, Picciolini E, De Leo V, Bonifazi M, Bernabei A. Effects of estrogens and androgens on erythrocyte antioxidant superoxide dismutase, catalase and glutathione peroxidase activities during the menstrual cycle. Journal of Endocrinology. 2000;**167**(3):447-452. DOI: 0022-0795/00/0167-447

[121] Mumford SL, Browne RW, Schliep KC, Schmelzer J, Plowden TC, Michels KA, Sjaarda LA, Zarek SM, Perkins NJ, Messer LC, Radin RG, Wactawski-Wende J, Schisterman E. Serum antioxidants are associated with serum reproductive hormones and ovulation among healthy women. Journal of Nutrition. 2016;**146**:98-106. DOI: 10.3945/jn.115.217620

[122] Lutoslawska G, Tkaczyk J, Panczenko-Kresowska B, Hubner-Wozniak E, Skierska E, Gajewski AK. Plasma TBARS, blood GSH concentrations, and erythrocyte antioxidant enzyme activities in regularly menstruating women with ovulatory and anovulatory menstrual cycles. Clinica Chimica Acta. 2003;**331**(1-2):159-163. DOI: 10.1016/S0009-8981(03)00085-8

[123] Cornelli U, Belcaro G, Rosaria M, Cesarone MR, Finco A. Analysis of oxidative stress during the menstrual cycle. Reproductive Biology and Endocrinology. 2013;**11**(1):74. DOI: 10.1186/1477-7827-11-74

[124] Iida T, Inoue K, Ito Y, Ishikawa H, Kagiono M, Teradaira R, Chikamura C, Harada T, Ezoe S, Yatsuya H. Comparison of urinary levels of 8-hydroxy-2′-deoxyguanosine between young females with and without depressive symptoms during different menstrual phases. Acta Medica Okayama. 2015;**69**(1):45-50

[125] Chung SC, Goldfarb AH, Jamurtas AZ, Hegde SS, Lee J. Effect of exercise during the follicular and luteal phases on indices of oxidative stress in healthy women. Medicine and Science in Sports and Exercise. 1999;**31**(3):409-413. DOI: 10.1097/00005768-199903000-00009

[126] Bell HK, Bloomer RJ. Impact of serum estradiol on postprandial lipemia, oxidative stress, and inflammation across a single menstrual cycle. Gender Medicine. 2010;**7**(2):166-178. DOI: 10.1016/j.genm.2010.03.001

[127] Brunelli E, Domanico F, La Russa D, Pellegrino D. Sex differences in oxidative stress biomarkers. Current Drug Targets. 2014;**15**(8):811-815. DOI: 10.2174/1389450115666140624112317

[128] Kowalska K, Milnerowicz H. Pro/antioxidant status in young healthy women using oral contraceptives. Environmental Toxicology and Pharmacology. 2016;**43**:1-6. DOI: 10.1016/j.etap.2016.02.006

[129] Kanaley JA, Ji LL. Antioxidant enzyme activity during prolonged exercise in amenorrheic and eumenorrheic athletes. Metabolism. 1991;**40**(1):88-92. DOI: 10.1016/0026-0495(91)90197-5

[130] Akova B, Surmen-Gur E, Gur H, Dirican M, Sarandol E, Kucukoglu S. Exercise-induced oxidative stress and muscle performance in healthy women: Role of vitamin E supplementation and endogenous oestradiol. European Journal of Applied Physiology. 2001;**84**:141-147

[131] Klapcinska B, Sadowska-Krepa E, Manowska B, Pilis W, Sobczak A, Danch A. Effects of a low carbohydrate diet and graded exercise during the follicular and luteal phases on the blood antioxidant status in healthy women. European Journal of Applied Physiology. 2002;**87**(4-5):373-380. DOI: 10.1007/s00421-002-0641-1

[132] Samsudeen N, Rajagopalan A. Effect of different phases of menstrual cycle on cardio-respiratory efficiency in normal, overweight and obese female undergraduate students. Journal of Clinical and Diagnostic Research. 2016;**10**(12):CC01-CC04. DOI: 10.7860/JCDR/2016/23080.8954

[133] Abdollahpor A, Khosravi N, Zahra NR. Effects of the menstrual cycle phase on the blood lactate responses and exercise performance in active women. European Journal of Experimental Biology. 2013;**3**(3):206-210

[134] Pestana ER, Salvador EP, Pereira GB, Mostarda CT, Leite RD, Silva CR, Carvalho WRG. Influence of the mid-follicular and late luteal phases on anaerobic power in university students. Sport Sciences for Health. 2017;**13**:281-286. DOI: 10.1007/s11332-016-0344-3

[135] Bruinvels G, Burden RJ, McGregor AJ, Ackerman KE, Dooley M, Richards T, Pedlar C. Sport, exercise and the menstrual cycle: Where is the research? British Journal of Sports Medicine. 2017;**51**(6):487-488. DOI: 10.1136/bjsports-2016-096279

5

Depression and Serotonergic Changes during the Climacteric and Postmenopausal Stages: Hormonal Influences

Rosa Isela García-Ríos, Armando Mora-Pérez and Cesar Soria-Fregozo

Abstract

Depression is a psychiatric disorder that affects a high percentage of women. Most of the depression disorders turn up during the premenopause and perimenopause stages when the hormonal oscillations make an impact in the brain function principally on the serotonergic system, which is related to neurobiology of depression. 5-HT1A and 5-HT2A receptors change on functionality and density in afferent areas related to emotional modulation and increased serotonin clearance, and the binding potential of serotonin transport has been related to the underlying mechanism of the depression during the climacteric or postmenopausal stage. Some findings have been proven on preclinical studies. These studies on animals have recognized how estrogen treatment activates intracellular signaling pathways as mitogen-activated protein (MAP)/extracellular signal-regulated kinase (ERK), tyrosine kinase brain-derived neurotrophic factor receptor (TrKB), insulin-like growth factor-1 receptor (IGF-1R), phosphatidylinositol 3-kinase (PI3)/serine/threonine-specific protein kinase (Akt), and metabotropic glutamate receptor 1 (mGluR1) which interact with the serotonergic system to allow establishment of the estradiol effects on mood regulation. Thus, the interaction between the woman's reproductive status and the serotonin changes could be useful to create prevention strategies, early diagnosis, and medical treatment of climacteric and postmenopausal women with depression, in order to improve their quality of life.

Keywords: depression, menopause, climacteric, 5-HT1A receptor, 5-HT2A receptor, estradiol

1. Introduction

Depression is one of the most common psychiatric disorders that affect approximately 4.84% people around the world, and it is considered to be one of the principal causes of disability worldwide [1]. According to the Global Burden of Disease study report in 2015 [2], the highest rates of disability-adjusted life years (DALYs) worldwide are established on women aged 15–49 years with 5.65%, followed by 50–69 years old women with 2.98% and 70 years old with 1.26%. DALYs represent the years of life that are adjusted by a certain level of disability experienced during a particular period of time, related to depressive disease. It supports studies which demonstrate that most of the depression disorder comes out during the premenopause and perimenopause stages.

During the beginning of menopausal stage or in the postmenopausal stage, women are more susceptible to suffer depression disorder with more severe and longer symptoms [3, 4]; severity of depression has been related to the ovarian hormone oscillating levels in the premenopause and very low levels in early postmenopause, specifically with estrogens [5].

The climacterium stage is a period of time that includes the perimenopause, premenopause, and menopause (see **Figure 1**); in this stage the women estrogenic oscillating, produces a dysfunction on the serotonergic neurotransmission system which is related to the high prevalence of depression in such stages compared with women in postmenopausal stage. However, this relationship seems to be controversial because not all the studies reported an increased prevalence of depression in the climacteric stage, when women's groups from different ethnic cultures, ages, school grade, and civil status, among others, were evaluated. These divergences on the clinical study results could be partially justified by different neurochemical changes related to the effects of estradiol on serotonergic system and the influence of these changes on the establishment of depression during the different stages of the climacteric period. For example, on early premenopausal stage, there is a decrease on the 5-HT1A autoreceptors in raphe, which is a brain structure responsible for the serotonin (5-HT) synthesis, and an increase on the 5-HT1A postsynaptic receptors located on the hippocampus (both receptors enable the antidepressant clinically effective, as the selective inhibitors of the serotonin, e.g., the fluoxetine) related to the high hormonal concentration compared with postmenopausal women [6].

				Climacterium						
				Premenopause		Perimenopause				
STAGE	REPRODUCTIVE				TRANSITION TO THE MENOPAUSE			POSTMENOPAUSE		
Phase	Early	Peak	Late		Early	Late	Menopause	Early		Late
Duration	Variable	Variable	Variable	Variable	Variable	1 - 3 years	1 year	1 year	3-6 year	Till the end of life

Figure 1. Classification of the reproductive phases of the woman. This classification is an abstract of the reproductive stage of women with their approximate during. Ovaries function markers and hormonal levels can help to make a correct classification. Modified from [57].

Thus, this can be related with the different antidepressant responses along the climacteric and postmenopausal stages.

The 5-HT2A receptors located on brain areas such as prefrontal cortex contribute on regulating the release of the 5-HT to areas that modulate the amygdala reactivity, brain structure involved to the emotional regulation. Treatment with 17β-estradiol for postmenopausal women increases the 5-HT2A receptors in prefrontal cortex [7]. However, the possible association between the establishment of depression in different climacteric and postmenopausal stages with the 5-HT2A receptor's activity has not been explored. Nevertheless, the preclinical data support the involvement of these receptors on the regulation of the depression disorder [8, 9].

On the other hand, in healthy postmenopausal women, there is a relation between personality features such as extroversion, aggressiveness, and neuroticism with the serotonin transporter (5-HTT). 5-HTT promotes polymorphism with "s" allele, which implies 5-HTT low expression and an increase in the impulsivity. Likewise, this trait is related with monoamine oxidase A (MAO-A) polymorphism that produces an increase of climacteric and depressive symptoms [10, 11]. In contrast, women under 50 years old with the "l" allele 5-HTT present a better antidepressant response and neural protection against the suicide attempt [12]; however, this response disappears when there is a low hormonal activity during menopausal stage [13].

Therefore, the main objective of this work is to collect and review scientific data not only clinical but also preclinical data that allow us to explain the knowledge about the impact of hormonal change experienced during climacteric and postmenopausal stages and how it affects serotonin neurotransmission that may contribute to the establishment of the depression disorder and the therapeutic response to antidepressant drugs.

2. Influence of hormones on the depression disorder establishment

Some researches point out a high vulnerability to suffer depression disorder on the women reproductive stage, related to the hormonal changes, as a decrease on the estradiol levels and an increase on the follicle-stimulating hormone (FSH) levels on the perimenopausal [3, 14, 15] throughout different reproductive stages it is set basically two different aspects about the hormonal influences, principally estradiol with the increasing risk to set out depressive symptomatology. The first one establishes that low hormonal concentrations on estradiol and progesterone during the earlier follicular stage of the menstrual cycle of the earlier productive stage of a woman are related to premenstrual dysphoric syndrome characterized among some other symptoms by depression and anxiety [16]. The second one suggests that oscillations on the hormonal levels on early stages of the menopause transition are determinant to increase the risk of having some depressive incidences. The same effect is observed on women who had been throughout menopause by surgical procedure, thus, became on the decrease of the hormonal levels, and also there is a surgical post-period where they show hormonal oscillations because the renal glands try to supply the hormonal lost, but it is important to mention that women who had been in a surgical procedure, such as oophorectomy on early age, indicate an increased probability to depression disease with severe and longer symptoms compared to women with a natural menopause [17].

There is a relationship at the establishment on depressive symptomatology with FSH or high luteinizing hormone (LH) levels and low inhibin B levels; this is a glycoprotein hormone secreted by teak and granulosa cells from the pre-antral and antral follicles that was responsible for the inhibition of FSH production at the level of the pituitary gland and a huge variability on estradiol levels, which occur during the menopause transition that includes women on the premenopause and perimenopause [2, 3]. Likewise, there is a FSH levels increasing and an abrupt fall of the estrogen levels after 12 months of menopause considered as early postmenopausal [18] pattern, which is independently from the sample analyzed on the late premenopausal and postmenopausal stage. Those hormonal variations are related to a rise on depression prevalence for 10 years before and 8 years after the last menstrual cycle and fall on the late postmenopausal period [4]. The above suggests that alterations in the feedback of the hypothalamic-pituitary-gonadal axis consequence of changes on the concentrations of ovarian hormone through the climacteric and postmenopausal stages, carry out a fundamental place on women's emotional stability, through the regulation of brain plasticity and neurochemical changes.

It has been established an association between a delay in appearance of menopause transition, in a period of two more years than average with 2% of decrease on the risk of a depression disease during the postmenopause, and also a reduction of the 50% to suffer depression disease on women who have menopause after 40 years old compared with early menopause on women before that age. It is suggested that those findings could be attributed to longer exposure to the endogenous estrogens that develop a neural protection and antidepressive effect [19]. This effect seems to be associated with the cerebral changes that induce the hormonal diminution according to the age of the woman.

The antidepressant effect on hormone replacement therapy (HRT) or estrogenic therapy on menopausal women is controversial. The estrogen supply such as 17β-estradiol (100 μg/day) has a lack of antidepressant effects on depressed women during the postmenopausal period on the late stage; it is to say that, 17 years after the menopausal stage, they show a FSH (≥40 pg/ml) and estradiol (≤19.7 pg/ml) hormonal concentrations [20]. This lack of antidepressant effect is also observed in postmenopausal women in the early phase, approximately 6 months to 3 years after menopause, with hormonal concentrations of FSH ≥ 35 pg/ml and estradiol ≤ 40 pg/ml, when 50 μg/day or 84 μg/day of estradiol was administered [7, 21]. The loss of estrogen efficacy against depression in women with postmenopausal may be associated with the downregulation of α- and β-estrogenic receptors at the brain level, caused by continued decrease of plasma estradiol concentrations. In contrast, antidepressant effects have also been reported in postmenopausal women with replacement treatments with bioidentical hormones (80% estriol/20% estradiol; 0.25 to 0.5 mg) and/or progesterone (20 to 60 mg), by transdermal injection in a volume of 1 ml/day for a period of 8 weeks. These women present an improvement in the depressive and anxiety symptoms according to Hamilton scales, at 2 months of treatment and annually until 36 months. Treatment with bioidentical hormones improved the health and quality of life of women without reports of adverse side effects. However, these women cursed postmenopausal, after an oophorectomy with a mean age of 52.3 ± 9.6 years and the time that elapsed since the surgery was not described, so it cannot be specified whether it was in the early or late stage of postmenopause [22]. This suggests that the type of molecule used for hormone replacement therapy and probably the age at which it is given could determine therapeutic success, a possibility that remains to be explored.

Changes in plasma levels of FSH on the establishment of depression in women with natural menopause are also seen in women with oophorectomy [23]; since the ovaries are removed, there is an abrupt cessation in the production of testosterone that is aromatized to estrogen and estradiol, which results in a dysfunction in the hypothalamic-pituitary-gonadal axis increasing FSH and LH levels, with the consequent decline of estradiol and progesterone levels [24]. These changes in hormone levels undergoing surgery take from 2 to 3 months to stabilize and are associated with a decrease in depressive symptoms [23]. Women undergoing menopause induced by surgeries such as hysterectomy and/or oophorectomy increase up to four times the probability to suffer postsurgery depression [25]. However, women who have undergone some depressive episode prior to surgery report a decrease in postoperative depressive symptomatology [25]. This may reflect a paradoxical effect. Some of the answers might be in the interrelation between estrogen and the serotonergic system.

3. Serotonergic alterations during the climacteric and postmenopause related with depression

A study by Stein et al. [6] detected an increase on 5-HT1A receptor levels in the hippocampus and a decrease in the dorsal nucleus raphe of premenopausal women at early ages (24.1 ± 2.6 years) compared to postmenopausal women (55.2 ± 4.8 years). In this same study, they identified higher concentrations of progesterone, estradiol, dehydroepiandrosterone sulfate (DHEAS), and cortisol in premenopausal women compared to postmenopausal women. This suggests that these hormones could be involved in the regulation of the expression of 5-HT1A receptors in different brain areas in women who travel through the climacteric, intervening in the establishment of depressive disorders of this stage, as well as in the different therapeutic responses to antidepressant drugs, and probably contributing to the effect of drug resistance, depending on the levels of receptors affected by oscillations on concentrations of hormones, mainly produced by the ovaries.

Studies made with positron emission tomography with [carbonyl-C11] WAY-100635 show that in the dorsal nucleus raphe, a structure highly involved in the regulation of serotonergic neurotransmission and therefore with a high density of 5-HT1A receptors, there is 1.5 times more 5-HT1A receptors in the luteal phase than in the follicular phase in healthy women, whereas this proportion is not observed in women with premenstrual dysphoric disorder [26], so a dysfunction like this could be a factor underlying to the establishment of depressive symptoms. Although Drevets et al. [27] reported a reduction in 5-HT1A receptors in the raphe (41.5%) and neocortical and limbic areas (25–33%) in depressed patients [27]. In this study the sex of the patients was not discriminated, and only from 4 to 7% of the patients were women and do not described the age neither conditions of the reproductive phase, so these results should be taken with reservation.

Moses-Kolko et al. [28] reported that in depressed women going through premenopause and postmenopause, there is a 15% decrease in 5-HT1A receptors in the orbitofrontal cortex compared to adult men with depression. The foregoing after performing an endocrine standardization to minimize the influence introduced by endogenous hormonal fluctuations and reproductive stage. They also detected an increase in the potential binding to 5-HT1A receptors in women, as age increases. They estimate that there is a 4.5% reduction per decade of age in the number of 5-HT1A receptors in the raphe in women. The 5-HT1A receptors have an age-dependent increase in neocortical regions in women, associated with decreased estrogen. In the same study, they identified that increase in 5-HT2A receptors is associated with the establishment of disorders such as neurosis, depression, suicide, and eating disorders [28], suggesting that age tends to reduce these receptors, since they are expressed in the neuropil of pyramidal neurons located mainly in the neocortex which are related to the release of glutamate and gamma-aminobutyric acid (GABA) regulating the postsynaptic excitatory impulses that project to the hippocampus and spinal cord neurons [29]. So, it is hypothesized that its reduction associated with age may be related to sleep disorder, cognition, and mood disorders [30].

4. Serotonergic changes associated to antidepressants and hormone replacement in the climacteric and postmenopause

The HRT in women undergoing climacteric, with 17β-estradiol by means of transdermal patches at a mean dose of 93 μg/day, causes an increase in plasma levels of estradiol from 14.7 pg/ml at baseline versus 176.5 pg/ml, after 10.2 weeks of treatment. This increase in estrogen levels has been related to the establishment of antidepressant effects after HRT [7]. However, several studies suggest that estrogens have the capability to produce a modulating effect on the serotonergic system that contributes to the establishment of the antidepressant effect (see **Table 1**).

In surgically postmenopausal women (58.4 age and 7.5 years after oophorectomy) and, therefore, with very low plasmatic concentrations of estradiol, the treatment with estradiol reduces the potential binding of 5-HTT in brain structures, such as in the amygdala, in the frontal cortex, and in various cortical regions. While the treatment with estradiol and testosterone reduces it in the parahippocampal gyrus, insular cortex, caudate nucleus, and thalamus [31]. Hence, the hormonal treatment reduces the efficiency of 5-HTT and increases the availability of 5-HT in the synaptic cleft on structures involved in the emotion modulation. This fact could be associated to an improvement in depressive symptomatology of these women measured with Beck Depression Inventory test [31]. However, some studies indicate that estrogen therapy in postmenopausal women does not produce antidepressant effects [21, 24], probably due to the downregulation of estrogenic receptors, associated with chronic decrease of

Changes associated to condition without pharmacological treatment

Condition (average age)	Serotonergic system	Hormonal changes	References
Premenopausal women (24.1 ± 2.6 years) vs. postmenopausal women (55.2 ± 4.8 years)	↑ 5HT1A receptor levels in the hippocampus ↓ 5HT1A receptor levels in the dorsal raphe	↑ Levels of progesterone, estradiol, dehydroepiandrosterone sulfate (DHEAS), and cortisol	[6]
Premenopausal depressed women (<50 years) Postmenopausal depressed women (>50 years)	↓ Postsynaptic 5-HT1A receptors in neocortical regions Increasing age was associated with↑ postsynaptic 5-HT1A receptor binding potential in neocortical regions Significant decline in 5HT2A receptor binding potential relative to age (8% per decade)	Low estradiol concentrations and low 5HT1A receptor binding potential	[28]

Changes associated to condition and estrogen replacement therapy

Condition (average age)	Serotonergic system changes	Regimen of treatment and/or changes associated to treatment	References
Surgically postmenopausal women (58.4 ± 4.7 years) Hysterectomy and bilateral oophorectomy	↓ The binding potential of 5-HTT in the amygdala, parahippocampal gyrus, insular cortex, and frontal cortex and in various cortical regions	Positive correlation between estradiol levels and the binding potential of 5-HTT in putamen, frontal cortex, and amygdala Negative correlation between testosterone levels and the binding potential of 5-HTT in the anterior cingulate cortex, hippocampus, caudate nucleus and thalamus	[31]
Postmenopausal women (54.5 years, 44–68 age range)	↑ 5-HT2A serotonergic receptors mainly in brain areas such as the right inferior prefrontal cortex, anterior cingulate cortex, and medial and inferior frontal gyrus	Transdermal patch (17β-estradiol, 0.075–0.15 mg; mean dose=0.084 mg for a mean of 10.2 weeks Negative correlation between estradiol levels and 5HT2A receptors	[7]
Postmenopausal women (55 ± 4.8)	No significant differences in 5-HT1A binding potential values	Combination 17β-estradiol valerate (Progynova® 21 mite; 2 mg/day, v.o.) and micronized progesterone (Utrogestan®, 200 mg/day, v.o.) for 67 ± 8 days Increase in estradiol and progesterone plasma levels	[56]
Female rats (2–3 months) Five postovariectomy days	↓ The time of 5-HT1A receptor desensitization of 7 days with fluoxetine and 2 days with estradiol + fluoxetine	17β-Estradiol-3-benzoate (0.01 mg/0.4 ml/kg, s.c.) plus fluoxetine (10 mg/2 l/kg, s.c.)	[37]
Female rats (2 months) Two months of postovariectomy	↑ 5-HT level in raphe	Estradiol benzoate (2.5 μg/kg/0.1 ml, s.c., day of ovariectomy; 5 μg/kg/0.1 ml, s.c., weekly; 20 μg/kg/0.1 ml, s.c. day of the test) + Progesterone (2 mg/kg/0.1 ml, s.c., 48 hours before the test)	[40]

Changes associated to condition and estrogen replacement therapy			
Condition (average age)	**Serotonergic system changes**	**Regimen of treatment and/or changes associated to treatment**	**References**
Female rats (1–2 months) 2–3 weeks of postovariectomy	Slowing of the 5-HT clearances, as well as an inhibition of the ability of fluvoxamine (SSRI antidepressant) to slow the clearance of 5-HT	Acute administration of both 17β-estradiol in the CA3 region of the hippocampus and systemic administration of estradiol benzoate (25 μg/100 μl, s.c., 48 hours before progesterone) + progesterone (500 μg/100 μl, s.c., 24 hours before the test)	[41]
Female rats (2–3 months) 2–3 weeks postovariectomy	Canceled the antidepressive-like effect of fluvoxamine (10 mg/kg) in forced swim test	Estradiol benzoate (25 μg/100 μl, s.c., 74–75 hours before the test and 24 hours before progesterone) + progesterone (500 μg/100 μl, s.c., 24 or 74–75 hours before the test)	[42]
Female rats (4 months) Two weeks of postovariectomy	Inhibits the 5-HTT	Estradiol (20 pmol) in the CA3 region of the hippocampus but not in 10 months in females, even at <40 pmol doses	[51]

5-HTT, serotonin transporter; 5-HT, 5-hidroxytriptamine; ↑, increase; ↓, decrease; SSRI, selective serotonin reuptake inhibitors

Table 1. Clinical and preclinical studies of the relation between serotonergic system and hormones.

concentrations of estradiol in the postmenopausal stage. This hypothesis is based on the fact that estrogenic antidepressant treatment on perimenopausal women produces therapeutic effects [32], probably because they still have considerable concentrations of estradiol, compared to postmenopausal women, which contribute that they do not present important neurochemical changes on estrogen receptors. In support, depressed postmenopausal women treated simultaneously with the combination of antidepressant serotonin-specific reuptake inhibitor drugs, such as fluoxetine with estrogen, showed significantly greater improvement of both mood and quality of life compared to fluoxetine monotherapy [33]. Pointing out that estrogen by itself probably does not produce antidepressant effects, the reduction that exerts on the potential binding of 5-HTT is enough to increase synaptic 5-HT concentration, a synergistic effect on serotonergic system of both estrogen and fluoxetine, which contributes to the establishment of the antidepressant effect. Paradoxically, the combination with tibolone, a synthetic steroid, does not produce synergistic antidepressant effects with fluoxetine [34]. The above suggests that substituents on steroid molecules could be a determinant in the potential interrelation in therapeutic efficacy between steroids and the serotonergic system.

On the other hand, some studies observed an increase on hypersensibility of postsynaptic 5-HT2A receptors on the basis of neurobiological depression [35, 36]. The 5-HT2A receptor is related to regulating the 5-HT release on the protection of neurons which are located on the prefrontal cortex, thus, to help the regulation easier to the amygdala's reaction and some other behaviors related. The administration of 150 mg/day of clomipramine for 3 weeks, tricyclic antidepressant, results a descend of 5-HT2A receptor's occupation on neocortex area, calculated by positron emission tomography (PET) which coincide with depression scores significantly improved, denoting the probability of the clomipramine's interaction with those receptors or may cause modified signal mechanism of these receptors [37].

There is a relationship with ovarian hormone and the 5-HT2A receptors. Kugaya et al. [7] developed a study on postmenopausal women, classified by the concentrations of FSH ≥30 UI/L. Those women were treated with 17β-estradiol HRT for almost 3 months; by PET that 5-HT2A serotonin receptors increased principally on brain areas such as prefrontal cortex and anterior cingulate cortex, related to increase of plasmatic estradiol density, this study did not mark any changes related to the effects on the mood but could be the result related to the test characteristics and the few subjects of study [7].

5. Preclinical studies of serotonergic changes associated with hormones and ovariectomy

Studies made in rodents have also shown the interrelation between estrogen and serotonergic system. Coadministration of estradiol with fluoxetine has been shown to contribute to 5-HT1A receptor desensitization [38], which is associated with antidepressant effect in humans and in rats evaluated in behavioral despair models [38]. In addition, this combination of estradiol with fluoxetine inhibits 5-HTT and increases de novo brain serotonin synthesis by activating tryptophan hydroxylase enzyme [39]. At the same time, it increases the number and sensitivity of the 5-HT1A receptors, mainly in the dorsal nucleus raphe of rats. This could be related to the antidepressant effect produced by estradiol.

It has also been detected that acute administration of estradiol on ovariectomized rats increased the turnover of serotonin, by increasing serotonin and its metabolite, 5-hydroxyindoleacetic acid (5-HIAA) in amygdale and striatum involved in the mood regulation. While chronic for 16 days, estradiol and progesterone administration has been found to increase serotonin mainly in the dorsal raphe of the ovariectomized rats [40].

Benmansour and collaborators' research group [41] has explored the signaling mechanisms involved in the interaction of estradiol and serotonergic systems in rats. Both acute administration of 17β-estradiol in the CA3 region of the hippocampus and systemic administration of estradiol benzoate cause slowing of the 5-HT clearances, as well as an inhibition of the ability of fluvoxamine to slow the clearance of 5-HT [41]. These effects are mediated by estrogen receptors α and β. The slowing of the 5-HT clearance was due to activation of β-estrogen and/or GPR30. Meanwhile, the blockade of fluvoxamine's inhibitory effect on 5-HT clearance was mediated by α-estrogen [42]. Both of them used different signaling mechanisms. The estradiol-induced slowing of serotonin clearance by means of activation of receptors of β-estrogen required MAPK/ERK1/2 signaling pathways and involved interactions both with tyrosine kinase BDNF receptor (TrKB) and insulin-like growth factor-1 receptor (IGF-1R). The effect of estradiol to prevention of the ability of fluvoxamine to slow serotonin clearance, through receptors of α-estrogen, required MAPK/ERK1/2 and PI3K/Akt signaling pathways as well as interactions with both IGF-1R and mGluR1 [43]. All these ways are etiologically implied to depression.

In this context, the ERK signaling cascade is activated by antidepressant clinically effective as fluoxetine [44] and the systemic blockade of the MAPK pathway in mice produced depressive-like behavior in several animal models of experimental depression as well as inhibits the antidepressant effect of desipramine and fluoxetine in the forced swim test, a main model of depression [45]. On the other hand, the action of BDNF, which has been implicated in the mechanism(s) of action of the antidepressant (see Ref. [46]), is mediated through its high-affinity tyrosine kinase receptor B (TrkB), whose activation is required for antidepressant-like effect [47].

The acute intraventricular administration of IGF-1 produced antidepressant-like effects in mice evaluated in the tail suspension and forced swim tests [48], an effect detected after 3 days of the administration with participation of 5-HT [49]. The antagonism of the mGluR produced antidepressant-like effects in the forced swim test, probably through the intracellular signaling pathways described above [50]. Therefore, there is evidence about the interaction with the estrogens and the serotonergic system on the regulation on the depression disorder not only removing them but also influencing them by the other neurotransmitter systems and other kinds of receptors.

We have already mentioned the difference between the plasmatic estradiol levels during the climacteric stage that is related to the establishment of the depression disease and the antidepressant responses. We have also mentioned that estradiol slows the clearance of 5-HT and at the same time disables the same effect produced by fluvoxamine per se. In this sense during the rat estrous cycle, it has been shown that both estrous and diestrus phases are characterized by low estradiol levels in comparison to the proestrous phase; the fluvoxamine increases the clearance time of 5-HT, but not in the proestrous phase [41]. Rats with 2–3 postovariectomy weeks, it is observed that fluvoxamine increases the clearance time of 5-HT, the same effect caused by the estradiol benzoate treatment. However, the pretreatment with estradiol benzoate blocks the fluvoxamine effect [41].

Additionally evaluated the estradiol effect on the 5-HTT functionality, through time a clearance of the 5-HT, in different ages and postovariectomy time identifying that microinjection of 20pmol of estradiol on CA3 region in the hippocampus to inhibit 5-HTT in young adult rats (4 months age) after 2 weeks from the postovariectomy, but had not effect in middle-age rats (10 months), even with the use of <40 pmol dosage. While fluvoxamine reduces the clearance of 5-HT on rats about 10 months aged with 2 weeks, 4 and 8 months postovariectomy the same way as the 4 months rats [51]. Additionally, they detected that 5 μg/day of estradiol for 2 weeks subcutaneously via implantation of osmotic minipumps produces antidepressant effects on forced swim test on 4-month aged rats but not in 10-month aged rats both with 2 weeks of postovariectomy. Nevertheless the dosage of estradiol for 10 μg/day produces an antidepressant effect after 2 weeks of the postovariectomy procedure, but not at 4 months of postovariectomy in 10-month aged rats. The same dosages produced the same antidepressant effect on older rats (14 months of age) after 2 weeks of postovariectomy. The authors conclude that the lack of an antidepressant effect in estradiol is due to the 4-month hormone withdrawal and not to an age effect. Also in the same study, they reported that 2 weeks of treatment with sertraline, an antidepressant selective serotonin reuptake inhibitors (SSRI), on rats from 4 to 10 months of age with 2 weeks, 4 months, and 8 months of postovariectomy produce antidepressant effect in the forced swim test. In this study, it is concluded that the age influences the potency of estradiol on the 5-HTT, but its effects were strongly reduced if the period of postovariectomy is longer. On the other hand, the treatment with sertraline inhibited the 5-HTT and produced antidepressant-like effects without affected either by age or length of hormonal depletion [51].

In support to clinics finding about 5-HT2A receptors above mentioned some animal studies it has been observed that the administration of 5-HT2A receptor antagonist, i.e., ketanserin (0.1 mg/kg, i.p., 14 days) produces antidepressant effects in forced swim test and anxiolytic effect in elevated plus-maze test both in the proestrous and estrous phases of estrous cycle, characterized by high concentrations of progesterone and estradiol. In contrast, produces anxiogenic effect in phases with reduce concentrations of estradiol [52]. It is suggested that 5-HT2A receptors play different roles on the modulation of anxiety and depression associated with the alterations of hormonal concentrations during the ovarian cycle. In contrast, ketanserin administered in the same doses (0.1 mg/kg, i.p.) for 7 days in male rats produces an antidepressant-like effect, and together with the antidepressant fluoxetine (5 mg/kg, i.p., 7 days), it potentiates the antidepressant effect in forced swim test [53]. This suggests that the effect of ketanserin on females goes beyond changes in hormonal concentrations, which requires exploration.

Previous searches suggest that different hormonal levels, which vary through different reproductive statuses on women, may cause some changes on serotonergic system. For example, density and potential binding of the 5-HT1A and 5-HT2A receptors, as well as the potential binding of the 5-HTT in different brain structures linked to the mood changes, may contribute to the depression establishment. Those disruptions on the serotonergic system may influence or modify negatively the success of therapeutic response treated with antidepressant drugs or HRT; there is one possibility that must be explored.

5.1. Pharmacological response prediction: 5-HT1A and 5-HT2A receptors

Pharmacological compounds that take action on 5-HT1A receptors such as SSRI are clinically effective antidepressants but require a period of 3–6 weeks of treatment to establish the therapeutic effects [54]. Additionally, 50 to 70% depressed patients respond to the first pharmacological treatment, and less than 40% get a total remission [54]. Combination of SSRI with 5-HT2A receptor antagonist makes the latency period shorter for the establishment of antidepressant effect [55]. This fact suggests that the stimulation of 5-HT1A receptors by SSRI and the inactivity of 5-HT2A receptors, which are part of the serotonin release on limbic areas, produce synergism effect. Therefore, the alteration in the expression of receptors in different brain areas, associated with variations of hormones such as estradiol, mainly in the stages of the climacteric, can influence the pharmacological response to antidepressants.

There are controversial data related to regulatory mechanism, which are exerted to antidepressant treatments on the 5-HT1A and 5-HT2A receptor density. A study developed by

Kranz et al. [56] did not detect differences on the 5-HT1A receptor density on structures such as the hippocampus, the frontal cortex, and the raphe on postmenopausal woman [56]. After the administration of HRT with 17β-valerate ester alone or combined with progesterone, no matter the fact exist, a significant increase of estradiol and progesterone, an effect that has been identified on postmenopausal women [28]. This suggests that plasma concentrations of estradiol that are still elevated in premenopausal women compared to postmenopausal women seem to determine the 5-HT 1A receptor expression on the estrogenic treatment response.

6. Final comments and conclusion

Variations in the levels of ovarian hormones that occur throughout the stages of climacteric and postmenopause severely impact women's mood. The depression is found mainly in the stages with continuous hormonal oscillations like perimenopause and premenopause. However, the relationship between hormonal and serotonergic systems in the climacteric and postmenopausal stages needs to be explored. The neurochemical and neurophysiological modification consequence of the oscillating hormonal levels leads to alterations in the cerebral neurotransmission functioning, mainly on the serotonergic system of the 5-HTT, 5-HT turnover, and 5-HT1A/5-HT2A receptors. This affects the pharmacological response to antidepressant treatments, both with estrogen therapy and with SSRI or tricyclic drugs in the different climacteric and postmenopausal stages.

The limitation on the studies have contributed to the establishment of these hypothesis emerged by the reduced length of women included in the studies and the wide range of ages which is used, because these incorporate women who are in different stages and different reproductive status and also women going through induced oophorectomy postmenopausal on early ages. Also, the lack of quantification of the hormonal levels, principally estradiol, FSH, and the ovarian function markers such as inhibin B, antral follicle count, anti-Müllerian hormone, and the estradiol levels. There is a direct relationship between advanced age and elevated serum basal levels which is associated with poor ovarian response. However, additional studies are needed to support these findings because it should let us categorize effectively those women on their reproductive stage. Thus, it allows us to establish a correct reciprocity between the serotonin changes and evaluated stages.

In addition, some limits in the imaging studies (e.g., PET), which are difficult to correct analysis on small brain structures or markers used, are not always selective to serotonin receptors, principally 5-HT2A receptors. It is also necessary to extend the researches related to serotonin changes on women with some depressant disorder, as major depression on all the reproductive stages, because some recent studies are only used to evaluate the symptomatology improvement on menopause, as somatic, urogenital, or physiologic symptomatology. On the last one, the symptomatology causes low motivation but without depression diagnosis, which limits the exploration of the neurochemical alterations that underlay to the depressive disorder on many different reproductive stages.

There are two areas that have been explored yet; the first one is nonsymptomatic women, thus, probably related to the hormonal levels through the reproductive stages and the correlation with brain serotonergic function, and also women through oophorectomies on early ages or ovarian failure (both under 40 years old). Women through an abrupt fall on ovarian hormone and some studies point out a high prevalence of depressive disorder longer and severe. Data may contribute to possible genetic factors, biological, psychosocial, and environmental, which are related to the establishment of the depressive disorder on different climacteric and postmenopausal stages.

In conclusion, depression associated to climacteric and postmenopausal stages involves changes in the serotonergic system, which includes an increase in the 5-HT clearance, turnover of 5-HT, and affinity of 5-HTT, as well as increased expression of 5-HT1A and 5-HT2A receptors in different brain regions (i.e., prefrontal cortex and hippocampus). All these changes seem to be a result of the oscillations in the ovarian hormone concentration characteristics of the climacteric and postmenopausal stages.

Conflicts of interest

The authors declare no conflicts of interest.

Acknowledgements

The present chapter was part of the postdoctoral activities linked to the strengthening of the quality of the national postgraduate that the first author made in the Centro Universitario de los Lagos of the University of Guadalajara with fellowships from the Consejo Nacional de Ciencia y Tecnología (CONACyT, CVU: 210315, SNI: 64200).

Author details

Rosa Isela García-Ríos[1]*, Armando Mora-Pérez[2] and Cesar Soria-Fregozo[2]

*Address all correspondence to: rosai_garios@yahoo.com

1 Department of Biomedics, University Center of Tonalá, University of Guadalajara, Tonalá, Jalisco, México

2 Laboratory of Psychobiology and Molecular Biology, University Center of Los Lagos, University of Guadalajara, Lagos de Moreno, Jalisco, México

References

[1] World Health Organization. "Depression", in Fact Sheet. 2015. Available online at: http://www.who.int/mediacentre/factsheets/fs369/en/[Accessed 10-September-2015]

[2] Cohen LS, Soares CN, Vitonis AF, Otto MW, Harlow BL. Risk for new onset of depression during the menopausal transition: The Harvard study of moods and cycles. Archives of General Psychiatry. 2006;**63**(4):385-390. DOI: 10.1001/archpsyc.63.4.385

[3] Freeman EW, Sammel MD, Liu L, Gracia CR, Nelson DB, Hollander L. Hormones and menopausal status as predictors of depression in women in transition to menopause. Archives of General Psychiatry. 2004;**61**(1):62-70. DOI: 10.1001/archpsyc.61.1.62

[4] Freeman EW, Sammel MD, Lin H, Nelson DB. Associations of hormones and menopausal status with depressed mood in women with no history of depression. Archives of General Psychiatry. 2006;**63**(4):375-382. DOI: 10.1001/archpsyc.63.4.375

[5] Ryan J, Burger HG, Szoeke C, Lehert P, Ancelin ML, Henderson VW, Dennerstein L. A prospective study of the association between endogenous hormones and depressive symptoms in postmenopausal women. Menopause. 2009;**16**(3):509-517. DOI: 10.1097/gme.0b013e31818d635f

[6] Stein P, Baldinger P, Kaufmann U, Christina RM, Hahn A, Höflich A, Kranz GS, Savli M, Wadsak W, Mitterhauser M, Winkler D, Kasper S, Lanzenberger R. Relation of progesterone and DHEAS serum levels to 5-HT1A receptor binding potential in pre- and postmenopausal women. Psychoneuroendocrinology. 2014;**46**:52-63. http://dx.doi.org/10.1016/j.psyneuen.2014.04.008

[7] Kugaya A, Epperson CN, Zoghbi S, van Dyck CH, Hou Y, Fujita M, Staley JK, Garg PK, Seibyl JP, Innis RB. Increase in prefrontal cortex serotonin 2A receptors following estrogen treatment in postmenopausal women. The American Journal of Psychiatry. 2003;**160**(8):1522-1524. http://dx.doi.org/10.1176/appi.ajp.160.8.1522

[8] Fedotova IUO, Platonova NA, Sapronov NS. 8-OH-DPAT modulates expression of 5-HT(1A)/5-HT(2A), 17beta-estradiol receptor mRNAs in ovariectomized rats in Porsolt test. Eksperimental'naia i klinicheskaia farmakologiia. 2006;**69**(3):53-57

[9] Yamada N, Araki H, Yoshimura H. Identification of antidepressant-like ingredients in ginseng root (Panax ginseng C.A. Meyer) using a menopausal depressive-like state in female mice: Participation of 5-HT2A receptors. Psychopharmacology (Berl). 2011;**216**(4):589-599. DOI: 10.1007/s00213-011-2252-1

[10] Stein MB, Campbell-Sills L, Gelernter J. Genetic variation in 5HTTLPR is associated with emotional resilience. American Journal of Medical Genetics Part B: Neuropsychiatric Genetics. 2009;**150B**(7):900-906. DOI: 10.1002/ajmg.b.30916

[11] Grochans E, Grzywacz A, Jurczak A, Samochowiec A, Karakiewicz B, Brodowska A, Starczewski A, Samochowiec J. The 5HTT and MAO-A polymorphisms associate with depressive mood and climacteric symptoms in postmenopausal women. Progress in Neuro-Psychopharmacology & Biological Psychiatry 2013;**45**:125-130. DOI: 10.1016/j.pnpbp.2013.05.007

[12] Gressier F, Verstuyft C, Hardy P, Becquemont L, Corruble E. Menopausal status could modulate the association between 5-HTTLPR and antidepressant efficacy in depressed women: A pilot study. Archives of Women's Mental Health. 2014;**17**(6):569-573. DOI: 10.1007/s00737-014-0464-1

[13] Baca-García E, Vaquero C, Diaz-Sastre C, Ceverino A, Saiz-Ruiz J, Fernández-Piquera J, de León J. A pilot study on a gene-hormone interaction in female suicide attempts. European Archives of Psychiatry and Clinical Neuroscience. 2003;**253**:281-285. DOI: 10.1007/s00406-003-0441-6

[14] Freeman EW, Sammel MD, Boorman DW, Zhang R. Longitudinal pattern of depressive symptoms around natural menopause. JAMA Psychiatry. 2014;**71**(1):36-43. DOI: 10.1001/jamapsychiatry.2013.2819

[15] Li RX, Ma M, Xiao XR, Xu Y, Chen XY, Li B. Perimenopausal syndrome and mood disorders in perimenopause: Prevalence, severity, relationships, and risk factors. Medicine (Baltimore). 2016;**95**(32):e4466. DOI: 10.1097/MD.0000000000004466

[16] de Zambotti M, Nicholas CL, Colrain IM, Trinder JA, Baker FC. Autonomic regulation across phases of the menstrual cycle and sleep stages in women with premenstrual syndrome and healthy controls. Psychoneuroendocrinology. 2013;**38**(11):2618-2627. DOI: 10.1016/j.psyneuen.2013.06.005

[17] Almeida OP, Marsh K, Flicker L, Hickey M, Sim M, Ford A. Depressive symptoms in midlife: The role of reproductive stage. Menopause. 2016;**23**(6):669-675. DOI: 10.1097/GME.0000000000000598

[18] Davis SR, Lambrinoudaki I, Lumsden M, Mishra GD, Pal L, Rees M, Santoro N, Simoncini T. Menopause. Natural Reviews Disease Primers. 2015;**1**:15004. DOI: 10.1038/nrdp.2015.4

[19] Georgakis MK, Thomopoulos TP, Diamantaras AA, Kalogirou EI, Skalkidou A, Daskalopoulou SS, Petridou ET. Association of age at menopause and duration of reproductive period with depression after menopause: A systematic review and meta-analysis. JAMA Psychiatry. 2016;**73**(2):139-149. DOI: 10.1001/jamapsychiatry.2015.2653

[20] Morrison MF, Kallan MJ, Ten Have T, Katz I, Tweedy K, Battistini M. Lack of efficacy of estradiol for depression in postmenopausal women: A randomized, controlled trial. Biological Psychiatry. 2004;**55**(4):406-412. http://dx.doi.org/10.1016/j.biopsych.2003.08.011

[21] Gleason CE, Dowling NM, Wharton W, Manson JE, Miller VM, Atwood CS, Brinton EA, Cedars MI, Lobo RA, Merriam GR, Neal-Perry G, Santoro NF, Taylor HS, Black DM, Budoff MJ, Hodis HN, Naftolin F, Harman SM Asthana S. Effects of hormone therapy on cognition and mood in recently postmenopausal women: Findings from the Randomized, Controlled KEEPS-Cognitive and Affective Study. PLoS Medicine. 2015;**12**(6):e1001833. DOI: 10.1371/journal.pmed.1001833

[22] Stephenson K, Neuenschwander PF, Kurdowska AK. The effects of compounded bioidentical transdermal hormone therapy on hemostatic, inflammatory, immune factors; cardiovascular biomarkers; quality-of-life measures; and health outcomes in perimenopausal and postmenopausal women. International Journal of Pharmaceutical Compounding. 2013;**17**(1):74-85

[23] Đoković DD, Jović JJ, Đoković JD, Knežević MŽ, Djukić-Dejanović S, Ristić-Ignjatović DI. Effects of hormone replacement therapy on depressive and anxiety symptoms after oophorectomy. Med Glas (Zenica). 2015;**12**(1):79-85

[24] Morrison JH, Brinton RD, Schmidt PJ, Gore AC. Estrogen, menopause, and the aging brain: How basic neuroscience can inform hormone therapy in women. Journal of Neuroscience. 2006;**26**(41):10332-10348. https://doi.org/10.1523/JNEUROSCI.3369-06.2006

[25] Mantani A, Yamashita H, Fujikawa T, Yamawaki S. Higher incidence of hysterectomy and oophorectomy in women suffering from clinical depression: Retrospective chart review. Psychiatry and Clinical Neurosciences. 2010;**64**(1):95-98. DOI: 10.1111/j.1440-1819.2009.02044.x

[26] Jovanovic H, Cerin A, Karlsson P, Lundberg J, Halldin C, Nordström AL. A PET study of 5-HT1A receptors at different phases of the menstrual cycle in women with premenstrual dysphoria. Psychiatry Research. 2006;**148**(2-3):185-193. DOI: 10.1016/j.pscychresns.2006.05.002

[27] Drevets WC, Frank E, Price JC, Kupfer DJ, Holt D, Greer PJ, Huang Y, Gautier C, Mathis C. PET imaging of serotonin 1A receptor binding in depression. Biological Psychiatry. 1999;**46**(10):1375-1387. http://dx.doi.org/10.1016/S0006-3223(99)00189-4

[28] Moses-Kolko EL, Price JC, Shah N, Berga S, Sereika SM, Fisher PM, Coleman R, Becker C, Mason NS, Loucks T, Meltzer CC. Age, sex, and reproductive hormone effects on brain serotonin-1A and serotonin-2A receptor binding in a healthy population. Neuropsychopharmacology 2011;**36**:2729-2740. DOI:10.1038/npp.2011.163

[29] Sharp T, Boothman L, Raley J, Queree P. Important messages in the 'post': Recent discoveries in 5-HT neurone feedback control. Trends in Pharmacological Sciences 2007;**28**:629-636. DOI: 10.1016/j.tips.2007.10.009

[30] Meltzer CC, Smith G, DeKosky ST, Pollock BG, Mathis CA, Moore RY et al. Serotonin in aging, late-life depression, and Alzheimer's disease: The emerging role of functional imaging. Neuropsychopharmacology. 1998;**18**:407-430. DOI: 10.1016/S0893-133X(97)00194-2

[31] Jovanovic H, Kocoska-Maras L, Rådestad AF, Halldin C, Borg J, Hirschberg AL, Nordström AL. Effects of estrogen and testosterone treatment on serotonin transporter binding in the brain of surgically postmenopausal women—A PET study. NeuroImage 2015;**106**:47-54. DOI: 10.1016/j.neuroimage.2014.11.003

[32] Soares CN, Almeida OP, Joffe H, Cohen LS. Efficacy of estradiol for the treatment of depressive disorders in perimenopausal women: A double-blind, randomized, placebo-controlled trial. Archives of General Psychiatry. 2001;**58**(6):529-534. DOI:10.1001/archpsyc.58.6.529

[33] Liu P, He FF, Bai WP, Yu Q, Shi W, Wu YY, He DJ, Xiao JH, Zheng Y, Liao QP. Menopausal depression: Comparison of hormone replacement therapy and hormone replacement therapy plus fluoxetine. Chinese Medical Journal. 2004;**117**(2):189-194

[34] Berlanga C, Mendieta D, Alva G, del Carmen Lara M. Failure of tibolone to potentiate the pharmacological effect of fluoxetine in postmenopausal major depression. Journal of Women's Health (2002). 2003;**12**(1):33-39. DOI: 10.1089/154099903321154121

[35] D'Haenen H, Bossuyt A, Mertens J, Bossuyt-Piron C, Gijsemans M, Kaufman L. SPECT imaging of serotonin2 receptors in depression. Psychiatry Research Neuroimaging. 1992;**45**:227-237. http://dx.doi.org/10.1016/0925-4927(92)90018-Y

[36] Stockmeier CA. Involvement of serotonin in depression: evidence from postmortem and imaging studies of serotonin receptors and the serotonin transporter Journal of Psychiatric Research. 2003;**37**(5):357-373. DOI:10.1016/S0022-3956(03)00050-5

[37] Attar-Lévy D, Martinot JL, Blin J, Dao-Castellana MH, Crouzel C, Mazoyer B, Poirier MF, Bourdel MC, Aymard N, Syrota A, Féline A. The cortical serotonin2 receptors studied with positron-emission tomography and [18F]-setoperone during depressive illness and antidepressant treatment with clomipramine. Biological Psychiatry. 1999;**45**(2):180-186. http://dx.doi.org/10.1016/S0006-3223(98)00007-9

[38] Li Q, Sullivan NR, McAllister CE, Van de Kar LD, Muma NA. Estradiol accelerates the effects of fluoxetine on serotonin 1A receptor signaling. Psychoneuroendocrinology. 2013;**38**(7):1145-1157. DOI: 10.1016/j.psyneuen.2012.11.005

[39] Kim SW, Park SY, Hwang O. Up-regulation of tryptophan hydroxylase expression and serotonin synthesis by sertraline. Molecular Pharmacology. 2002;**61**(4):778-785. https://doi.org/10.1124/mol.61.4.778

[40] Cone RI, Davis GA, Goy RW. Effects of ovarian steroids on serotonin metabolism within grossly dissected and microdissected brain regions of the ovariectomized rat. Brain Research Bulletin. 1981;**7**:639-644. http://dx.doi.org/10.1016/0361-9230(81)90111-8

[41] Benmansour S, Piotrowski JP, Altamirano AV, Frazer A. Impact of ovarian hormones on the modulation of the serotonin transporter by fluvoxamine. Neuropsychopharmacology. 2009;**34**(3):555-564. DOI: 10.1038/npp.2008.23

[42] Benmansour S, Weaver RS, Barton AK, Adeniji OS, Frazer A. Comparison of the effects of estradiol and progesterone on serotonergic function. Biological Psychiatry. 2012;**71**(7):633-641. DOI: 10.1016/j.biopsych.2011.11.023

[43] Benmansour S, Privratsky AA, Adeniji OS, Frazer A. Signaling mechanisms involved in the acute effects of estradiol on 5-HT clearance. The International Journal of Neuropsychopharmacology. 2014;**17**(5):765-777. DOI: 10.1017/S146114571300165X

[44] Mercier G, Lennon AM, Renouf B, Dessouroux A, Ramaugé M, Courtin F, Pierre M. MAP kinase activation by fluoxetine and its relation to gene expression in cultured rat astrocytes. Journal of Molecular Neuroscience 2004;**24**:207-216. DOI: 10.1385/JMN:24:2:207

[45] Duman CH, Schlesinger L, Kodama M, Russell DS, Duman RS. A role for MAP kinase signaling in behavioral models of depression and antidepressant treatment. Biological Psychiatry 2007;**61**:661-670. DOI: 10.1016/j.biopsych.2006.05.047

[46] Schmidt HD, Duman RS. The role of neurotrophic factors in adult hippocampal neurogenesis, antidepressant treatments and animal models of depressive-like behavior. Behavioural Pharmacology 2007;**18**:391-418. DOI: 10.1097/FBP.0b013e3282ee2aa8

[47] Saarelainen T, Hendolin P, Lucas G, Koponen E, Sairanen M, MacDonald E, Agerman K, Haapasalo A, Nawa H, Aloyz R, Ernfors P, Castren E. Activation of the TrkB neurotrophin receptor is induced by antidepressant drugs and is required for antidepressant-induced behavioral effects. Journal of Neuroscience. 2003;**23**:349-357. DOI: 0270-6474/02/220349-09

[48] Malberg JE, Platt B, Rizzo SJ, Ring RH, Lucki I, Schechter LE, Rosenzweig-Lipson S. Increasing the levels of insulin-like growth factor-I by an IGF binding protein inhibitor produces anxiolytic and antidepressant-like effects. Neuropsychopharmacology. 2007;**32**:2360-2368. DOI: 10.1038/sj.npp.1301358

[49] Hoshaw BA, Hill TI, Crowley JJ, Malberg JE, Khawaja X, Rosenzweig-Lipson S, Schechter LE, Lucki I. Antidepressant-like behavioral effects of IGF-I produced by enhanced serotonin transmission. European Journal of Pharmacology. 2008;**594**:109-116. DOI: 10.1016/j.ejphar.2008.07.023

[50] Pomierny-Chamioło L, Poleszak E, Pilc A, Nowak G. NMDA but not AMPA glutamatergic receptors are involved in the antidepressant-like activity of MTEP during the forced swim test in mice. Pharmacological Reports. 2010;**62**(6):1186-1190

[51] Benmansour S, Arroyo LD, Frazer A. Comparison of the antidepressant-like effects of estradiol and that of selective serotonin reuptake inhibitors in middle-aged ovariectomized rats. Frontiers in Aging Neuroscience 2016;**8**:311. DOI: 10.3389/fnagi.2016.00311

[52] Fedotova IuO. Behavioral effects of m-CPP and ketanserine during ovarian cycle in female rats. Eksperimental'naia i klinicheskaia farmakologiia. 2010;**73**(11):6-9

[53] Pilar-Cuéllar F, Vidal R, Pazos A. Subchronic treatment with fluoxetine and ketanserin increases hippocampal brain-derived neurotrophic factor, β-catenin and antidepressant-like effects. British Journal of Pharmacology. 2012;**165**(4b):1046-1057. DOI: 10.1111/j.1476-5381.2011.01516.x

[54] Gaynes BN, Jackson WC, Rorie KD. Major depressive disorder in the primary care setting: Strategies to achieve remission and recovery. The Journal of Family Practice. 2015;**64**(9):S4–S15

[55] Pandey DK, Bhatt S, Jindal A, Gautam B. Effect of combination of ketanserin and escitalopram on behavioral anomalies after olfactory bulbectomy: Prediction of quick onset of antidepressant action. Indian Journal of Pharmacology. 2014;**46**(6):639-643. DOI: 10.4103/0253-7613.144935

[56] Kranz GS, Rami-Mark C, Kaufmann U, Baldinger P, Hahn A, Höflich A, Savli M, Stein P, Wadsak W, Mitterhauser M, Winkler D, Lanzenberger R, Kasper S. Effects of hormone replacement therapy on cerebral serotonin-1A receptor binding in postmenopausal women examined with [carbonyl-^{11}C]WAY-100635. Psychoneuroendocrinology 2014;**45**:1-10. DOI: 10.1016/j.psyneuen.2014.03.004

[57] Harlow SD, Gass M, Hall JE, Lobo R, Maki P, Rebar RW, Sherman S, Sluss PM, de Villiers TJ; STRAW 10 Collaborative Group. Executive summary of the Stages of Reproductive Aging Workshop + 10: addressing the unfinished agenda of staging reproductive aging. Menopause. 2012;**19**(4):387-395. DOI: 10.1097/gme.0b013e31824d8f40

6

Psychological and Social Aspects of Menopause

Iqbal Afridi

Abstract

Menopause is one of the age-related phases of physiological transition of females. There is robust research and information regarding its biological aspects specially its endocrine base, yet the psychosocial aspect is quite interesting and debatable due to its variability among different cultures and climates. There are certain subthreshold response in form fear and loss of reproductive life to no more ability to reproduce and a feeling of loss of femininity. The period of menstruation simulated to reproductive age or fertility is around half of their lives; therefore, loss of fertility or reproductive life may be a source of stress specially among tribes where long reproductive age period is desired on the cultural belief that this will lead to a large family size that is considered as a symbol of success. Psychological factors such personal or inter-psychic (personality, self-esteem, and coping skills) and intra-psychic (relationship issues and social support) may contribute in the onset, course, and repose to perimenopausal period. There are certain psychiatric conditions such as anxiety, depressive disorder, and premenstrual dysphoric syndrome related to premenopausal period that must be screened. Before embarking on pharmacological treatment, psychosocial intervention especially lifestyle modifications must be offered to avoid complications.

Keywords: menopause, psychosocial, women, depression, anxiety

1. Introduction

As female grows old with passing years, she undergoes different phases of life, from childhood to adulthood. Her body keeps on changing at all levels; may it be anatomical, physiological, and hormonal with the years of aging. Menopause is just another phase of life like puberty. It is the time when ovaries stop producing eggs any more.

Menopause is a Latin word where *"Meno"* means month and *"pause"* means to stop. Various terms have been used for menopause in different languages as *"Haiz ka band hona"* in Urdu, *"alssnn yas"* in Arabic.

It is neither a disease, an illness, a pathology, nor a state of being not well but just a normal physiological phenomenon of aging among females from transition of reproductive life to no more ability to reproduce. It has no impact on sexuality of a female. This transition occurs with some changes in hormones of female endocrine system predominantly estrogen leading to menopausal symptoms.

For women, the menopausal period is considered the climacterium, the middle adulthood; a period in life characterized by decreased biological and physiological functioning and may lead to psychosocial disturbance in form of interpersonal relationships [1]. It may start anywhere from the 40s to the early 50s but generally occurs between 47 and 53 years [1].

Considering the onset of menopausal age, one must keep in mind the difference between days per year in various calendars such as a lunar year of 354 days used by Muslims as compared to the solar year of 365 despite the fact that the later also known as Gregorian calendar is widely in use, but ancient calendars are also used by a significant number of peoples who belong to certain regions and religions, in the form of the Julian calendar, the Islamic calendar, etc.

The menopausal condition has been analog in men as andropause. For men, the climacterium has no clear demarcation; male hormones stay fairly constant through the 40s and 50s and then begin to decline [1].

All women will not experience menopause in the same way in terms of their onset and symptoms. Apart from a normal response or may be a positive feeling in the form of relief from pain or at least the burden of the management of menstruation each month, many premenopausal women have concerns that they will experience mental instability, sudden signs of aging, and diminution of sexuality at this time. Culture, health, previous experience of mood problems, lifestyle, and whether menopause onset is a natural, surgical, or chemotherapy-induced, will all impact on menopausal symptoms. Increased risk for psychiatric morbidity is seen in women who experienced early menopause or surgical menopause [2]. According to study of Bernice Neugarten, the famous American psychologist who is specialized in adult development and the psychology of aging, more than 50% of females described menopause as an unpleasant experience, some believed that their lives had not changed in any significant way, and many women experienced no adverse effects while some reports feeling sexually free after menopause of any worry of becoming pregnant.

2. Psychological factors

2.1. Personal psychological vulnerability

Large epidemiological studies have shown that the years usually associated with natural menopause, that is 45–55, are not associated with increased psychiatric morbidity or more utilization of health services by women [2–5]. Various personal factors of an individual female may affect her menopausal experience. Such as follows:

- Past experience of mood disorders.
- Negative attitude to menopause and aging: women with more negative attitudes toward the menopause in general report more symptoms during the menopausal transition [6].
- Life events, personality, and coping.
- Self-esteem: women with a low self-esteem used to have more severe menopausal complaints [7].

2.2. Life stressors

They may include the following:

- Lack of social support
- Unemployment
- Surgical menopause
- Poor overall health status

2.3. Interpersonal relationships

Social interpersonal relationships also have their impact on a person's life and general well-being. They constitute a major social support in a woman's life and help her in managing stressors and problems in life with influencial effect on psychological health. They may include the following:

- Relationship with a partner
- Relationship with children
- Relationship with friends/social support

Menopause could be a stressful transition due to various beliefs related to fertility and a gradual diminishing role or role shifts in society. Depression at menopause has been attributed to the *Empty Nest Syndrome.* A phenomenon observed with depression that occurs in some men and women when their youngest child is about to leave home. Many women, however, report an enhanced sense of well-being and enjoy opportunities to pursue goals postponed because of child rearing [1].

3. Social factors

Education and socioeconomic statuses are also important factors found to influence the intensity and symptoms of menopause [8]. The influence of psychological factors, lifestyle, body image, interpersonal relationships, role, and sociocultural factors in predicting levels of depression and anxiety in the menopause cannot be ignored.

Role, social factors, and culture have a great impact on menopausal symptoms, as few studies have shown rates of depressive symptoms and hot flashes or sweats were significantly lower among Japanese women than females of American and Canadian population [9]. Such variations across cultures may reflect differences in

- Beliefs and expectations regarding menopause and aging
- Status and roles of women in a particular society
- Sensitivity to specific symptoms
- Biology, diet, and health behaviors

In developing countries where there is low literacy rate, it has been observed that females expect conception even after menopause, and this may be because the success of woman was considered to be related to production of more children, particularly males.

The factors that must be considered while dealing with menopausal women are the following:

1. The variation in reproductive period, i.e., from onset of menses (also termed "menarche)" to menopause.
2. Variation in life expectancy among different countries, e.g., life expectancy of woman is as low as 50.8 years in Sierra Leone and as high as 86.8 years in Japan.

As reproductive life could vary significantly among the various countries, we may consider average menarche age as 13 years and age of menopause as 51 years, and on calculating the reproductive period of women in developing country with average life expectancy of 50 years, they would have reproductive life that is 74% of their total life in comparison to women of developed country with life expectancy of 86 years who would have reproductive life constituting only 44% of their life from birth.

With the above fact, the period of menstruation is simulated to reproductive age or fertility is around half of their lives; therefore, loss of fertility or reproductive life may be a source of stress specially among tribes, where long reproductive age period is desired on the cultural belief that this will lead to a large family size that is considered as a symbol of success.

4. Secondary effects on mood/psychiatric morbidity and menopause

Popular psychiatric nosology such as the WHO International Classification of Diseases (ICD-10) and Diagnostic and Statistical Manual of Mental *Disorders* (DSM-5) is also ambiguous about this condition; therefore, insurance for its management need to be addressed. ICD-10 has a variety of coding for menopause and related menopausal disorders as shown in **Figure 1**.

Menopause is not a time of high risk for psychiatric illness but may be a time of psychological stress for women. Some women will experience psychological symptoms during the perimenopausal years [10]. Since mild emotional symptoms occur in many women during

N95	**Menopausal and other perimenopausal disorders** *Excl.:* excessive bleeding in the premenopausal period (N92.4) postmenopausal: • osteoporosis (M81.0) • osteoporosis ◦ with pathological fracture (M80.0) • urethritis (N34.2) premature menopause NOS (E28.3)
N95.0	**Postmenopausal bleeding** *Excl.:* that associated with artificial menopause (N95.3)
N95.1	**Menopausal and female climacteric states** Symptoms such as flushing, sleeplessness, headache, lack of concentration, associated with menopause *Excl.:* those associated with artificial menopause (N95.3)
N95.2	**Postmenopausal atrophic vaginitis** Senile (atrophic) vaginitis *Excl.:* that associated with artificial menopause (N95.3)
N95.3	**States associated with artificial menopause** Post-artificial-menopause syndrome
N95.8	**Other specified menopausal and perimenopausal disorders**
N95.9	**Menopausal and perimenopausal disorder, unspecified**

Figure 1. ICD-10 coding for menopause and related disorders.

the perimenopausal years, it is important to establish whether the symptoms are of sufficient severity and duration to constitute major depression, generalized anxiety disorder, or panic disorder. Psychological distress is usually seen more in females with disturbed sleep [11]. Sleep could be disturbed in midlife due to psychosocial stressors of life or as a result of symptoms of menopause like hot flushes (also termed as "flashes") and night sweats. Female reproductive hormones and rapid changes in their levels may influence neurotransmitters in the brain, particularly the serotonin and gamma amino butyric acid systems. Estrogen modulates serotonin to increase serotonin presynaptic reuptake, modulates norepinephrine levels, decreases monoamine oxidase levels, affects dopamine turnover, increases brain excitability, affects endorphin levels, and possibly interacts with gamma amino butyric acid [12]. Progesterone is found to increase monoamine oxidase levels. In high doses, progesterone has an anesthetic effect and may decrease brain excitability through an interaction with the gamma amino butyric acid system [12]. The drop in estrogen levels during perimenopause and menopause can lead to hot flashes that disturb sleep. This can lead to anxiety, fears, and mood swings [1].

The greater frequency of symptoms during the years prior to the end of the menses and the reduction of symptoms once menopause has occurred suggest that emotional symptoms are related to changing hormone levels rather than low hormone levels [12].

Research has shown that reproductive hormones produced during menopause contribute to mood alterations, such as depression [13]. Menopausal status, however, remains an independent predictor of depressive symptoms [14]. Some women experience anxiety and depression, but women who have a history of poor adaptation to stress are more predisposed to the menopausal syndrome [1].

The two most common psychiatric conditions are anxiety and depression. Therefore, all the general physicians and gynecologists must ask two screening questions for each of these conditions from women of perimenopausal age, as suggested by experts, given in **Figures 2** and **3** (*in Urdu—for developing countries where Urdu language is medium of communication).

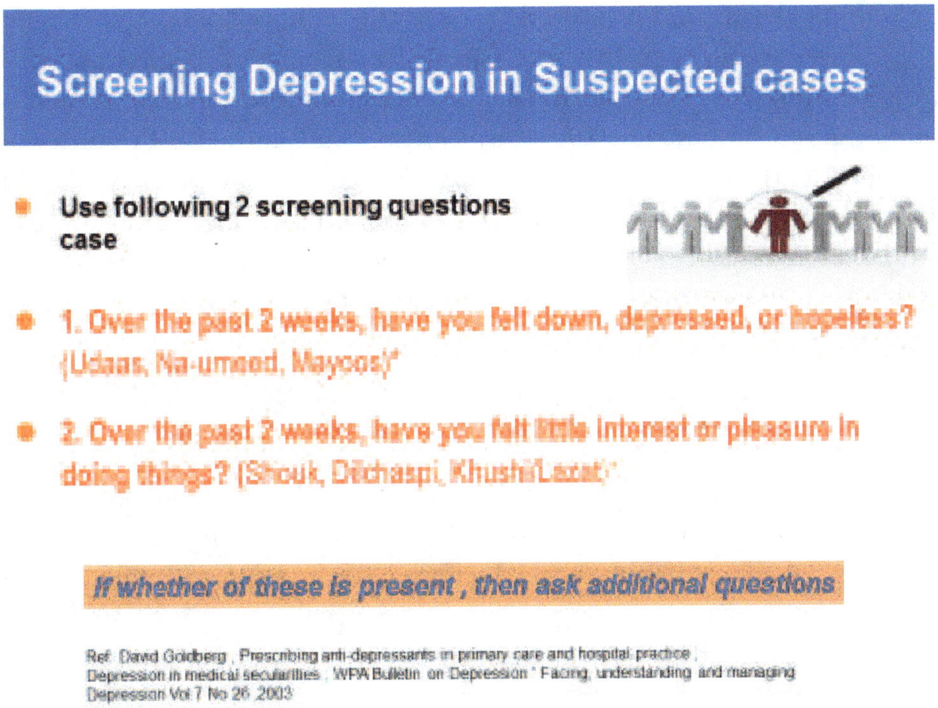

Figure 2. Screening questions for depression among perimenopausal cases (Urdu).

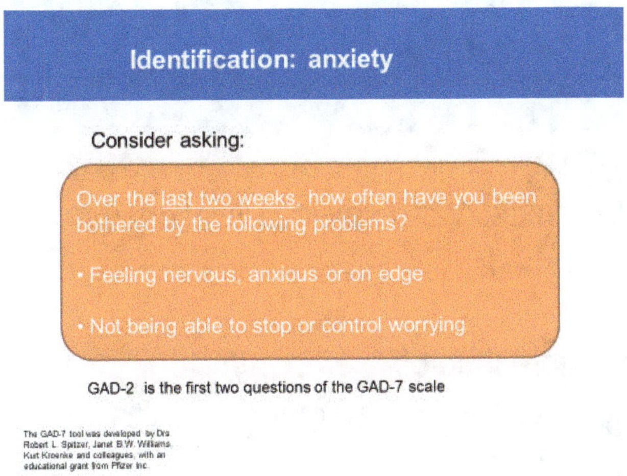

Figure 3. Screening questions for anxiety among perimenopausal cases.

4.1. Depression and the menopause

The changes that occur in hormone levels along with general health, shifts, and stresses of family life in a woman's menopausal years as a whole effect the onset of depression among them [15]. According to a study at Harvard on Moods and Cycles constituting premenopausal women aged 36–44 years with no history of major depression with a follow-up of these women for 9 years to detect new onsets of major depression. Clinically significant depressive symptoms likely to develop among perimenopausal women were twice as common than women who had not yet gone under menopausal transition [16].

Typical symptoms of depression include depressed mood, anhedonia, and fatigue. Reaching diagnosis of Depressive Disorder, two internationally recognized criteria are of ICD-10 and DSM-5. Symptoms should be there for at least 2 weeks and leading to poor social or occupational functioning and condition should not be due to any substance use. Presence of at least two typical expressions with two common symptoms constitutes the criteria of Major Depressive Disorder (F32) according to International Classification of Diseases version 10 (ICD-10), while presence of at least one typical and five or more common symptoms constitute criteria to diagnose Depressive Disorder in Diagnostic and Statistical Manual (DSM). List of Symptoms is shown in **Figure 4**.

4.2. Anxiety and the menopause

Women who are more anxious experience greater extent of menopausal symptoms. Many of the symptoms of anxiety and menopause coincide like sweating, palpitations (increased heart rate), restlessness, sleep disturbance, which may confuse some. But no correlations have been found in between hormonal changes during menopause with incidence of anxiety disorder. Other psychosocial factors may contribute in development of anxiety among females of midlife.

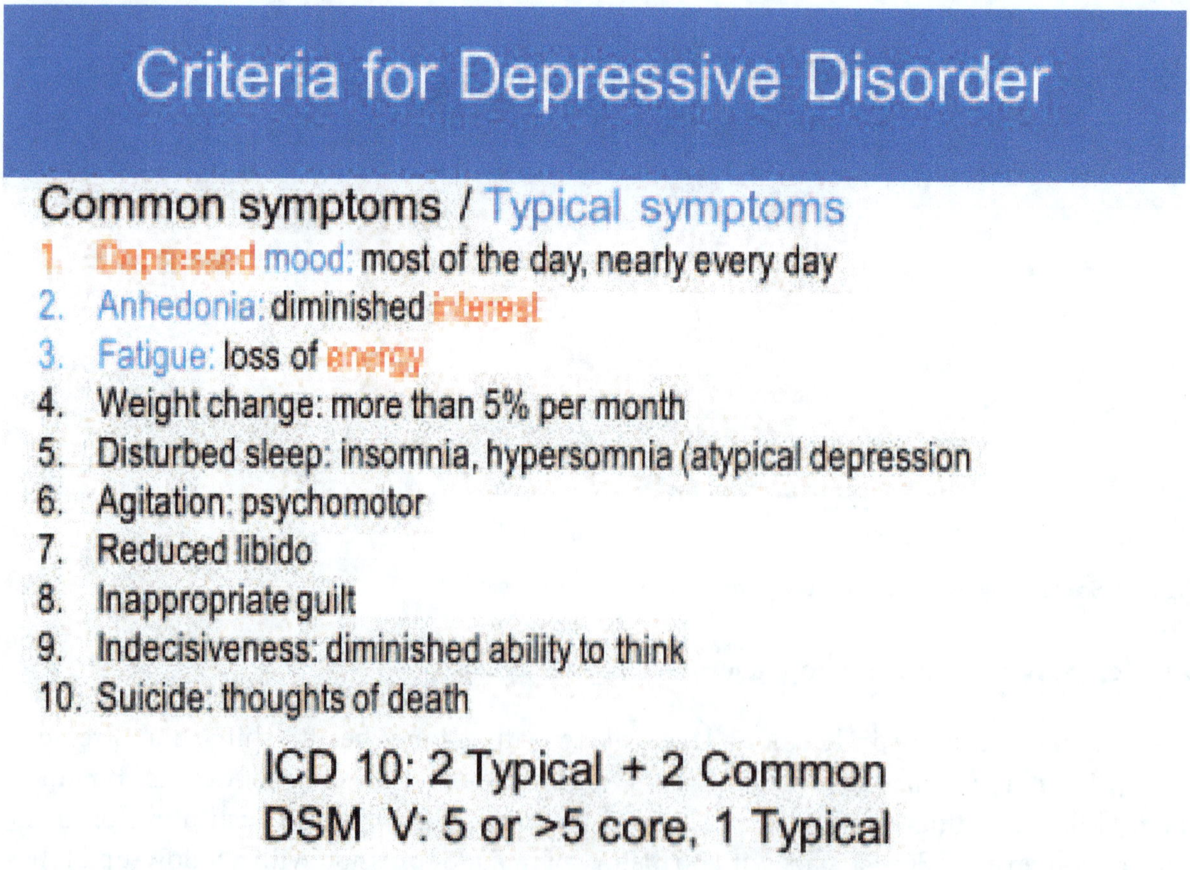

Figure 4. ICD-10 and DSM diagnostic criteria for depressive disorder.

Symptoms of anxiety include the following:

- apprehension
- irritability
- impatience
- fearfulness
- restlessness
- difficulty concentrating
- trouble falling asleep
- increased frequency of urination
- hyperventilation
- sweating, especially in the palms
- muscle tension

The symptoms of anxiety and depression may sometimes coincide and may be present simultaneously so if asked what are the defining symptoms of anxiety and depression? The clear difference and presentation of symptoms have been described in **Figure 5** with various differences and the similarities of anxiety and depressive disorder.

Anxiety & Anxiety Disorder	Depression
Feeling of fear, apprehension and excessive anxiety energy	Feeling of emptiness, deep sadness or misery, loss of hope
Physical feelings of agitation, muscle tension and symptoms of anxiety eg. heart symptoms, nausea, dissociation, diarrhoea, breathing difficulties etc	Slowing down of physical movement and lack of physical energy
General sense of being tense and rigid	Physical body slumped
May be a perfectionist and is concerned about the results of activities (can lead to poor performance)	Loss of interest and ambition (can lead to poor performance)
May fear death but not focused on suicide (Suicide thoughts come only when Depression is a secondary effect of anxiety disorder)	Suicidal thoughts present in deep depression

Figure 5. Features that differentiate anxiety and depression.

4.3. Other psychiatric conditions

Apart from anxiety and depressive disorder, the other psychiatric conditions that have been linked to menopause are premenstrual dysphoric syndrome and surprisingly a rare condition Trichotillomania discussed as under.

Premenstrual dysphoric syndrome: it is a condition of changing mood with changes in hormone levels every month before menstruations.

Anecdotally, many cases as they approach to menopause report that their symptoms of premenstrual dysphoric syndrome worsen at onset of perimenopause and alleviate with menopause [17].

Trichotillomania (hair-pulling disorder) symptoms may worsen at perimenopause [17].

5. Biopsychosocial aspects in management of symptoms of menopause

The art of assessing menopausal symptoms and menses may be threatening in some culture; therefore, reaching this condition needs proper working and skills which are less cumbersome because in general females are sensitive about aging process and loss of fertility.

5.1. Pharmacological interventions

5.1.1. Hormone replacement therapy

Estrogen and androgen alone or in combination of both is found to be more effective in improving symptoms in nonclinically depressed perimenopausal and menopausal women according to meta-analysis [18] of various studies on effects of hormone replacement therapies on mood. Progesterone had a much smaller effect, and when combined with estrogen, reduced the positive effects of the estrogen. The most robust effect was noted with androgen, either alone or in combination with estrogen.

Studies have shown that combined estrogen-progestin drugs (e.g., premarin) cause small increases in breast cancer, heart attack, stroke, and blood clots among menopausal women. Studies of the effects of estrogen alone in women who have had hysterectomies (because estrogen alone increases the risk for uterine cancer) are ongoing [1].

5.1.2. Antidepressants

Depression during perimenopause and menopause is treated in much the same way as depression that strikes at any other time.

Although symptoms of depression are relieved by a majority of antidepressants including SSRIs such as Fluoxetine, Paroxetine, SNRIs, e.g., venlafaxine, des-venlafaxine, and TCA as amitriptyline, but desvenlafaxine (the dual serotonin and norepinephrine reuptake inhibitor) is used popularly, off label, for symptoms of depression with menopause despite the fact that the US Food and Drug Administration (FDA) has denied an application for its use for the treatment of moderate-to-severe vasomotor symptoms such as hot flashes associated with menopause.

A meta-analysis shows that desvenlafaxine was associated with a statistically significant reduction in the number and severity of daily moderate-to-severe hot flashes. The number of nighttime awakenings because of hot flashes was also significantly decreased. However, the rate of desvenlafaxine treatment discontinuation because of adverse events was significantly higher than placebo-treated women and the risk ratios of adverse events such as asthenia, hypertension, anorexia, constipation, diarrhea, dry mouth, nausea, dizziness, insomnia, somnolence, and *mydriasis* (the dilation of the pupil) were very high [19].

5.2. Nonpharmacological interventions

5.2.1. Lifestyle modifications

A healthy lifestyle can help to reduce symptoms of menopause

1. Exercise

- Being physically active helps with hot flushes, stress, and mood
- Exercise has beneficial effects on hot flashes, well-being, Body Mass Index (BMI) and Coronary Heart Diseases risks [20]
- Activities that stimulate the brain can help rejuvenate memory such as doing crossword puzzles, longhand mathematics, and reading books.

2. Diet

- A nutritious diet helps with fatigue and moodiness.
- A healthy diet, low in fat, high in fiber, with plenty of fruits, vegetables, and whole-grain foods.
- Intake of foods with phytoestrogen.

    Phytoestrogens are estrogen-like substances found in some cereals, vegetables, legumes (including soy), and herbs. They might work in the body like a weak form of estrogen. The first widely attributed health benefit of phytoestrogen consumption was relief from vasomotor perimenopausal symptoms, including hot flushes and night sweats. Moderation is a likely key and the incorporation of real foods, as opposed to supplements or processed foods to which soy protein is added, is probably essential for maximizing health benefits [21]. Consumption of 30 mg/day of soy isoflavones reduces hot flashes by up to 50% [22].

- Ensure enough calcium and vitamin D intake on regular basis

- Avoid smoking and alcohol, as it is known to make hot flushes worse
- Foods that should be avoided in menopause
    - Caffeine
    - Spicy foods

5.2.2. Social support

- Social interactions with family and community, nurturing relationship, and healthy emotional support from friends are very effective means. A professional help from a counselor and mental health professional is quite effective and must be readily available. Misconception as described by individuals as potentially difficult, embarrassing, and stigmatized leading to fear and avoidance in some individuals at developing countries must be addressed.

Author details

Iqbal Afridi

Address all correspondence to: driqbalafridi@yahoo.com

1 Department of Psychiatry & Behavioural Sciences, JPMC (Jinnah Postgraduate Medical Centre), Karachi, Pakistan

2 JSMU (Jinnah Sindh Medical University), Karachi, Pakistan

3 Pakistan Psychiatric Society, Pakistan

4 TAC (Technical Advisory Committee), PMRC, Islamabad, Pakistan

5 JPMC, Pakistan

References

[1] Sadock BJ, Sadock VA, Ruiz P. Kaplan & Sadock's Synopsis of Psychiatry; Behavioral Sciences/Clinical Psychiatry, 11th ed. Philadelphia: Wolters Kluwer; 2015

[2] McKinlay JB, McKinlay SM, Brambilla D, et al. The relative contributions of endocrine changes and social circumstances to depression in mid-aged women. Journal of Health and Social Behavior. 1987;**28**:345-363

[3] Hallstrom T, Samuelson S. Mental health in the climacteric: The longitudinal study of women in Gothenburg. Acta Obstetricia et Gynecologica Scandinavica. 1985;**13**:130-135

[4] Kaufert PA. A health and social profile of the menopausal woman. Experimental Gerontology. 1994;**29**:343-350

[5] Nicol-Smith L. Causality, menopause, and depression: A critical review of the literature. BMJ. 1996;**313**:1229-1232

[6] Ayers B, Forshaw M, Hunter MS. The impact of attitudes towards the menopause on women's symptom experience: A systematic review. Maturitas. 2010 Jan;**65**(1):28-36

[7] RosemeierHP, Schultz-ZehdenB. Psychological aspects of menopause. In: FischlFH, ed. Menopause-Andropause: Hormone Replacement Therapy Through The Ages. Gablitz: Krause & Pachernegg GmbH. 2001

[8] Dennerstein L. Wellbeing, symptoms and the menopausal transition. Maturitas. 1996;**23**: 147-157.

[9] Avis N, Kaufert PA, Lock M, McKinlay SM, Vass K. The evolution of menopausal symptoms. Baillieres Clinical Endocrinology and Metabolism. 1993;**7**:17-32

[10] Diana C. Depression and emotional aspects of the menopause. BCMJ. 2001 Oct:**43**(8); 463-466

[11] Bromberger JT, Meyer PM, Kravitz HM, et al. Psychologic distress and natural menopause: A multiethnic community study. American Journal of Public Health. 2001 Sep; **91**(9):1435-1442

[12] Pearlstein TB. Hormones and depression: What are the facts about premenstrual syndrome, menopause, and hormone replacement therapy? American Journal of Obstetrics and Gynecology. 1995;**173**:646-653

[13] Gordon JL, Girdler SS, Meltzer-Brody SE, Stika CS, Thuston RC, Clark CT, et al. Ovarianhormone fluctuation, neurosteroids, and HPA axis dysregulation in perimenopausal depression: A novel heuristic model. American Journal of Psychiatry. 2015 Mar; **172**(3):227-236.

[14] Bromberger JT, Schott LL, Kravitz HM, Sowers M, Avis NE, Gold EB, et al. Longitudinal change in reproductive hormones and depressive symptoms across the menopausal transition: Results from the Study of Women's Health Across the Nation (SWAN). Archives of General Psychiatry. 2010 Jun;**67**(6):598-607

[15] Kaufert PA, Gilbert P, Tate R. The Manitoba project: A reexamination of the link between menopause and depression. Maturitas. 1992;**14**:143-155

[16] Cohen LS, Soares CN, Vitonis AF, Otto MW, Harlow BL. Risk for new onset of depression during the menopausal transition: The Harvard study of moods and cycles. Archives of General Psychiatry. 2006;**63**:385-390

[17] American Psychiatric Association. Diagnostic and statistical manual of mental disorders (5th ed.). Arlington, VA: American Psychiatric Publishing. 2013

[18] Zweifel JE, O'Brien WH. A meta-analysis of the effect of hormone replacement therapy upon depressed mood. Psychoneuroendocrinology. 1997;**22**:189-212

[19] Berhan Y, Berhan A. Is desvenlafaxine effective and safe in the treatment of menopausal vasomotor symptoms? A meta-analysis and meta-regression of randomized double-blind controlled studies. Ethiopian Journal of Health Sciences. 2014 Jul;**24**(3):209-218

[20] Dennerstein L, Lehert P, Guthrie JR, et al. Modeling women's health during the menopausal transition: A longitudinal analysis. Menopause: Journal of the North American Menopause Society. 2007;**14**(1):53-62

[21] Patisaul HB, Jefferson W. The pros and cons of phytoestrogens. Frontiers in Neuroendocrinology. 2010 Oct;**31**(4):400-419

[22] Kurzer MS. Soy consumption for reduction of menopausal symptoms. Inflammopharmacology. 2008 Oct;**16**(5):227-229

7

Premenstrual Syndrome

Preye Fiebai, Avwebo Ochuko Ukueku and
Rosemary Ogu

Abstract

Approximately 80–90% of women experience some symptoms in the premenstrual period at some point in their reproductive years. Teenagers often present with moderate to severe symptoms, while women in the fourth decade of life appear to have worse symptoms with the severity of the disease worsening with increasing age up until menopause. Obesity and smoking have also been identified as risk factors. Symptoms could be physical, psychological, emotional, environmental and/or behavioral and affect the ability to perform normal daily activities as well as adversely affect interpersonal relationships. Though several theories have been propounded, the exact cause of premenstrual syndrome is unknown. Management of this disorder requires a multi-disciplinary approach involving the general practitioner, the general gynecologist or a gynecologist with a special interest in PMS, a mental health professional (psychiatrist, clinical psychologist or counselor), physiotherapist and dietician.

Keywords: menstruation, psychosomatic menstrual syndrome, girls

1. Introduction

A syndrome is a group of symptoms and/or signs associated with a medical disease or disorder, often occurring concurrently. Premenstrual syndrome (PMS) can be defined as a group of physical and emotional symptoms and signs usually occurring within the last 14 days of the menstrual cycle, that is, from ovulation to the onset of menstruation, of sufficient severity to result in deterioration of interpersonal relationships and affect normal activities [1]. The symptoms span a range of medical specialties; from the gynecological to the psychiatric. PMS is included as a diagnostic category in the 10th edition of the International Statistical Classification of Diseases and Related Health Problems (ICD) with its' more "severe" form,

Premenstrual Dysphoric Disorder (PMDD), included in the 5th edition of the Diagnostic and Statistical Manual for Mental Disorders (DSM) [1, 2].

Premenstrual syndrome became a recognized medical disorder over the last century. It was initially thought to be an 'imagined' disease all in the heads of 'crazy' women [3]. Later it was presumed that the female reproductive organs had complete control over the woman and energies diverted from reproductive organs caused suboptimal functioning as such women involved in manual labor required more treatments than those who only exercised their brains [4]. Till date, symptoms of PMS are often viewed with skepticism or used in mockery of the female sex or the idealism of gender equality such that many females who suffer from this condition are unwilling to seek help or even admit to having difficulty managing the psychological symptoms associated with their menstrual cycles. This chapter methodology derives from a synthesis of the available literature under the MESH search term premenstrual and focus group discussion of women attending a tertiary health facility in Southern Nigeria.

Premenstrual syndrome was named by a British physician Katharina Dalton in 1953 [5]. PMS psychological symptoms had been described as early as the time of the ancient Greeks, but it wasn't until 1931 that this disorder was recognized by the medical community. This diagnosis was made popular by a paper presented at the New York Academy of Medicine by Robert T. Frank titled "Hormonal Causes of Premenstrual Tension" [6]. Robert Frank theorized that excess estrogen levels were the cause of symptoms experienced by affected women. In 1981, Dalton served as the chief defense medical expert in a murder trial in London. She successfully argued that the defendant was not responsible for murdering her lover because she suffered from severe PMS. This trial caught the attention of different viewers in the United States and brought publicity to PMS. PMS or the "disease of the 1980s" became a media event. More importantly, PMS acquired medical legitimacy, "after years of telling women their problems were 'all in the head,' the proportion of doctors who accepted PMS as a real disease reached critical mass" [7].

2. Epidemiology

Approximately 80–90% of women experience some symptoms in the premenstrual period at some point in their reproductive years. However, only 20% of these women meet the diagnostic criteria for PMS, of these; 10% are severely affected and 3–8% have PMDD [1].

Teenagers often present with moderate to severe symptoms, 14–88% of teenage girls are affected, with the older teenagers more likely to have symptoms than the younger teenagers. PMS and PMDD are associated with a higher risk of Anorexia nervosa, Bulimia nervosa and substance abuse. It is also more likely to occur in women who have suffered some form of abuse (emotional, physical or sexual) in early life or are presently in abusive relationships [8, 9].

Women in the fourth decade of life appear to have worse symptoms, and the severity of the disease tends to worsen with increasing age up until menopause. There is also an increased risk of hypertensive disorders in affected patients later in life.

There is evidence of genetic predisposition to the disease as women whose mothers suffered from PMS are at higher risk of having the disease, and also monozygotic twins have a 93% rate of PMS compared with 44% in dizygotic twins [9]. Symptoms also vary with race; while black women often experience a higher prevalence of food cravings than white women, the white women often experience a higher prevalence of mood swings and weight gain [10].

Obesity and smoking have also been identified as risk factors for this condition. Women with body mass index more than 30, are three times more likely to have PMS than non-obese women and women who smoke are more than two times likely to present with severe symptoms [10, 11].

3. Clinical presentation

PMS symptoms tend to occur in a cyclic pattern from ovulation to onset of menstruation. Symptoms could be physical, psychological/emotional, environmental and/or behavioral [12, 13]. Over 200 symptoms have been described. Symptoms and signs tend to affect a patient's ability to perform normal daily activities and adversely affect their interpersonal relationships. Occasionally it results in violence in the home and broken marriages as well as loss of a woman's economic means in society. In a focus group discussion carried out among women attending a tertiary health facility in Southern Nigeria, premenstrual syndrome was viewed as a curse because of its myriad of symptoms.

Physical symptoms include the following:

Headaches

Acne

Breast tenderness

Abdominal bloating

Diarrhea or constipation

Joint and muscle pains

Fatigue

Weight gain (from fluid retention)

Swelling of the extremities

Dysmenorrhea

Change in bowel habits

Frequent urination

Hot flashes or cold sweats

General aches or pains (malaise)

Nausea and vomiting

Allergic reactions

Upper respiratory tract infections

Palpitations

Unusual food cravings

Low tolerance for noise, odors or light

Psychological/emotional symptoms include the following:

- Anxiety symptoms such as:

  Difficulty sleeping

  Tense feelings

  Irritability

  Clumsiness

  Mood swings

  Panic attacks

  Paranoia

- Depressive symptoms such as:

  Depressed mood and affect

  Angry feelings for no reason

  Feelings that are easily upset

  Poor concentration

  Memory loss

  Feelings of low self-worth

  Violent feelings and/or action

  Crying spells

  Social withdrawal

  Changes in appetite

  Changes in libido

Mental health disorders are worsened or exacerbated by PMS. These include depression and anxiety disorders. Other medical conditions whose symptoms may be worsened by PMS include; myalgic encephalomyelitis or chronic fatigue syndrome, irritable bowel syndrome and bladder pain syndrome. Health problems such as asthma, allergies and migraines may also worsen with this disease. Patients with PMS may also experience heavy menstrual bleeding and early menopause.

4. The pathophysiology of premenstrual syndrome

The exact cause of premenstrual syndrome is unknown and is the subject of much ongoing research. Several theories have been proposed; from sex hormones interactions to neurotransmitters interactions in the central nervous system. Older theories that have proven to be incorrect include estrogen excess or withdrawal, progesterone deficiency (these were the initial sex hormones theories), pyridoxine (vitamin B6) deficiency, alteration of glucose metabolism, fluid-electrolyte imbalances. Current research provides some evidence supporting the following etiologies:

4.1. Sex hormone

Symptoms of premenstrual syndrome begin following ovulation and resolve with menses, and because they only affect women in reproductive age, it is assumed that the female gonadal hormones (estrogen and progestogen) have a role in the pathophysiology of the disease. This is underscored by the facts that symptoms are less common in women with surgical oophorectomy or drug-induced ovarian hypofunction, such as with gonadotropin-releasing hormone (GnRH) agonists. Moreover, women with anovulatory cycles rarely report PMS symptoms. For these reasons, research of PMS pathophysiology has focused on the sex steroids, estrogen and progesterone. However, no propounded theory so far has borne fruit.

4.2. Serotonin deficiency

It is postulated that patients with PMS suffer from lower serotonin level in the luteal phase, which may or may not be as a result of the various interactions of the sex hormones. It has been proven that patients most affected by symptoms of PMS have differences in serotonin levels when compare to others. This evidence supports a role for serotonergic system dysregulation in the pathophysiology of PMS. Moreover, trials of serotonergic treatments have shown symptom reduction in women with PMS, symptoms respond to selective serotonin reuptake inhibitors (SSRIs), which increase the levels of circulating serotonin.

4.3. Central nervous system interaction

Estrogen and progesterone are neuroactive steroids and influence the central nervous system (CNS) neurotransmitters: serotonin, noradrenaline, and γ-aminobutyric acid (GABA). The predominant action of estrogen is neuronal excitability, whereas progestogens are inhibitory. Women with PMS have exaggerated responses to normal levels of these hormones, and rapid changes in the levels of these hormones as is experienced in the luteal phase of the menstrual cycle promote the development of symptoms.

4.4. Nutrient deficiencies

Magnesium and calcium deficiencies have been hypothesized to be causes of PMS symptoms. Studies evaluating supplemental therapies have shown improvement in symptoms.

4.5. Psychosocial theory

The psychosocial theory postulates that PMS is a conscious demonstration of a woman's conflict with her femininity and motherhood. It suggests that the premenstrual physical changes remind the woman that she is not fulfilling her traditional role of incubating, nurturing, and rearing a child. This theory is highly subjective and scientifically unprovable.

4.6. Sociocultural theory

The sociocultural theory postulates that PMS is a manifestation of a conflict between the societal expectation of the dual role of a woman as both a productive part of the workforce and a mother. It suggests that PMS is a cultural expression of women's dissatisfaction with their traditional roles in society.

4.7. Cognitive and social learning theory

This theory suggests that the onset of menstrual bleeding is an adverse psychological outcome for some women and PMS is a display of maladaptive coping strategies in other to reduce immediate stress.

5. Diagnosis of premenstrual syndrome

Diagnosis of PMS can often be difficult because may medical and psychological conditions mimic the symptoms, and there are no laboratory tests to confirm the diagnosis. Women with PMS usually present with complaints from multiple systems, and these symptoms display temporal association with the menstrual cycle luteal phase. Symptoms must begin at least 5 days (American College of Obstetricians and Gynecologists [ACOG] criteria) [8] or 1 week (DSM-IV-TR) before menses, and remit within 4 days (ACOG criteria) or a few days (DSM-IV-TR) after menses onset [2]. Evaluation of women complaining of PMS symptoms includes prospective daily symptom rating for at least two or three menstrual cycles.

A menstrual diary could be used to record the onset and duration of symptoms of PMS for 2–3 cycles; this not only helps the physician make the diagnosis but also increases the patient's awareness of her body and moods. She is thus, better at coping with her symptoms. The Endicott Daily Record of Problem Severity chart or the Daily Symptom Rating are tools that can be used to assess the frequency and severity of symptoms described in the luteal phase as against those experienced in the follicular phase of the menstrual cycle [14].

A within-cycle increase from follicular to luteal phase score of at least 20–50% is necessary to confirm a diagnosis of PMS. This is calculated by subtracting the follicular score from the luteal score, divided by the luteal score and multiplied by 100 (luteal score – follicular score/luteal score × 100).

A physical examination may identify some of the physical symptoms and signs of the disease. In certain instances, PMS symptoms may be an exacerbation of underlying primary psychiatric condition(s). Thus, a psychiatric evaluation may help rule out other common psychiatric conditions such as depression, dysthymia, and anxiety disorders. Additionally, other medical conditions that have a multisystem presentation should be considered. These include hypothyroidism, systemic lupus erythematosus, endometriosis, anemia, fibromyalgia, chronic fatigue syndrome, fibrocystic breast disease, irritable bowel syndrome, and migraine. Laboratory studies should include complete blood count, thyroid function tests and gynecological hormone profile.

6. Premenstrual dystrophic disorder (PMDD)

This is a condition in which a woman has severe depressive symptoms, tension and irritability before menstruation. It is a more severe form of PMS that affects a small percentage of women within reproductive age resulting in remarkable disability and loss of function. Symptoms are of sufficient severity as to interfere with work or school, social activities, interpersonal relationships and quality of life. Patients complain of similar symptoms as seen in PMS but of increased severity. Most symptoms of PMDD are similar to symptoms of a major depressive disorder (MDD). These symptoms, however, are cyclic and disappear with the onset of menses. The most common symptoms of PDMM are irritability, limited concentration, sleep disturbance, mood lability and marked depressed mood. Similarities to MDD are highlighted below.

- Markedly depressed mood. A symptom of MDD is depressed mood most of the day, nearly every day.
- Decreased interest in usual activities. One criterion for MDD is markedly diminished interest or pleasure in all activities.
- Lethargy, fatigability or lack of energy. Similarly, patients with MDD have fatigue or loss of energy.
- Hypersomnia or insomnia—also symptoms of MDD.

7. Diagnosis

The Diagnostic and Statistical Manual of Mental Disorders, 5th edition established 7 criteria for diagnosis of PMDD [2] (A–G).

7.1. Criterion A

In Criterion A in most menstrual cycles during the past year, 5 out of 11 symptoms listed must be present (including one of the first four) in the last 1–2 weeks before the onset of menses and disappear in the week post-menses. These symptoms are as follows:

1. Marked lability (mood swings)
2. Marked irritability or anger
3. Marked depressed mood
4. Marked anxiety or tension
5. Decreased interest in usual activities
6. Difficulty in concentration
7. Lethargy and marked lack of energy
8. Marked change in appetite (overeating or special food cravings)
9. Hypersomnia or insomnia
10. Feeling overwhelmed or out of control
11. Physical symptoms (e.g. breast tenderness, bloating, weight gain or swelling of extremities etc.)

7.2. Criterion B

One of the following symptoms must be present:

1. Marked affective lability
2. Marked irritability or anger or increased interpersonal conflicts
3. Marked depressed mood, feelings of hopelessness or self-deprecating thoughts
4. Marked anxiety tension and/or feelings of being keyed up or on edge.

7.3. Criterion C

One or more of the following symptoms must be present additionally, to reach a total of five symptoms when combined with Criterion B.

1. Decreased interest in usual activities (e.g. work, school, hobbies, friends)
2. Subjective difficulty in concentrating
3. Lethargy, easy fatigability, or marked lack of energy
4. Marked change in appetite (overeating or specific food cravings)
5. Hypersomnia or insomnia

6. Feeling overwhelmed or out of control
7. Physical symptoms (e.g. breast tenderness, bloating, weight gain or swelling of extremities)

Note: the symptoms in criteria A–C must be met for most of the menstrual cycles in the preceding year.

7.4. Criterion D

The symptoms are associated with clinically significant distress or interference with work, school, usual social activities or relationship with others (e.g. avoidance of social activities, decreased productivity and efficiency at work, school, or home).

7.5. Criterion E

The disturbance is not merely an exacerbation of the symptoms of another disorder, such as a major depressive disorder, panic disorder, persistent depressive disorder (dysthymia) or a personality disorder (although it may occur concurrently with any of these disorders).

7.6. Criterion F

Prospective daily ratings during at least two symptomatic cycles should confirm Criterion A. (Note: the diagnosis may be made provisionally prior to this confirmation).

7.7. Criterion G

The symptoms are not attributable to the physiological effects of a substance, (e.g. substance abuse, a medication, or other treatment) or another medical disorder (e.g. hyperthyroidism).

8. Management

8.1. Patient education/counseling

PMS may cause significant distress for patients especially the adolescents and as such providing patients with adequate information on the disease including alternative therapies is imperative. Management of this disorder requires a multi-disciplinary approach involving the general practitioner, the general gynecologist or a gynecologist with particular interest in PMS, a mental health professional (psychiatrist, clinical psychologist or counselor), physiotherapist and dietician.

8.2. Life style and dietary changes

Treatment of PMS is majorly according to the severity of symptoms [8, 12, 13, 15]. Regular exercise and dietary restrictions often reduce symptoms. Obese patients should be encouraged to join a weight management program. Dietary modification is often a part of the overall treatment regime. Patients are encouraged to consume smaller meal portions high in carbohydrates. Patients should be counseled to avoid salt, caffeine, alcohol and simple or refined sugars. Exercise and physical activities cause a release of endorphins which improve general health, nervous tension and anxiety.

8.3. Behavioral anger and stress management therapies

This may help patients cope and or regain control during times of heightened emotions. A variety of methods may be employed. These include; emotional support from family and friends, individual and couples' therapy, self-help support groups, anger management courses, stress management classes, as well as cognitive-behavioral therapy. Our clients described emotional support from family and friends as very helpful. Relaxation techniques such as yoga, biofeedback and self-hypnosis are also be helpful.

8.4. Supplements

These include but are not limited to calcium and magnesium supplements, vitamin E and B6, and polyunsaturated fatty acids (omega-3 and omega-6). Some alternative medicines/herbal supplements have been used to ease PMS symptoms with varying reports of success. These include; Black cohosh, Chaste berry (or vitex agnus-castus), Evening Primrose oil, St John's Wort and Dandelion. Research has shown that for these remedies to be effective, they need to be taken for at least two consecutive cycles. However, some of these remedies may be toxic and cause liver damage at high doses.

8.5. Medications

Various medications have been used to address the moderate to severe symptoms of PMS including:

Diuretics: These are often given to eliminate excess fluid. For example, spironolactone is widely used to treat swelling of the hands, feet and face.

Hormonal therapies: Some women benefit from combined oral contraceptives. The newer formulations (drospirenone-containing COCPs) control the fluctuations of the sex hormones reducing symptoms of PMS. The Mirena Intrauterine System releases low doses of progesterone and suppresses ovulation reducing the symptoms of PMS; however, it may initially induce PMS-like symptoms. Depo-Provera has a similar mechanism of action. Percutaneous estradiol combined with cyclical progestogens has been found to be useful in managing both physical and psychological symptoms of PMS.

Gonadotrophin-releasing hormone (GnRH) analogues and agonists: These are ovarian hormone suppressors, by suppressing the release of the sex hormones from the ovaries, they reduce the symptoms of PMS. GnRH analogues are highly effective in treating symptoms of severe PMS. An example of a GnRH analogue is danazol, and a GnRH agonist is goserelin. However, use of these therapies for greater than 6 months is associated with increased risk of osteoporosis and irreversible virilizing effects; therefore, in women receiving GnRH analogues for more than 6 months, add-back hormone therapy should be given. COCPs should be given or tibolone is recommended.

Analgesics and anti-prostaglandins: These are commonly used to treat menstrual cramps, headaches, breast tenderness and pelvic discomfort. Non-steroidal anti-inflammatory drugs like ibuprofen, naproxen and mefenamic acid have been very useful. However, long-term use may predispose patient to gastric ulcers.

Antidepressants: These increase levels of neurotransmitters and excitatory chemical in the brain (e.g. serotonin, GABA, opioids). They help treat mood disturbances associated with PMS. Examples include; fluoxetine and paroxetine.

Selective serotonin reuptake inhibitors (SSRIs) and selective noradrenaline reuptake inhibitors (SNRIs): These are mood stabilizers with antidepressant effects. There increase the levels of serotonin and noradrenaline in the brain, both of which tend to decrease in the luteal phase in women with PMS.

8.6. Bilateral oophorectomy

In extreme cases, especially when the patient's quality of life is affected as seen in PMDD, and knowing the disease worsen with age, patients may be counseled for a bilateral oophorectomy and hysterectomy. This is especially recommended for patients who have completed their reproductive careers or patients who have severe symptoms unresponsive to all other therapies. It, however, tilts the women into early menopause with its problems as such hormone replacement therapies (HRT) should be considered. Bilateral oophorectomy without removal of the uterus will necessitate the use of a progestogen as part of HRT which carries the risk of PMS-like symptoms.

9. Conclusion

Premenstrual syndrome is a disease very prominent among women of reproductive age. It is not to be dismissed, taken for granted or treated with skepticism. There are therapies to end the sufferings of affected women. It is essential that we treat these women in other to promote their health, the health of the family and to sustain the economic productivity of women in our communities.

Author details

Preye Fiebai[1,2], Avwebo Ochuko Ukueku[2] and Rosemary Ogu[1,2*]

*Address all correspondence to: rosemary.ogu@uniport.edu.ng

1 University of Port Harcourt, Port Harcourt, Nigeria

2 University of Port Harcourt Teaching Hospital, Port Harcourt, Nigeria

References

[1] O'Brien S, Rapkin A, Dennerstein L, Nevatte T. Diagnosis and management of premenstrual disorders. BMJ. 2011;**342**:d2994

[2] American Psychiatric Association. Diagnostic and Statistical Manual of Mental Disorders (DSM-V). 5th ed. Washington, DC: APA; 2013

[3] Lane D. The curse of PMS. In: Evening Echo. Thomas Crosbie Holdings; July 2011. p. 11

[4] Martins E. Premenstrual syndrome, work, discipline and anger. In: Holmstrom N, editor. The Socialist Feminist Project: A Contemporary Reader in Theory and Politics. New York (USA): NYU Press; 2002. pp. 63-72

[5] Greene R, Dalton K. The premenstrual syndrome. BMJ. 1953;**1**:1007-1014

[6] Frank RT. The hormonal causes of premenstrual tension. Arch Neurol Psychiatry. Nov 1 1931;**26**(5):1053-1057

[7] Figert AE. Is PMS real? PMS as a scientific and cultural artifact. In: Women and the Ownership of PMS: The Structuring of a Psychiatric Disorder. 2nd ed. New Brunswick, USA: Transaction Publishers; 2007. pp. 6-7

[8] American College of Obstetricians and Gynecologists, ACOG. Premenstrual Syndrome (PMS). Washington, DC: ACOG; 2015. Available from: https://www.acog.org/Patients/FAQs/Premenstrual-Syndrome-PMS [cited 7/25/18]

[9] Dickerson LM, Mazyck PJ, Hunter MH. Premenstrual syndrome. American Family Physician. Apr 2003;**67**(8):1743-1752

[10] Bradshaw KD. Chapter 13. Psychosocial issues and female sexuality. In: Schorge JO, Schaffer JI, Halvorson LM, Hoffman BL, Bradshaw KD, Cunningham FG, editors. Williams Gynecology. 3rd ed. China: McGraw-Hill Companies Inc; 2008. pp. 625-629

[11] Khajehei M. Aetiology, diagnosis and management of premenstrual syndrome. Journal of Pain Relief. 2015;**4**:193

[12] Steiner M, Pearlstein T, Cohen LS. Expert Guidelines for the treatment of severe PMS, PMDD and comorbidities: The role of SSRIs. Journal of Women's Health (Larchmt). 2006;**15**(1):57-69

[13] Green LJ, O'Brien PMS, Panay N, Craig M, on behalf of the Royal College of Obstetricians and Gynaecologists. Management of premenstrual syndrome. Green-top guideline No. 48 February 2017. BJOG. 2017;**124**:e73-e105

[14] Endicott J, Nee J, Harrison W. Daily record of severity of problems (DRSP): Reliability and validity. Arch Womens Ment Health. Jan 2006;**9**(1):41-49

[15] Rapkin AJ, Lewis EI. Treatment of premenstrual dystrophic disorder. Women's Health. 2013;**9**(6):537-556

8

Normal Menstrual Cycle

Barriga-Pooley Patricio and Brantes-Glavic Sergio

Abstract

Normal menstrual cycle represents a coordinated serial event, repeated month by month, at regular intervals, in which the hypothalamus participates along with the secretion of GnRH, the pituitary gland secreting follicle stimulating hormone and luteinizing hormone (LH), and the ovary which responds to those hormones, recruiting a dominant follicle and secreting estradiol and inhibin A. Estradiol stimulates endometrial proliferation and production of cervix mucus. A peak of estradiol triggers discharge of LH, responsible for ovulation and posterior secretion of progesterone by the corpus luteum, which in turn, involutionates 14 days later if it does not receive the stimulation of hCG (pregnancy). Normal menstrual cycles last 28 ± 7 days, being accepted a fluctuation of ±2 days in the same woman, as a normal pattern, what is described as a regular cycle. Normality of these events would allow to achieve a successful embrionary implantation in the case of looking for pregnancy. For this it is required that an adequate ovule to be fertilized is reached by a capacitated spermatozoon, during the ovulatory stage. Spermatozoon can survive as long as 5 days at feminine genital tractum, but the ovum is possible to be fecundated only during 12–24 hours. Fecundation occurs at the distal third of the fallopian tube and the fecundated zygote arrives in the state of a morula, to be implanted at the endometrium 4 days later. Once the state of blastocyst is reached, it is detached from its shaggy area (hatching) and it is implanted in a receptive endometrium when the window of implantation is open (days 7–9) postovulation. The first marker of pregnancy is the detection in maternal blood of β-hCG. No more than the 25% of fertile couples exposed to pregnancy can achieve gestation at the month of exposure.

Keywords: menstrual cycle, fertility, concepcional cycle

1. Definition of normality

Menstrual cycle lasts 28 ± 7 days. Just a third of patients have cycles every 28 days and 82% fluctuations among 22 and 32 days [1].

A cycle is known as regular when the frequency has a variation of no more than 2 days. The lasting of each cycle is calculated since the first day of menstruation until the previous day of next menstruation. The cycle frequency is regulated by the hypothalamus-pituitary-gonadal axis; hormones such as follicle stimulating hormone (FSH) and luteinizing hormone (LH) must reach their effectors at the ovarian level where a dominant follicle must be recruited and developed, secrete estradiol, in enough amounts to obtain endometrial receptivity but also participating directly in a feedback-regulated control of the cycle.

Cycles show more irregularity in the extremes of the reproductive lifespan, during the first 2 years from the menarche and during the perimenopausal transition. The ovarian cycle has two stages separated by ovulation, the first, from the beginning of the cycle to ovulation, is called the follicular or proliferative phase. The second, between ovulation and the next menstruation, is called the luteal phase or secretory phase.

The follicular phase is characterized by the maturation of the follicle containing an ovule and a retinue of follicular cells, which are responsible for transforming androstenedione into estradiol, which in turn is released and, among many other actions, stimulates endometrial renewal.

The luteal phase, named because the follicular cavity that left the ovule after hatching, is transformed into a corpus luteum and continues to produce estrogen, but it also releases important amounts of progesterone. The luteal phase is preceded by a significant increase in LH, and ovulation marks its onset; then, it lasts ±14 fairly constant days when comparing different women. During this phase, the average total body temperature of women is constantly 0.5°C higher than in the follicular phase.

If there is no embryo implantation, the endometrium is detached giving rise to menstrual flow, which has normal volume parameters, up to 80 mL, in duration, 3–8 days, content, absence of clots and symptoms, and absence of pain.

It is considered that the conserved cyclicity expresses that the hypothalamic-pituitary-gonadal axis is healthy. The ovaries do not alternate to ovulate.

2. Important concepts

Ovarian reserve: *it corresponds to the number of follicles that a woman has and it is defined during fetal life and then the number of follicles goes slowing down gradually.*

When is born, each woman counts with a fixed number of ova, which are getting lost with the past of years (atresia) Delaying maternity is nonrecommendable, since at higher age the risk of not having ovum of a good quality at the moment when a pregnancy is planned.

In a woman fertility, among 38–40 years is lower than at 25–30 years. Atresia of oocytes is a continuous process that never stops not even with the use of anovulatory or pregnancy.

Oocyte atresia: *it is the mechanism of follicular apoptosis that seems to contribute to the selection of optimal ovules.* During the early fetal stage, about 7,000,000 oocytes are formed in the ovary.

Before birth, the ovular reserve has been reduced to one-third by mechanisms of apoptosis (programmed death).

At birth, only 1–2 million oocytes remain in the ovary and during puberty, there are usually 300,000 available for eventual ovulation. In fact, they will only ovulate between 400 and 500 throughout the lifespan. Then, through the female reproductive life, between the periods of puberty and menopause, about 250,000 follicles will be destined to die, reaching less than 1000 during perimenopause (**Figure 1**).

Sex steroids—estrogens and progesterone: Estrogens are steroid hormones produced by the granulosa follicle, the corpus luteum, and the placenta (if there is pregnancy). Its synthesis comes from cholesterol molecules. Progesterone is synthetized by corpus luteum and placenta, if there is pregnancy.

Of the estrogens, the most potent is estradiol. The actions they develop are:

- *Female genital apparatus*: they stimulate the growth and development of the female sexual organs and the proliferation of the endometrium during the sexual cycle.
- *Breast*: they favor the growth of the mammary ducts and are, in part, responsible for the development of the mammary gland during puberty.
- *Bone*: they regulate the osteoclastic activity and stimulate the osteoblastic activity, in such a way that they are essential to maintain adequate bone mineralization.

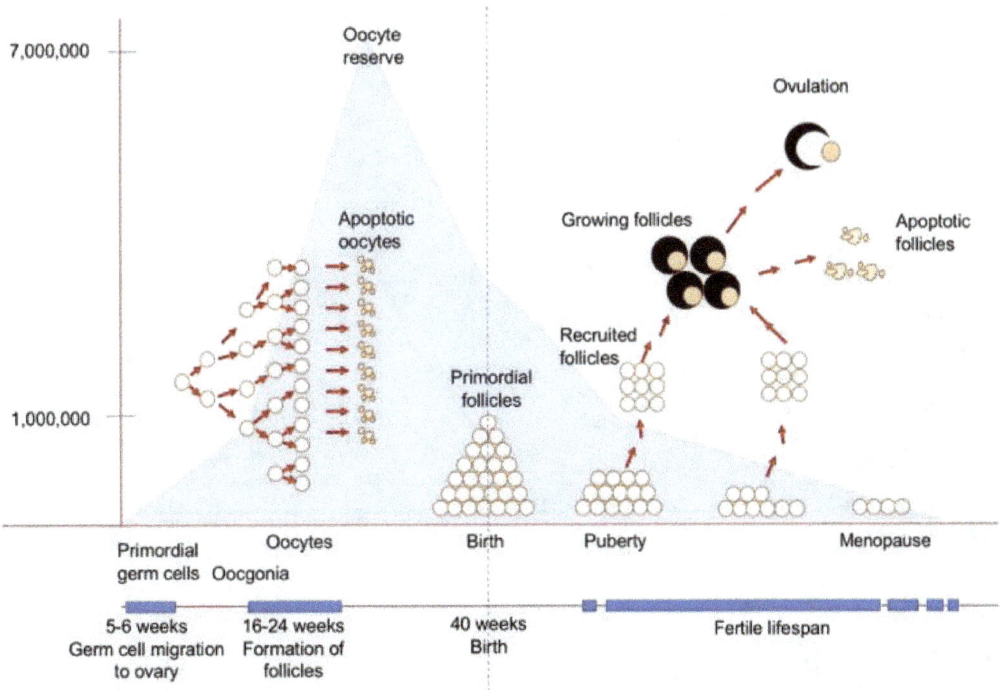

Figure 1. The number of oocytes in any woman comes defined at the moment of birth and slow down inevitably during her life during her life from 1 to 2 million at the moment of birth at 300,000 to go decreasing through her life 25,000 at 37–38 years and near 500 during the postmenopause.

- *Cardiometabolic*: estrogen relaxes the smooth muscle of arterioles, increases HDL cholesterol, and lowers LDL cholesterol, which has been associated with the lower incidence of cardiovascular disease that women have in relation to men, especially before menopause.

Progesterone is also a steroid hormone. It is responsible for the progestational changes of the endometrium. On the breasts, progesterone stimulates the development of the lobes, being its action complementary to that of the estrogens. Progesterone is thermogenic and contributes to the increase in basal temperature experienced by some women after ovulation.

3. Follicular phase

Follicular phase begins the very first day of menstruation. The development of ovarian follicles, named folliculogenesis, begins at the last days of menstrual cycle before the release of mature follicle during ovulation (**Figure 2**).

When a pregnancy did not occur, the release of inhibin A and sex steroids are reduced by the end of the functional period of the corpus luteum. Both falls contribute to reduce the release of FSH by feedback at the central level, which is dependent on pulsatility of hypothalamic GnRH. This is how FSH increases during the last days of the menstrual cycle (**Figures 3** and **4**) [2].

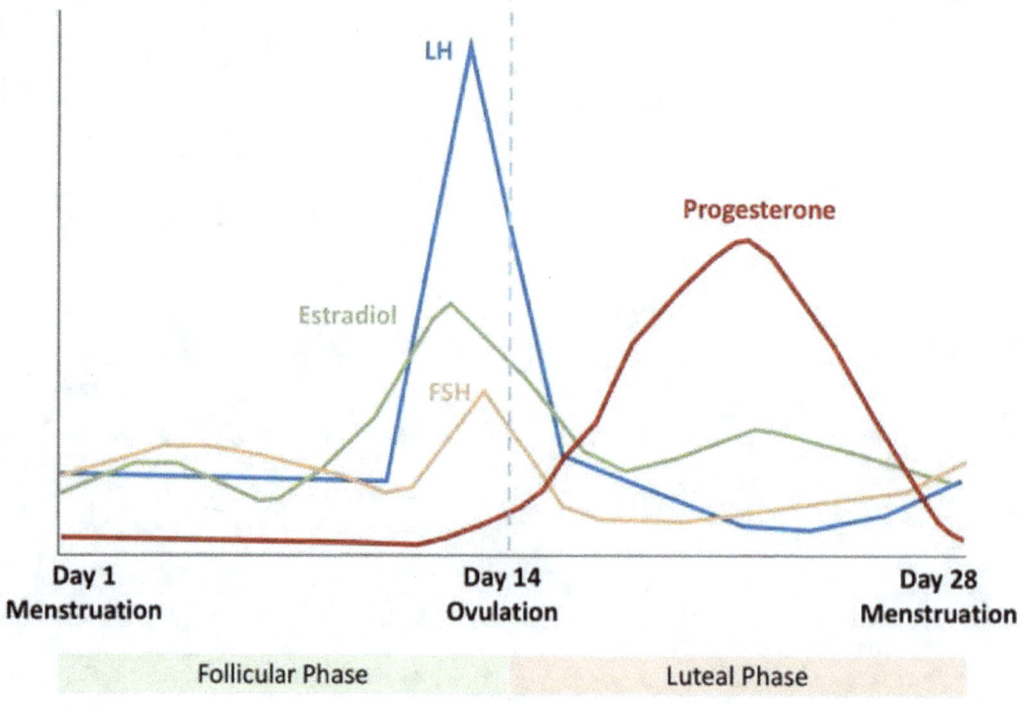

Figure 2. The menstrual cycle has two phases, follicular phase and luteal phase. The follicular phase begins with menstruation. The follicle stimulating hormone (FSH) increases released by the anterior pituitary gland and stimulates follicular growth and estradiol production. The 17 beta-estradiol produced by the follicles exerts negative feedback on the FSH. Estradiol continues to increase due to the growth of the dominant follicle. The LH increases sharply to trigger ovulation. Immediately after ovulation, the luteal phase begins. The corpus luteum produces progesterone and 17 beta-estradiol concentrations of progesterone and estradiol decrease, menstruation begins a new cycle, unless a pregnancy has been established.

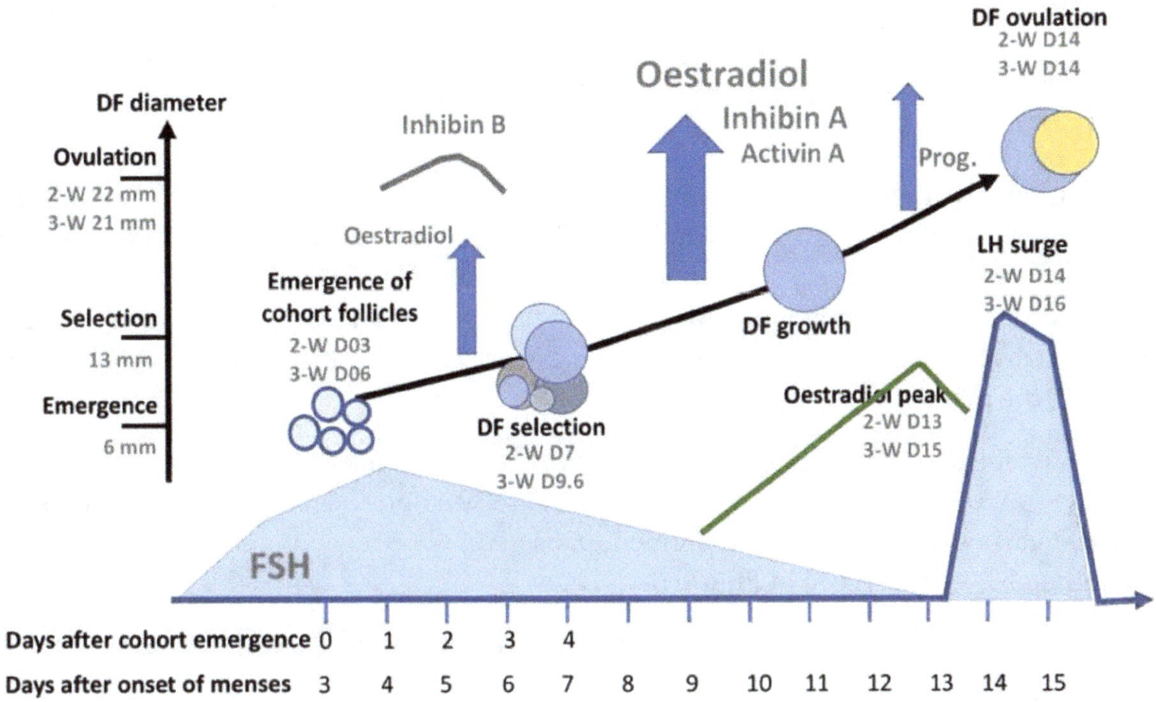

Figure 3. Dynamic scheme of follicular activity and the changes in gonadotropins, steroids, and inhibins during follicular phase of menstrual cycle.

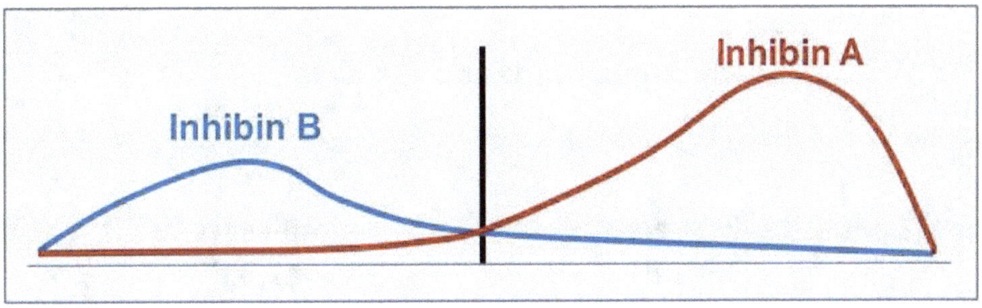

Figure 4. The level of inhibin changes through menstrual cycle. Inhibin B dominates follicular phase during the cycle while inhibin A dominates luteal phase.

The progressive elevation of FSH allows many follicles to be recruited simultaneously. Nevertheless, only some persist, in such a way that an approximate 99% of the cycles, only a dominant follicle will be destined to ovulate, during the next menstrual cycle.

The remaining 1% has codominance, that is two dominant follicles, which eventually can generate a double ovulation at the risk of a multiple pregnancy.

In women from 19 to 42 years, follicular phase has an average duration of 14.6 days, however, to be precise on each woman in what step of the cycle she is very difficult because of the following reasons:

- Duration of menstrual cycle is very changing, even among young women of similar ages, with variations described from 25 to 34 days.

- Changes that normally occur during the fertile lifespan, between the menarche to menopause. Some women may have long and irregular cycles, many times associated to abundant uterine bleeding, at the first 2 years after to menarche and 4–6 years that precede menopause.
- Besides there is a wide range of presentation for both phases of the cycle, the follicular phase may last from 10 to 23 days and luteal phases could last between 7 and 19 days. Only 10% of women with a cycle of 28 days shows follicular and luteal phase of 14 days. The variability depends more on follicular phase, which vary ±3–7 days with time, depending on the estrogen take off (ETO), at the beginning of the middle follicular phase on each cycle, which is the main explanation for the duration of cycles.
- Finally, despite of normal length in their cycles, 7% of women of 25–39 years may show anovulation, even though is more frequent to observe shorter cycles or longer ones, especially in early postmenarche and premenopause (60% between 10 and 14 years and 34% older than 50 years) as seen in **Figure 5**.
- Other environmental, ethnic, or even socioeconomic factors may affect the duration of the cycle and bleeding.

At the development of dominant follicle (DF), three steps have been described namely, **recruiting, selection,** and **dominance** (**Figure 6**). Recruiting stage is developed during the days 1–4 of menstrual cycle.

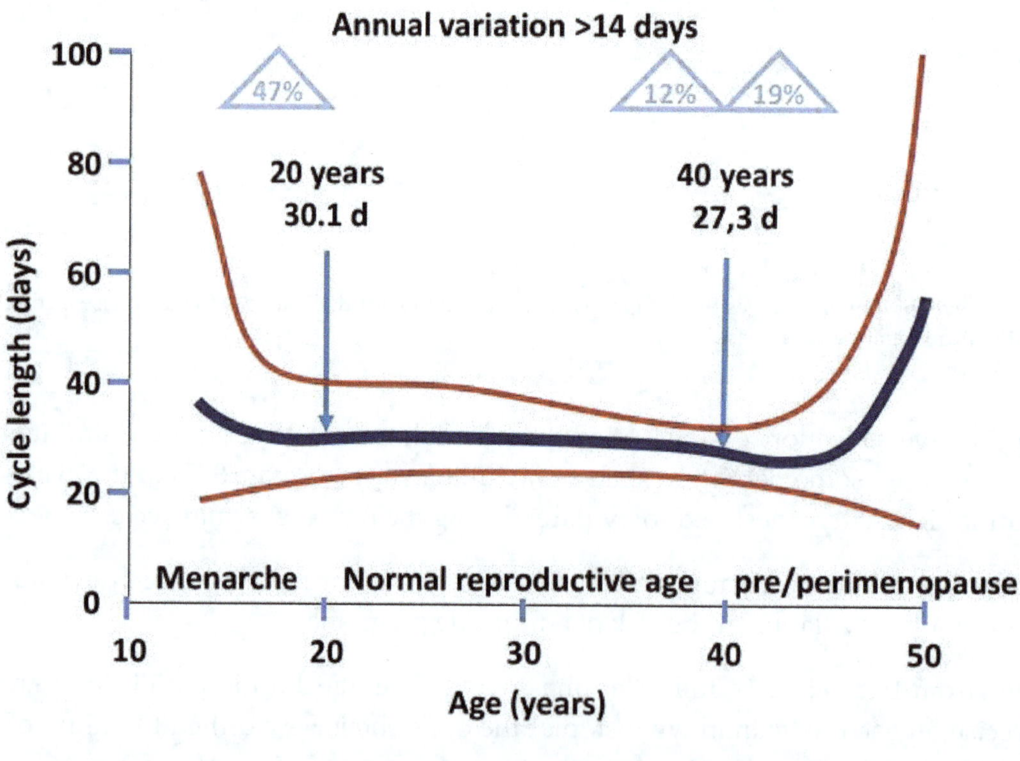

Figure 5. Menstrual cycle lasting variation according to age. Graphic shows the average lasting of the cycle and the range (percentiles 95 and 5) yrs. = years, d = days. Triangles indicate the group of age in the percentage of women with more than14 days of variation of a cycle during a year. From Mihm et al. [3].

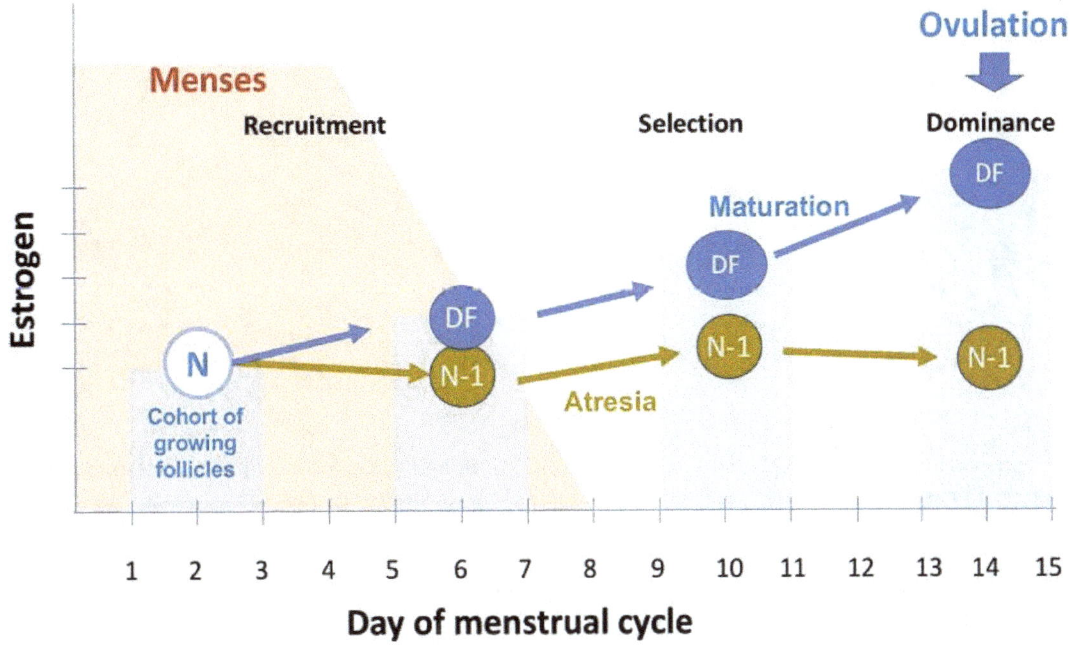

Figure 6. Time lapse of recruiting, selection, and ovulation of dominant follicle (DF) with the beginning of atresia in the other follicles of the group. Adapted from Hodgen [4].

During the follicular phase, FSH is responsible for recruitment among those follicles that remain available. Between days 5 and 7 of the cycle, follicular selection normally occurs, to allow only one follicle, the dominant follicle (FD) to ovulate and the rest to experience atresia. Anti-müllerian hormone (AMH), which is secreted in the granular layer, also participates in the selection of FD. On day 8 of the cycle, the FD promotes its own growth, suppressing the maturation of the other ovarian follicles.

During the follicular phase, estradiol plasma levels are higher along with the growth of the number of granulosa cells and the growth of the DF. FSH receptors are found exclusively in the cell membrane of granulosa cells. The increase in FSH during the late luteal phase induces its own FSH receptors and eventually increases the secretion of estradiol by the granulosa cells by transforming androstenedione, which diffuses from the theca cells (**Figure 7**).

It is important to point out that the increase in the numbers of receptors of FSH is due to an increase in the population of granulosa cells and not to an increase of the concentration of receptors of FSH on them. Each granulosa cell has 1500 receptors of FSH at secondary stage of follicular development, and the number of receptors of FSH stays constant during the rest of DF growing.

The increase in estradiol secretion also upregulates their own receptors, increasing the total of estradiol receptors (ER) in the granulosa cells. On the other hand, in the presence of estradiol, FSH stimulates the formation of LH receptors in the same cells, which allows the secretion of small amounts of progesterone and 17-hydroxyprogesterone (17 OHP) that would exert positive feedback on the pituitary gland. Already sensitized by the increase of estrogen, thus allowing the release of luteinizing hormone (LH) and achieve its peak. FSH also stimulates many steroidogenic enzymes such as aromatase and 3β-hydroxysteroid dehydrogenase (3β-HSD).

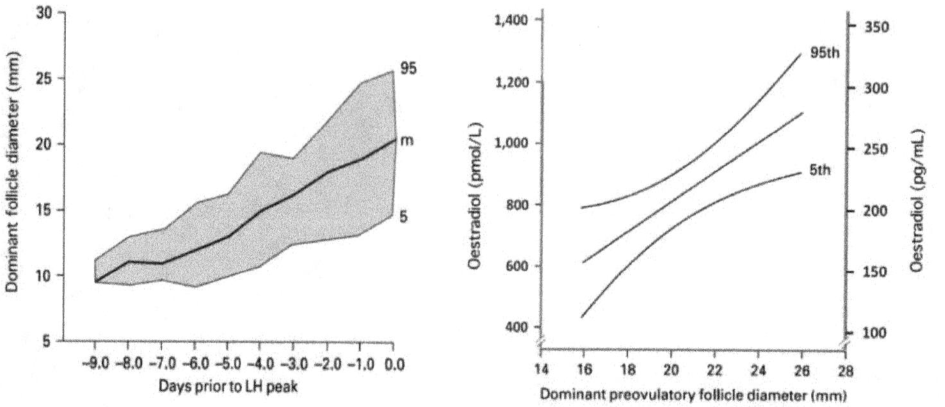

Figure 7. Diameter of dominant follicle (DF) days prior to LH peak and plasma concentration of estradiol per follicle diameter (curved lines are 95th and 5th percentiles). Adapted from Macklon and Fauser [5].

There are other signaling pathways that impact the differentiation of theca cells, not only LH but also insulin-like 3 (INSL3) that appear to modulate LH-mediated androgen biosynthesis and increased follicle cell apoptosis and luteal regression, bone morphogenetic proteins (BMPs) produced by granulosa cells, and/or oocytes who antagonized the effects of LH and INSL3, the circadian clock genes, androgens, and estrogens and (2) theca-associated vascular, immune and fibroblast cells, as well as the cytokines and matrix factors that play key roles in follicle growth [6].

At **Table 1**, production rates are presented for sexual steroids during follicular phase, luteal phase at the moment of ovulation.

Differently from granulose cells, LH receptors are localized at theca cells during all of the stages of menstrual cycle. LH receptors stimulates granuloma's cells. LH stimulates the production of androstenedione and at a lesser level the production of testosterone at the theca cells.

Androstenedione is then transported to the cells of granulosa where it is aromatized, and finally, it becomes estradiol 17-β-hydroxysteroid dehydrogenase type I. This is known as the

Sex steroids*	Early follicular	Preovulatory	Mid-luteal
Progesterone (mg)	1	4	25
17α-Hydroxyprogesterone (mg)	0.5	4	4
17α-Hydroxyprogesterone (mg)	7	7	7
Androstenedione (mg)	2.6	4.7	3.4
Testosterone (μg)	144	171	126
Estrone (μg)	50	350	250
Estradiol (μg)	36	380	250

*Values are expressed in milligrams or micrograms per 24 hours.
From Baird and Fraser [7].

Table 1. Production rate of sex steroids in women at different stages of the menstrual cycle.

hypothesis of two cells and two gonadotropins of the regulation of synthesis on the ovary (**Figure 8**).

The normal follicular phase has been divided in two stages: (a) early and (b) middle and (c) late, to allow a better comprehension of the endocrine events that will be finally responsible of ovulation.

Early follicular phase (days 1–4): it begins with the first day of menstruation. Follicular recruitment occurs due to the elevation of FSH, as a consequence of the decrease in estradiol, progesterone, and inhibin A released by the corpus luteum of the previous cycle, allowing the number of LH receptors to increase in the cells of the teak and the granulosa. The plasma levels of estradiol tend to remain low at this stage (**Figure 1**).

Medium follicular phase (days 5–7): as the recruitment and growth of follicles induced by FSH progress, estradiol increases slowly in a progressive manner thanks to the increased activity of CYP19, an FSH-dependent aromatase that is present in granulosa cells. The follicle that achieves the highest number of FSH receptors may aromatize more estradiol and become the dominant follicle. The other follicles, with fewer receptors for FSH, suffer atresia. For estrogen synthesis, it is necessary for the thecal cells to produce androgens, under the stimulus of LH, and for these to diffuse to the granulosa cells. Simultaneously, two glycoproteins, activin and inhibin, are produced in the theca and granulose, with local actions. Inhibin B exerts a negative hypophyseal feedback effect, where it potentiates the effect of estradiol and inhibits the synthesis and release of FSH [9, 10]. This would be a mechanism to achieve dominance giving an advantage to the follicle that has greater

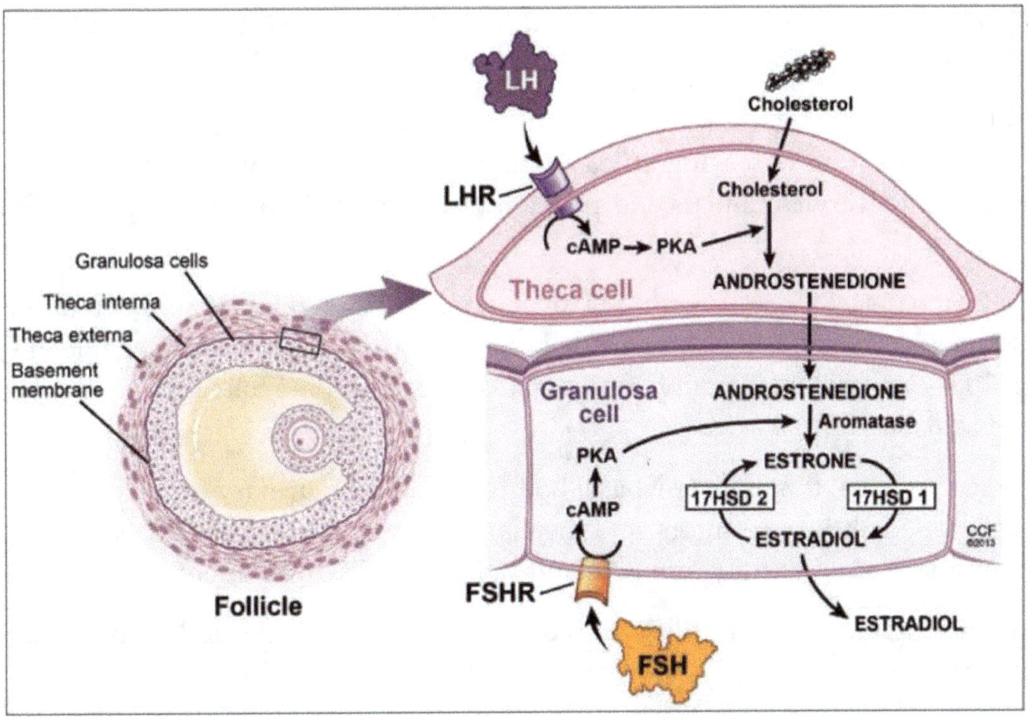

Figure 8. Two cells and two gonadotropins, on the regulation and the synthesis of estrogens at the ovary. From: Doshi and Agarwal [8].

development. The estrogen take-off (ETO) marks the successful establishment of the dominance of a follicle.

The FD develops its internal theca and increases receptivity to LH, which stimulates the production of androgens by degrading molecules of cholesterol to progesterone and from this to dehydroepiandrosterone, androstenedione, and testosterone.

At the end of this phase, the granulosa-theca complex of the FD has almost complete functionality to enter the late follicular phase.

Late follicular phase (days 8–12): this period is characterized by the elevation of estrogens that come from the DF, reaching its maximum values between 40 and 50 hours, before an elevation of FSH that precedes the ovulatory peak of LH. This preovulatory follicle reaches an average diameter of 15–20 mm.

3.1. Follicular phase and fertility

The moment of greatest likelihood of successful fertilization is intercourse on the day before ovulation. However, the potentially fertile period, which depends on sperm survival, can extend from 5 days before ovulation. Those pregnancies that have been obtained after day 14, are associated with later ovulation, a normal variability in the duration of the follicular phase depending on the time of the ETO.

It is believed that cycles of 30–31 days and 5 days of bleeding would have a higher probability of pregnancy [11], perhaps due to better quality of the DF, good function of the corpus luteum and optimal endometrial receptivity. The moment of the fertile window is quite variable. It has been reported that a significant number of women with regular menstrual cycles can be in their fertile window before day 10 or after day 17, of their menstrual cycle [12]. However, it seems that the possibility of pregnancy is low when the cycles are short, less than 25 days [13].

In clinical practice, to determine the fertility potential of a given cycle, indirect methods are used, which require observing at least one of the three primary signs of fertility (basal body temperature, cervical mucus and position of the cervix), known as methods based on symptoms.

There are kits to detect the increase in LH, which occurs 24–36 hours before ovulation named ovulation predictor kits (OPK). Those urine-based ovulation test kits are available in versions standard OPKs, digital OPKs or advanced digital OPKs, but some saliva-based ovulation tests are available also.

Computerized devices that interpret basal body temperature, urinary test results, or changes in saliva are called fertility monitors, and there are different types: urine-based fertility monitors, perspiration-based fertility monitors and saliva-based fertility monitors.

In the monitoring of assisted fertility procedures, effective follicular follow-up with ultrasonography is preferred.

In infertility treatments, ovulation inducers are used that increase endogenous levels of FSH or eleven therapeutically by administering FSH parenterally, which manages to rescue multiple follicles from atresia. So, this patient has a higher risk of multiple ovulation. It is interesting to note that when rescuing follicles from atresia, the follicular endowment remains the same, so that follicles will not be depleted in an accelerated manner.

3.2. Follicle types

At born, woman count with primordial follicles (PF), each surrounded by one layer of cells of granulosa and are detained at the pro phase of the first meiotic division.

During adolescence, the woman has antral follicles that depend on FSH. On average, this follicle takes 14 days to mature to preovulatory FD. They are derived from a recruitment process that is independent of FSH and is mainly regulated by the anti-müllerian hormone (AMH), which is produced by the granulosa cells of the follicles in early development and inhibits the transition from the primordial to the primary follicular stage [14]. AMH levels can be measured in serum and used to measure the follicular reserve (**Figures 9 and 10**).

Primordial follicles (PF) are independent of FSH. Their average life is 60–65 days, then they are transformed in to preantral follicles (PAF), also independent of FSH, and are surrounded by many layers of granulosa's cells and also by theca cells. In this process, many primordial follicles suffer atresia (**Figure 11**).

Due to the presence of 5α-reductase, the early preantral and antral follicles produce more androstenedione and testosterone compared to the estrogen rate. 5α-reductase is the enzyme responsible for converting testosterone to dihydrotestosterone (DHT). Once testosterone has been reduced by 5α, DHT cannot be aromatized.

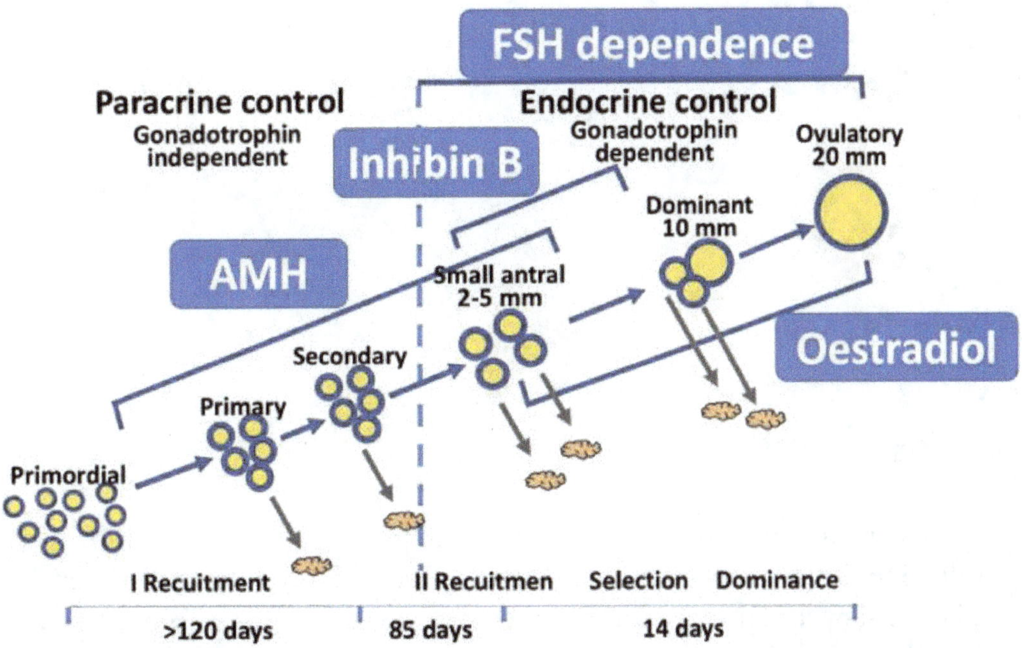

Figure 9. AMH is involved in the paracrine control of recruitment in the first stage, when the process is still independent of gonadotropins. AMH can not only reflect the number of early antral follicles in the process of development, but also those in earlier stages. Adapted from Ref. [1].

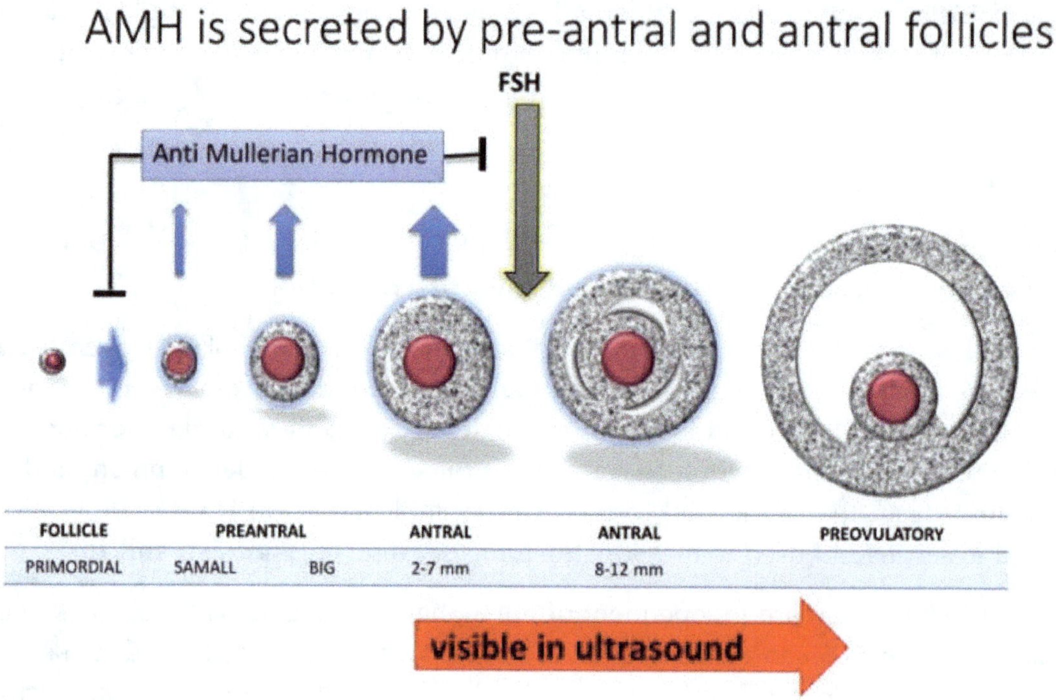

Figure 10. Clinical witnesses of the follicular development in stage pre- and postdependence of FSH: AMH and ultrasound, respectively. Adapted from Ref. [15].

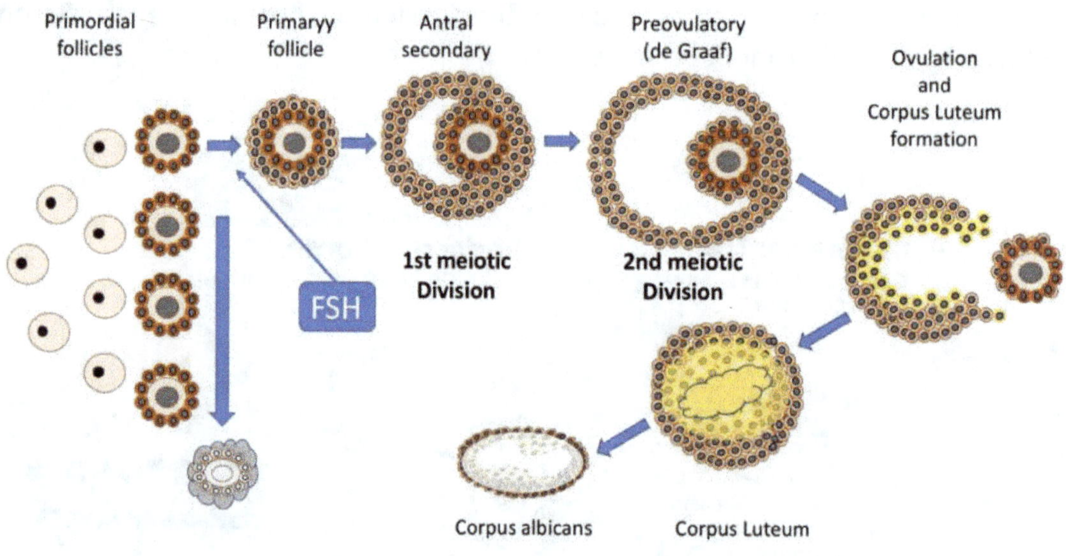

Figure 11. Follicular dynamics and illustration of folliculogenesis process.

With the increase in age in women, the involution of granulosa cells decreases the levels of inhibin production. Because of this, when a woman approaches menopause her FSH levels become higher, a sign that her ovarian reserve has decreased. On the other hand, the perimenopausal follicles are of the worst quality, half have chromosomal alterations.

As mentioned, the development of the preantral follicle is independent of FSH, so any follicle that grows beyond this point will require an interaction.

Secretion of gonadotropin is regulated by the releasing hormone of gonadotropin (GnRH), steroidal hormones, and diverse peptides released by dominant follicle.

Among substances that can be found al follicular liquid there are steroids, pituitary hormones, plasmatic proteins, proteoglycans, and ovarian factors nonsteroidal, which regulate the micro environment of the ovary and the steroidogenesis of the granulosa.

Factors of growing such as the insulin growth factors 1 and 2 (IGF1, IGF2) and the epidermal growth factor (EGF) would have an important role at the development and maturity of oocytes. Concentration of ovarian steroids is higher at follicular liquid compared to plasmatic concentrations.

There are two population of antral follicles: **big follicles**, which measure more than 6 mm diameter, and **little follicles**, less than 8 mm. In big follicles, concentrations of FSH are higher. Estrogen and progesterone are higher as well, while prolactin concentration is lower. Inside little follicles, prolactin and androgen levels are higher in comparison to big antral follicles.

In addition, as mentioned, FSH increases during the early follicular phase and then begins to decrease until the ovulation phase, except in the short preovulatory peak. In contrast, LH is low in the early follicular phase and begins to increase in the middle follicular phase due to positive feedback of increasing levels of estrogen.

To achieve positive feedback of LH release, plasma estradiol should be greater than 200 pg/ml, for at least 48 hours. The gonadotropins are secreted in a pulsatile manner in the anterior pituitary, with a frequency and widening of pulses that change according to the phase of the menstrual cycle (**Figure 12**).

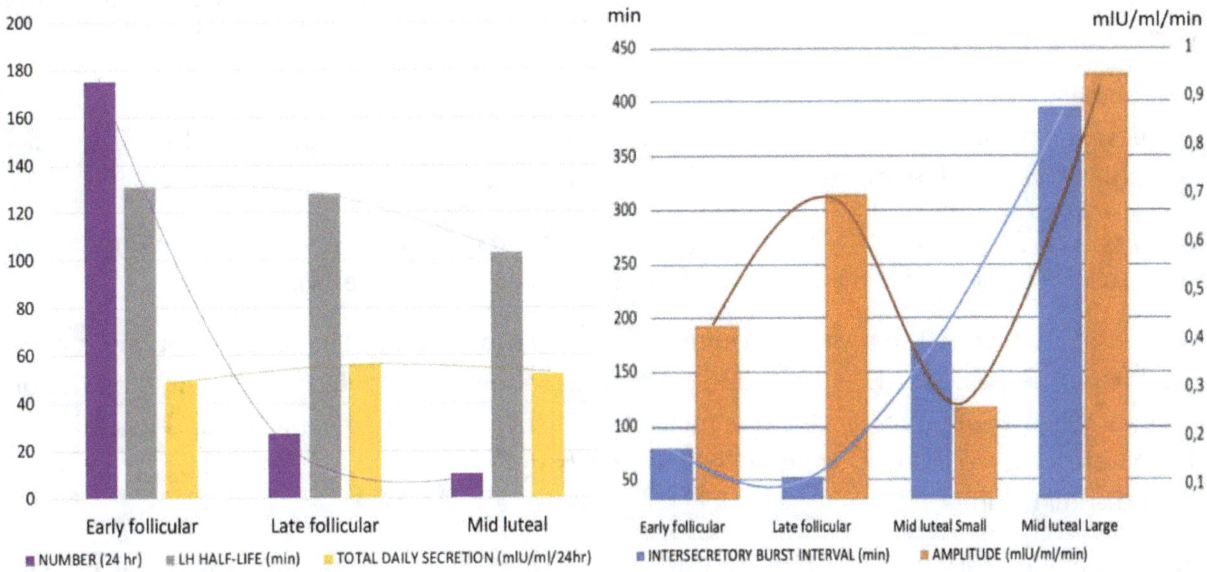

Figure 12. Pulses of LH throughout a normal cycle. Number of pulses per 24 h decreases, but total daily secretion and LH half-life are stable. The intersecretory burst interval becomes longer as the cycle progresses, being very long in the luteal phase, whereas the pulse amplitude of LH shows a dichotomous behavior, with small and high waves. Adapted from data of Sollenberger et al. [16].

During early follicular phase, secretion of LH occurs to a frequency of pulse from 60 to 90 minutes with a widening of pulse constant but variations on number of pulses intersecretory burst interval and pulse amplitude [16]. During late follicular phase, previous to ovulation, frequency of pulse increases and widening may be beginning to increase. Most of women have widening of pulse of LH beginning to increase after ovulation.

Once menstruation is produced, levels of FSH begin to decrease due to negative retro alimentation on inhibin B produced by developing follicle.

4. Ovulation

Hatching occurs 10–12 hours after peak of LH (**Figure 8**). Augmentation of LH is generated by significative raising of estradiol, with levels between 200 and 450 pg/mL, produced at the preovulatory follicle.

The critical concentration of estradiol needed to initiate positive feedback requires that the dominant follicle reach a size >15 mm in diameter. The increase in LH occurs 34–36 hours before ovulation and is a very reliable predictor of ovulation (**Figure 9**). This increase in LH is responsible for the luteinization of granulosa cells that stimulates the synthesis of progesterone and also estradiol. In addition, the LH increase resumes the second meiotic division and the chromosomal reduction in the oocyte with the release of the first polar corpuscle.

Estradiol levels decrease abruptly immediately before peak of LH. This can be due to regulation to down of LH from its own receptor or due to direct inhibition of estradiol synthesis because of progesterone.

Progesterone also participates in the stimulation of the increase in FSH in the middle of the cycle (**Figure 13**).

This increase in FSH would produce the release of oocytes from their follicular junctions, to stimulate the plasminogen activator and increase the LH receptors in the granulosa. The exact mechanism responsible for the post ovulatory fall is unknown.

Decrease in LH would occur as the consequence of the loss of positive retro alimentation of estrogens the inhibitory retro alimentation of progesterone (**Figure 14**).

It takes 36 hours from the peak of estrogen until ovulation occurs. The time to ovulation measured from the peak of LH is 12 hours; considering the time of detection in urine, ovulation will take place at 24 hours since LH is measured in the urine. The hormone hCG is similar to LH and can be used as an exogenous hormone to trigger ovulation, which will occur 36 hours after administration.

During the ovulatory period, progesterone and prostaglandins are secreted inside the follicle, as well as proteolytic enzymes. This results in digestion and rupture of the follicular wall allowing hatching, commonly called ovulation [18].

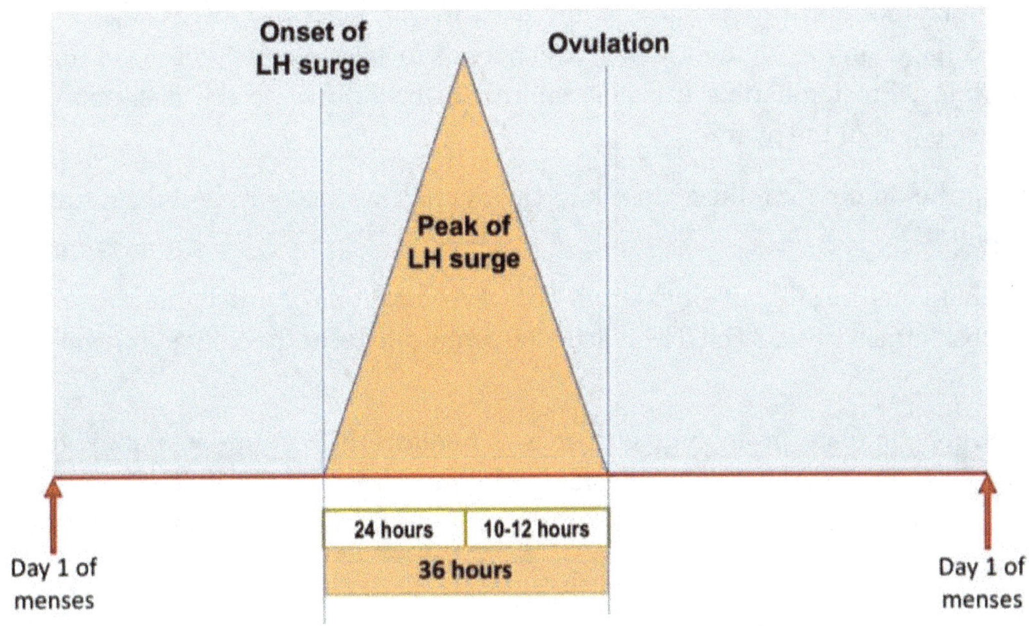

Figure 13. Increase of LH precedes ovulation in 36 hours. Peak, on the other side, precedes ovulation in 10–12 hours.

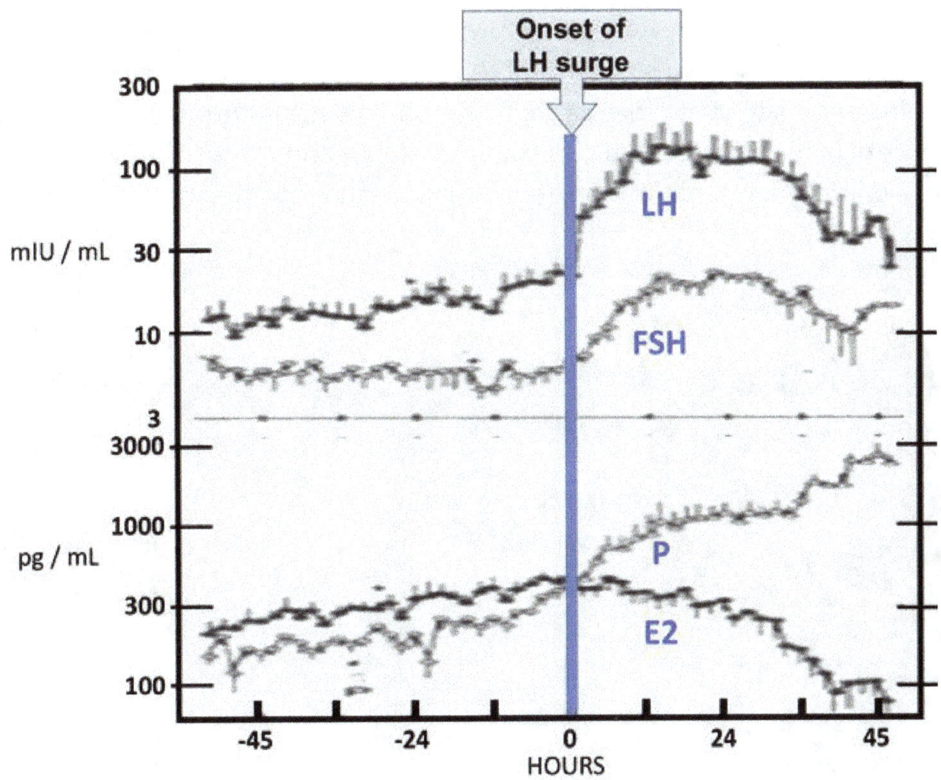

Figure 14. Changes in ovarian gonadotropins and steroids in the middle of the cycle, just before ovulation. The beginning of the increase of LH is at time. 0 time. Abs: E2, estrogen; P, progesterone. Adapted from Hoff et al. [17].

Proteolytic enzymes and prostaglandins are activated in response to LH and progesterone and digest collagen in the follicular wall, which leads to an explosive release of the cumulus-oocyte complex. Prostaglandins can also stimulate the release of oocytes, stimulating the smooth muscle within the ovary.

The point of the dominant follicle closest to the ovarian surface where the rupture occurs is called a "stigma."

All the mechanisms are still not elucidated. The concentrations of prostaglandins E and F and hydroxyeicosatetraenoic acid (HETE) reach a maximum level at the follicular level just before ovulation.

Prostaglandins stimulate proteolytic enzymes, whereas HETE stimulates angiogenesis and hyperemia. The use of high doses of prostaglandin inhibitors could hinder the follicular rupture, causing what is known as luteinized unruptured follicle syndrome, and can be observed in fertile and infertile women.

Consequently, it should be recommended to women in search of pregnancy and especially that with fertility problems, avoid the intake of inhibitors of prostaglandin synthesis, and inhibitors of cyclooxygenase (COX), in fact, are being investigated as an alternative to morning after pill in emergency contraception [19, 20].

For ovulation to occur, a series of complex molecular mechanisms that commence after the gonadotrophin surge must be given. These include intracellular signaling, gene regulation, and remodeling of tissue structure in each of the distinct ovarian compartments, which can be summarized in (a) ovulatory mediators that exert effects through the cumulus cell complex, (b) convergence of ovulatory signals through the cumulus complex co-ordinates the mechanistic processes that control oocyte maturation and ovulation, and (c) other multiple inputs, including

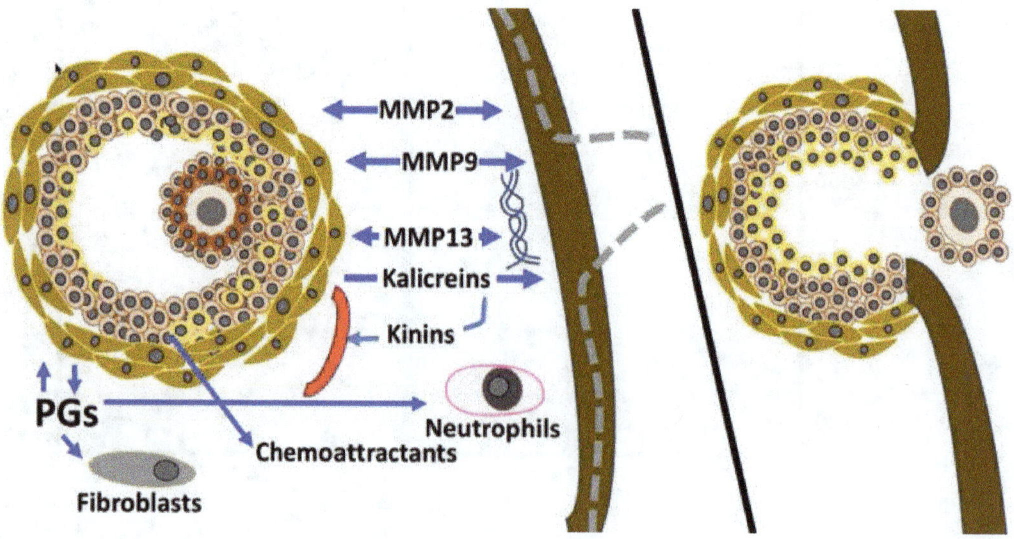

Figure 15. Proposed mechanisms at follicular rupture. LH stimulates the expression of genes in granulosa cells (PR, PGS-2) that control the activation of matrix metalloproteinases (MMPs), leading to the breakdown and remodeling of extracellular matrices and the surface epithelium to allow rupture of the follicle and extrusion of the oocyte (ovulation). Modified from Richards et al. [22].

endocrine hormones, immune and metabolic signals, as well as intrafollicular paracrine factors from the theca, mural and cumulus granulosa cells, and the oocyte itself. Therefore, healthy and meiotically competent oocytes and the coordination and synchronization of endocrine, paracrine, immune, and metabolic signals acting mainly through the cumulus compartment exert control on oocyte maturation, developmental, and ovulation process [21].

Mechanisms suggested implied in follicle rupture [22] are shown in **Figure 15**.

5. Luteal phase

This phase lasts 14 days in most women after ovulation. The granulosa cells that are not released with the oocyte acquire a vacuolated appearance and a characteristic yellow color due to the concentration of a carotenoid called lutein and the incorporation of fat drops. No other function has been described for lutein than being a powerful antioxidant.

The luteinized cells combine with the newly formed theca-lutein cells together with the surrounding stroma; thus, originates the transitory endocrine organ that secretes progesterone, known as the corpus luteum, whose main function is to prepare the endometrium, already proliferated by the action of follicular phase estrogens, for the implantation of the fertilized egg.

The endometrium expresses adhesion molecules that make it receptive to the blastocyst and between days 7 and 9 from ovulation, a period of maximum efficiency known as the window of implantation is established; after day 9, implantation is not possible, which is why it is called the refractory phase.

Eight or nine days after ovulation, at the time when implantation is expected, maximum vascularization is reached, the basal lamina dissolves, and the capillaries invade the granulosa cell layers in response to the secretion of angiogenic factors, both from the granulosa and from the theca cells, in harmony with the maximum levels of plasma progesterone and estradiol.

The survival of the corpus luteum depends on the continuous stimulation of LH, but estradiol metabolites, acting via paracrine-autocrine pathways, affect angiogenesis or LH-mediated events also [23].

The function of the corpus luteum decreases at the end of the luteal phase unless chorionic gonadotropin appears due to an eventual pregnancy. If pregnancy does not occur, the corpus luteum undergoes luteolysis. Under the action of estradiol and prostaglandins, it forms a scar tissue called *corpus albicans* [24].

As noted, estrogen levels increase and decrease twice during the menstrual cycle, increase during the middle follicular phase, and then decrease rapidly after ovulation, followed by a further increase during the middle luteal phase, in parallel with the increase in serum levels of progesterone and 17α-hydroxyprogesterone, all falling at the end of the menstrual cycle (**Figure 1**).

The mechanism of how the corpus luteum regulates steroid secretion is not known exactly. It may be determined in part by the pattern of LH secretion, changes in its receptor, or variations in the levels of enzymes that regulate the production of steroid hormones. The amount of granulosa cells formed during the follicular phase and the levels of LDL cholesterol that surround it may also play a role in the regulation of steroid synthesis by the corpus luteum.

There are at least two types of luteal cells, large and small.

Both produce progesterone but with differences. Large cells come from granulosa, are more active in steroidogenesis, produce large amounts of progesterone, and although they have numerous LH receptors, they do not elevate progesterone secretion in response to LH or cAMP. Instead, they possess receptors for PGF2a and respond to this hormone with activation of at least two second messengers. Activation of protein kinase C (PKC) decreases progesterone's secretion.

As a result of the binding of PGF2a to its receptor, the concentration of free intracellular calcium increases, which seems to be related to the induction of apoptosis and cell death.

The large cells are influenced by other autocrine and paracrine factors, such as inhibin, relaxin, and oxytocin (**Figure 16**). The small cells are derived from the theca, contain receptors for LH, and respond to LH or cAMP by increasing the secretion of progesterone by 5–15 times [25, 26].

The synthesis of progesterone by the corpus luteum is essential for the establishment and maintenance of pregnancy.

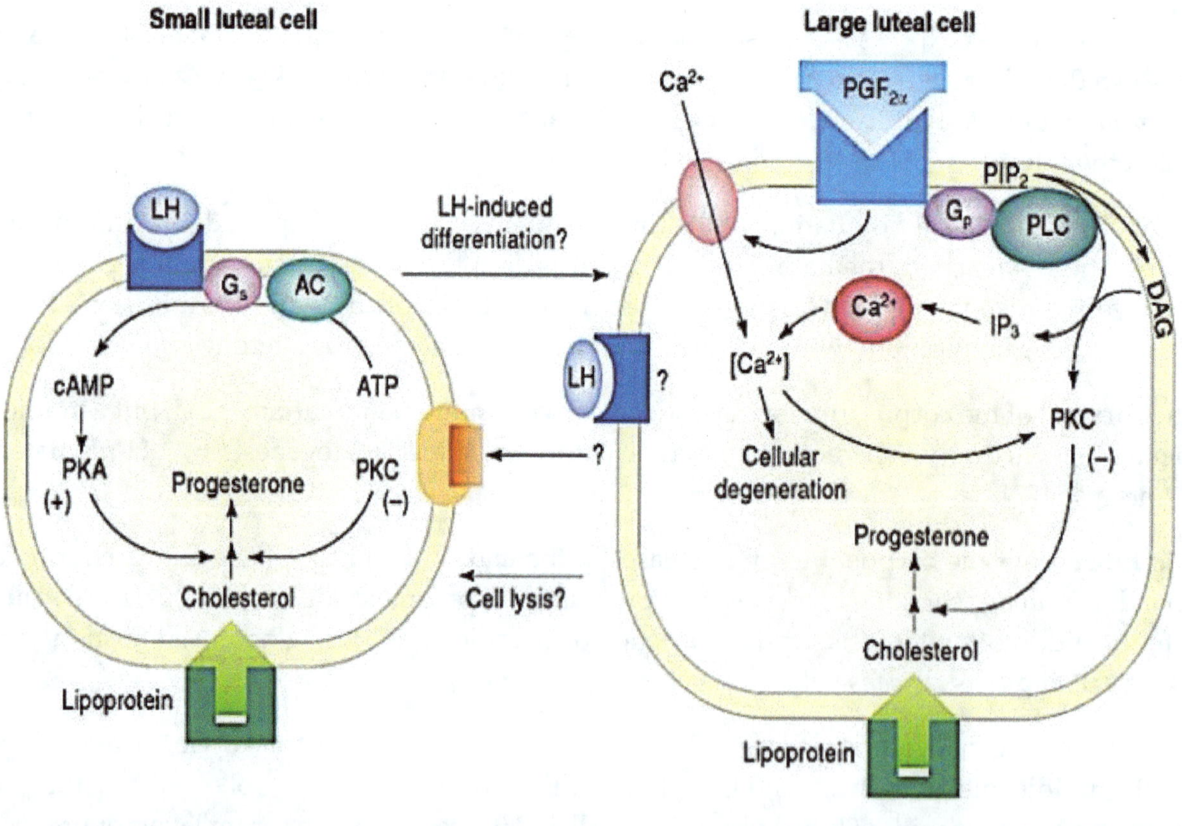

Figure 16. Regulation of small luteal cells (left) and large (right). In small luteal cells, the binding of LH to its receptor activates the second messenger protein kinase A (PKA) pathway, which stimulates the synthesis of progesterone. In large cells, the LH that binds to its receptor does not increase the intracellular concentrations of cAMP nor the synthesis of progesterone, but the binding of PGF2a to its receptor activates PKC, which inhibits the synthesis of progesterone and causes an influx of calcium that leads to cell degeneration. AC: adenylate cyclase, DAG: diacylglycerol, IP3: inositol 1,4,5-trisphosphate, PIP2: phosphatidylinositol 4,5-bisphosphate, and PLC: phospholipase C. From Niswender [25].

In addition to luteinization, that is, the conversion of an ovulatory follicle into the corpus luteum and luteal regression to allow a new cycle, there are also mechanisms of luteal maintenance and rescue to sustain pregnancy.

Humans preferably use circulating LDL cholesterol for steroidogenesis although the corpus luteum has the ability to synthesize its own cholesterol, in smaller amounts [27].

Inside the cells, lipid steroid precursors are found as free cholesterol. There is also esterified cholesterol that accumulates within the rough endoplasmic reticulum and as cytoplasmic lipid droplets or lipoprotein particles. These fatty acid esters of cholesterol cannot replace free cholesterol as a structural ingredient of the plasma membrane nor serve as direct substrates for the production of steroids. They are hydrolyzed by a neutral cholesterol ester hydrolase (NCEH), also known as hormone-sensitive lipase, because their activity is tightly regulated in steroidogenic tissues by FSH, LH, and hCG.

Progesterone secretion and estradiol during luteal phase is tightly connected with the pulses of secretion of LH (**Figure 12**). The frequency and widening of secretion of LH during follicular phase regulates the function of the posterior luteal phase and is concordant with the function of LH during luteal phase.

The frequency and widening of the pulses of secretion of pituitary LH affect the secretion of progesterone and estradiol during the luteal phase (**Figure 12**).

The half-life of the corpus luteum can be reduced with the continuous administration of LH during any of the phases, follicular or luteal, as if the LH concentration is lower or its pulses are reduced.

The luteal phase can suffer shortening also if the levels of FSH are inadequate or low, during the follicular phase, conditioning the development of a smaller corpus luteum.

The function of the corpus luteum begins to decrease 9–11 days after ovulation. The mechanism by which the corpus luteum undergoes involution (luteolysis) is partially elucidated. Prostaglandin F2α would have a luteolytic action, through the synthesis of endothelin-1 that inhibits steroidogenesis and stimulates the release of a growth factor, the tumor necrosis factor alpha (TNFα) oxytocin, and vasopressin and would produce a luteotropic effect through an autocrine/paracrine mechanism.

The ability of LH to negatively regulate its own receptor may also play a role at the end of the luteal phase; thereby, the involution of the corpus luteum must be caused by a decrease in the sensitivity of the LH receptors, rather than by a pulsatile secretion of it. Finally, the matrix metalloproteinases would also play a role in luteolysis and, therefore, in the fall of progesterone levels.

6. Menstruation

In the absence of pregnancy, the levels of progesterone and estradiol begin to decrease as a result of the corpus luteum decreasing. The fall of progesterone increases in degree of coiling and the constriction of the spiraled arterioles. This finally produces tissue ischemia due to decreased blood flow from the superficial, spongy, and compact endometrial layers. After the fall of serum concentrations of ovarian steroids, matrix metalloproteinases play a key role in the onset of menstrual bleeding in the human endometrium, by inducing the degradation of the extracellular matrix of this mucosa [28]. Endometrial prostaglandins cause contractions of the uterine smooth muscle and detachment of degraded tissue.

The release of prostaglandins may appear due to instability of the lysosomal membranes in the endometrial cells. The magnitude of this effect is such that inhibitors of prostaglandin synthesis can be used as a therapy in women with excessive uterine bleeding. Menstrual flow is composed of detachment of endometrial tissue, red blood cells, inflammatory exudates, and proteolytic enzymes.

Two days after the start of menstruation and while the shedding of the endometrium still occurs, the estrogen produced by the new growing follicles begins to stimulate the regeneration of the superficial layers of the endometrium. The estrogen secreted by the growing follicles causes a long constriction of the vessel facilitating the formation of a veil over the denuded endometrial vessels.

The average duration of menstruation is 4–6 days, but the normal range can be 2–8 days. As mentioned above, the average amount of bleeding loss is 30 ml and more than 80 ml is considered abnormal. A few years ago, a classification has been generalized to describe the abnormalities of bleeding suggested by the International Federation of Gynecology and Obstetrics [29].

6.1. Types of endometrium at echographies

The characteristics of the endometrium in gynecological ultrasound change depending on the period of the menstrual cycle, presenting different thicknesses according to the stage of the menstrual cycle (**Figure 17**).

Endometrium type 0, postmenstrual: it is characterized because only a fine refractive line can be seen. It is the endometrium typical of postmenopause, postpartum, or after a uterine scraping. Most postmenopausal women are between 3 and 5 mm thick, but it is normal up to 8 mm if there has been no unexpected bleeding.

Endometrium type 1, preovulatory: trilaminar endometrium, refers to the observation of three refractive lines. This stage corresponds to the proliferative or estrogenic phase. In an early follicular stage, the size of the endometrium is between 3 and 4 mm thick, while in the stage close to ovulation, it can reach 9–11 mm.

Endometrium type 2, postovulatory: in this stage, the progesterone matures the already proliferated endometrium, especially in its glandular and vascular structures, thickening the endometrium. The ultrasound image becomes whiter to the extent that it contains more water and glycogen. This layer of refringency represents most of the endometrium toward the end of the luteal phase.

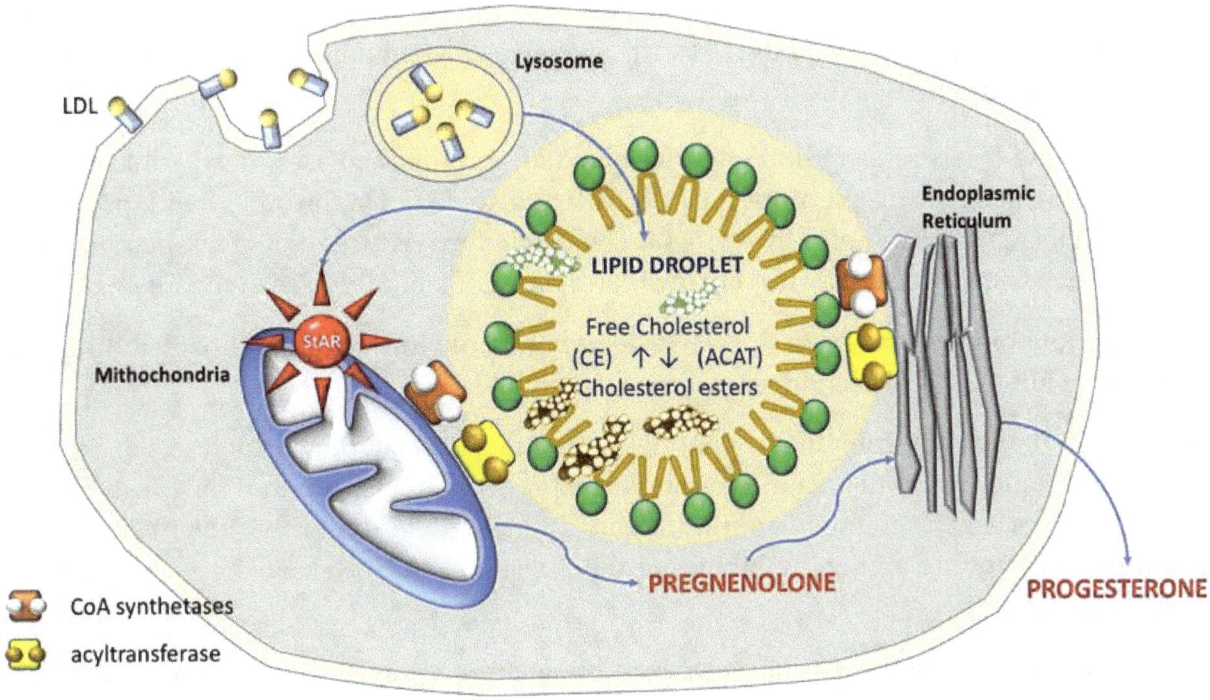

Figure 17. The main substrate for human steroidogenesis is LDL cholesterol: it is incorporated by endocytosis and stored as free cholesterol or as ester. Esterified cholesterol is hydrolyzed cholesterol esterases (CE) and transported as free cholesterol to the mitochondria. It passes from the outer mitochondrial membrane to the internal membrane, with the concurrence of the steroidogenic acute regulatory protein (StAR), peripheral type benzodiazepine receptors and endozepine. In mitochondria, cholesterol is converted to pregnenolone by cytochrome P450scc, which is transported out of the mitochondria and converted to progesterone by 3b-hydroxysteroid dehydrogenase, D5, D4 isomerase (3b-HSD), which is present in the smooth endoplasmic reticulum (The cell nucleus is not shown.)

Endometrium type 3, premenstrual: in this stage, there is only one large refractive line and corresponds to the late secretory phase.

6.2. Endocrine regulation of the menstrual cycle

When the gonadal axis has reached maturity, the neurons of the preoptic area and the infundibular and arcuate nuclei in the hypothalamus secrete GnRh in a pulsatile fashion, every 60–90 minutes, to the pituitary portal system.

Frequency and amplitude are essential to produce and maintain the effect on the gonadotropic cells of the anterior part of the pituitary gland, which consists of releasing both LH and FSH. The secreted amounts of each will depend not only on the pulsatility of GnRH, but also on the positive and negative feedbacks mechanisms of sex steroids.

In general, estrogen sensitizes and counter-regulates FSH, at both levels, the hypothalamus and the adenohypophysis, selectively modulated by other factors such as inhibins A and B. LH is sensitive to positive feedback, while there are estrogens in the late follicular phase and in the luteal phase, but the feedback becomes negative when estrogen levels fall at the end of the cycle.

Recent evidence indicates that the administration of progesterone in the late well-estrogenized follicular phase does not prevent the LH surge, which is of great importance because it would have no interference with ovulation [30, 31].

Relatively, low levels of estradiol, in early follicular and luteal phases, decrease kisspeptin expression, which reduces the amplitude of GnRH pulses [32]. On the other hand, progesterone would increase the dynorphin expression, which in turn reduces that of kisspeptin. These changes have been associated with the lower frequency of GnRH pulses in the luteal phase.

Other modulators that stimulate the pulsatile secretion of GnRH are glutamate and norepinephrine, while GABA and endogenous opioids inhibit it.

Neurokinin B and dynorphin neuropeptides act in an auto-synaptic fashion in the arcuate/infundibular nucleus, so that an increase in the expression of neurokinin B (NKB) stimulates the secretion of and, therefore, of GnRH, while an increase in dynorphin (Dyn) expression decreases kisspeptin secretion by inhibiting the pulsatility of GnRH. This system is known as KNDy [33].

At the beginning of the menstrual cycle, estradiol levels are low and FSH levels are slightly elevated. This ratio manages to recruit follicles and as that happens, not only estradiol increases but also inhibin A, due to the empowerment of FD, which generates a continuous decrease in FSH in the follicular phase.

The concentrations of FSH reach the maximum levels on the day when the FD is defined, followed by a slow decrease during the follicular phase, from day 5 to 13, reaching a nadir and then a peak just before ovulation (**Figure 14**). There comes a time when estradiol levels are such that they trigger the peak of FSH and LH, producing ovulation.

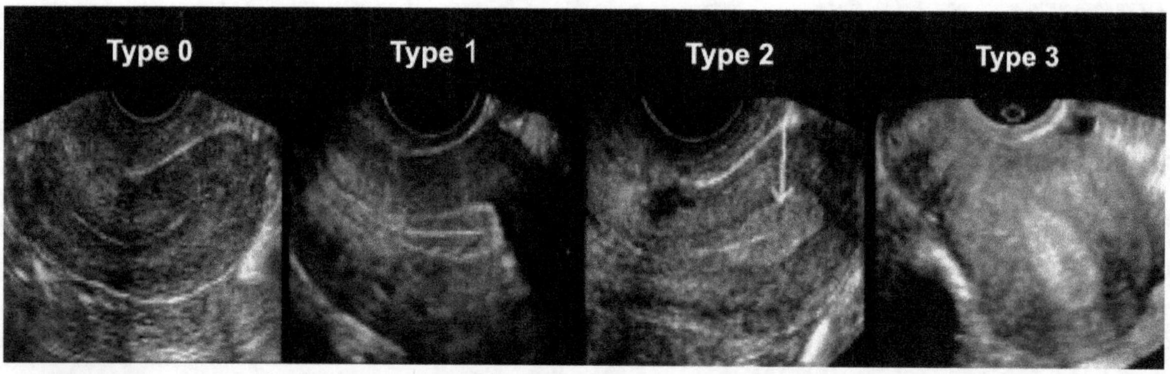

Figure 18. Types of endometrium in transvaginal ultrasound. The endometrium was classified into four types (0, 1, 2, and 3) according to the appearance of the myometrium-endometrium and endometrium-endometrium interfaces, the texture, and the thickness of the functional layer. Type 0: smooth, thin as a pencil line; type 1: trilaminar structure with an iso- or hypoechoic functional layer; type 2: also trilaminar, but the myometrium-endometrium interfaces are thicker than those of type 1; and type 3: thick and homogeneous echogenic image. The type of endometrium correlates with the day of the menstrual cycle. Ultrasound is defined on day 0 as the day of the follicle break. Type 0 is usually found on day −11, during and immediately after menstruation. Type 1 is observed during the middle follicular phase and until day +2. Types 2 and 3 are observed after the ovulatory days. The endometrium increases more thickness during the preovulatory phase (average +5.5 mm), and in the luteal phase, the average is +2.6 mm.

As the luteal phase advance in time, inhibin A, estradiol, and progesterone fall together with the increase in activin A. FSH increases in the transition from the luteal phase to the next follicular phase, beginning 4 days before menstruation, a stage in which inhibin B increases during follicular recruitment.

The concentration of activin A secreted by the follicles increases in the second half of the luteal phase [34] (**Figure 18**), decreases at the beginning of the follicular phase, increases during the early follicular phase, and then increases during the middle follicular phase in parallel with estradiol and inhibin A (**Figure 19**).

In older women, FSH is higher, even during nadir, and the increase occurs early during the luteal phase. Recruitment of a group of follicles begins early, but the selection of DF is altered and can either advance or delay. The result is the variability of the cycle at the expense of a variable follicular phase, called "lag phase," which ends when the ETO is produced [35].

The ETO is when the estradiol overt elevation is achieved, which marks the selection of the FD. If an FD capable of ovulating was not achieved, the woman can go through a hyperestrogenic state without establishing a corpus luteum, so at the endometrial level, the cycle is hormonally monophasic. This is the pathophysiological basis that explains the monophasic hyperestrogenism that affects approximately one-third of women in perimenopause (**Figure 20**).

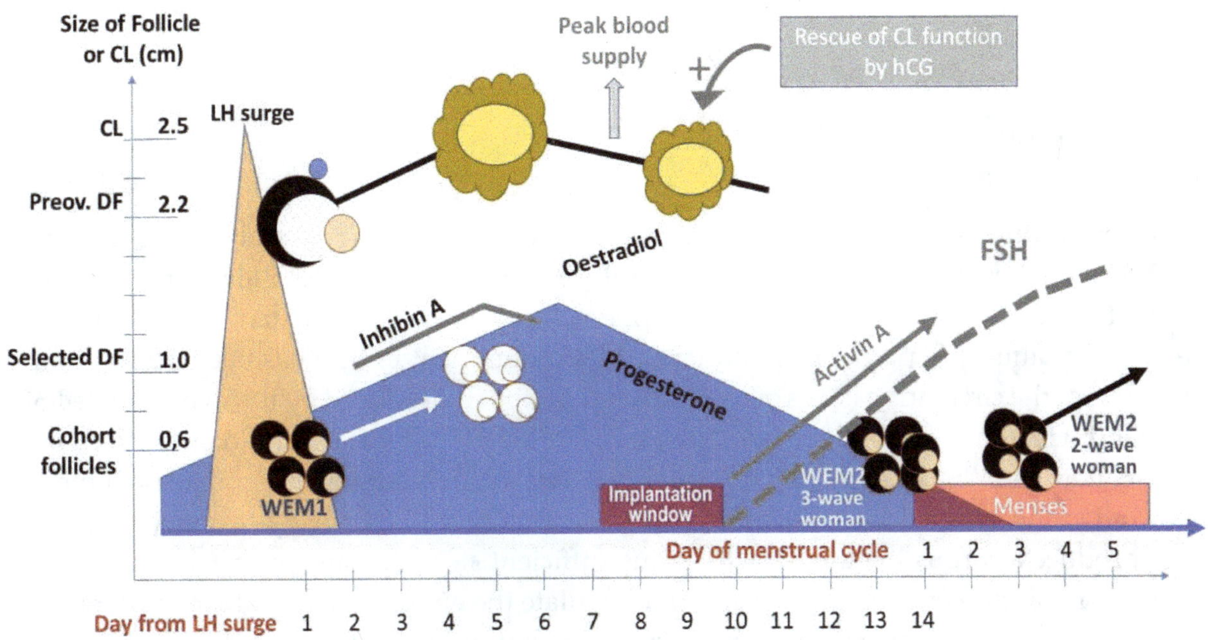

Figure 19. Scheme composed shows luteal events, follicular ones and hormonals during luteal phase of woman CL = corpus luteum; DF = dominant follicle; WEM1–3 = wave emergency 1, 2, or 3 at the cycle; the waves of follicle of light gray color indicates the low frequency of the principal waves (selection of DF) during luteal phase or early follicular ones in women of 2 or 3 waves. The estradiol rise in the follicular phase begins after the emergence of the ovulatory DF and becomes more rapid following DF selection, and occurs earlier in women with 2 versus 3 follicle waves per cycle. After ovulation, estradiol concentrations increase to the mid-luteal phase (days 7–9 after ovulation) and then decline, and this is due to luteal estradiol secretion and is unaffected by minor or major anovulatory waves. Adapted from Macklon and Fauser [5].

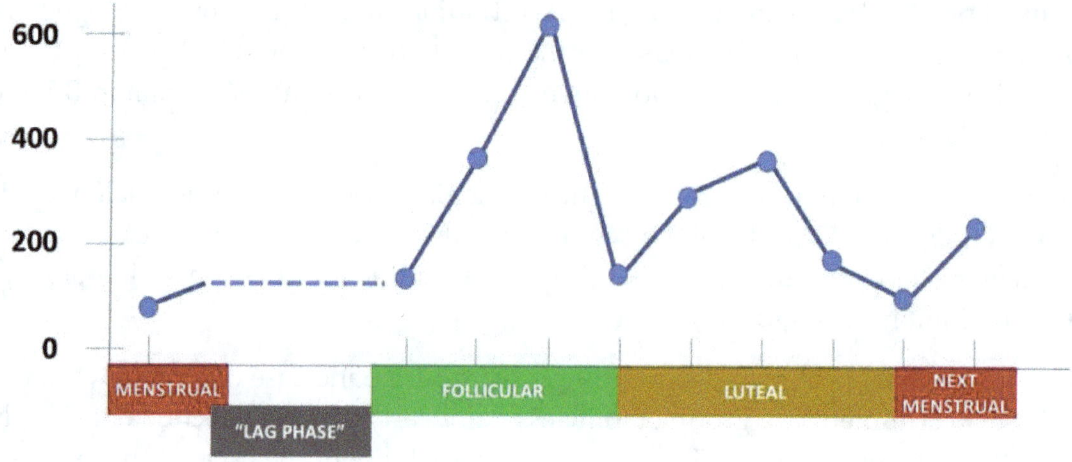

Figure 20. The variability in perimenopause depends on the lag phase, a delayed recruitment process. Adapted from Hale et al. [35].

A chronic negative energy imbalance reduces the pulsatility of LH, generates atresia of FD and, consequently, anovulation and amenorrhea. Weight loss is associated with a reduction in LH pulses, which generates functional, reversible hypothalamic amenorrhea. On the contrary, the pulsatility of LH is increased in adolescents with irregular cycles or in women with polycystic ovary syndrome, associated with anovulation also, but here the selection of DF is absent.

7. Conclusion

Human reproduction depends on the integrity of a system of intracrine and paracrine signals within the ovaries, in which those recruited follicles that have reached a level of differentiation that make them sensitive to the endocrine control of the other distant and great actor, the hypothalamus axis participate pituitary. Once a dominant follicle has been achieved, the elevations of the circulating levels of estradiol and inhibin B produced by it will modulate FSH levels and will allow, on the one hand, the atresia of the other follicles, and on the other, they will facilitate the LH surge, necessary to trigger ovulation. After hatching, the surrounding theca and granulosa cells from the follicular bed abandoned by the newly ovulated egg interact to produce a corpus luteum, which retains sufficient steroidogenic properties to produce progesterone at the concentration required to regulate the endometrium, till the implantation of a fertilized egg. If pregnancy does not occur, since the end of the luteal phase, gonadotropic changes are prepared to allow the development of a follicular recruitment phase.

Being such a complex process, dependent on so many variables and exposed to so many actions, reactions and interferences, the sequences of the menstrual cycle are remarkably predictable within not very wide ranges of variability. In general, the duration standards of each cycle, 25–35 days, coincide with the ovulation presumption criteria accepted for women with ovulatory anomalies such as in the polycystic ovarian syndrome. The detailed understanding of the mechanisms allow to improve the efficiency in the clinical management when it is intended to give assistance to obtain a pregnancy, as well as to avoid it when the goal is contraception, or to correct bleeding anomalies that may result from ovulatory disorders with luteal insufficiency. There are still many aspects to investigate.

Author details

Barriga-Pooley Patricio[1]* and Brantes-Glavic Sergio[2]

*Address all correspondence to: pbarriga@uft.cl

1 Obstetrics and Gynaecology Department, School of Medicine, Finis Terrae and San Sebastian Universities, Santiago, Chile

2 Depto Ginecología y Obstericia, Universidad de Chile, Santiago, Chile

References

[1] Reed BG, Carr BR. The normal menstrual cycle and the control of ovulation. In: De Groot LJ, Chrousos G, Dungan K, Feingold KR, Grossman A, Hershman JM, et al., editors. Endotext [Internet]. South Dartmouth (MA): MDText.com, Inc.; 2000 (ver 2018 Aug 5.)

[2] Welt CK, Pagan YL, Smith PC, Rado KB, Hall JE. Control of follicle-stimulating hormone by estradiol and the inhibins: Critical role of estradiol at the hypothalamus during the luteal-follicular transition. The Journal of Clinical Endocrinology and Metabolism. 2003 Apr;**88**(4):1766-1771. DOI: 10.1210/jc.2002-021516

[3] Mihm M, Gangooly S, Muttukrishna S. The normal menstrual cycle in women. Animal Reproduction Science. 2011;**124**(3-4):229-236. DOI: 10.1016/j.anireprosci.2010.08.030

[4] Hodgen GD. The dominant ovarian follicle. Fertility and Sterility. 1982;**38**:281-300

[5] Macklon NS, Fauser BC. Aspects of ovarian follicle development throughout life. Hormone Research. 1999;**52**(4):161-170. DOI: 10.1159/000023456

[6] Richards JS, Ren YA, Candelaria N, Adams JE, Rajkovic A. Ovarian follicular theca cell recruitment, differentiation, and impact on fertility: 2017 update. Endocrine Reviews. Feb 1 2018;**39**(1):1-20. DOI: 10.1210/er.2017-00164

[7] Baird DT, Fraser IS. Blood production and ovarian secretion rates of esuadiol-17β and estrone in women throughout the menstrual cycle. The Journal of Clinical Endocrinology and Metabolism. 1974;**38**:1009-1017

[8] Doshi SB, Agarwal A. The role of oxidative stress in menopause. Journal of Midlife Health. 2013;**4**(3):140-146. DOI: 10.4103/0976-7800.118990

[9] Groome NP, Illingworth PJ, O'Brien M, Pai R, Rodger FE, Mather JP, et al. Measurement of dimeric inhibin B throughout the human menstrual cycle. The Journal of Clinical Endocrinology and Metabolism. 1996;**81**(4):1401-1405. DOI: 10.1210/jcem.81.4.8636341

[10] Welt CK, Martin KA, Taylor AE, Lambert-Messerlian GM, Crowley WF Jr, Smith JA, et al. Frequency modulation of follicle-stimulating hormone (FSH) during the luteal-follicular transition: Evidence for FSH control of inhibin B in normal women. The Journal of Clinical Endocrinology and Metabolism 1997;**82**(8):2645-2652. DOI: 10.1210/jcem.82.8.4138

[11] Small CM, Manatunga AK, Klein M, Feigelson HS, Dominguez CE, McChesney R, et al. Menstrual cycle characteristics: Associations with fertility and spontaneous abortion. Epidemiology. 2006 Jan;**17**(1):52-60

[12] Wilcox AJ, Dunson D, Baird DD. The timing of the "fertile window" in the menstrual cycle: Day specific estimates from a prospective study. BMJ. 2000;**321**(7271):1259-1262. DOI: 10.1136/bmj.321.7271.1259

[13] Wise LA, Mikkelsen EM, Rothman KJ, Riis AH, Sørensen HT, Huybrechts KF, et al. A prospective cohort study of menstrual characteristics and time to pregnancy. American Journal of Epidemiology. 2011;**174**(6):701-709. DOI: 10.1093/aje/kwr130

[14] La Marca A, Broekmans FJ, Volpe A, Fauser BC, Macklon NS, ESHRE Special Interest Group for Reproductive Endocrinology–AMH Round Table. Anti-Mullerian hormone (AMH): What do we still need to know? Human Reproduction. 2009 Sep;**24**(9):2264-2275. DOI: 10.1093/humrep/dep210

[15] Broekmans FJ, Visser JA, Laven JS, Broer SL, Themmen AP, Fauser BC. Anti-Müllerian hormone and ovarian dysfunction. Trends in Endocrinology and Metabolism. 2008 Nov;**19**(9):340-347. DOI: 10.1016/j.tem.2008.08.002

[16] Sollenberger MJ, Carlsen EC, Johnson ML, Veldhuis JD, Evans WS. Specific physiological regulation of luteinizing hormone secretory events throughout the human menstrual cycle: New insights into the pulsatile mode of gonadotropin release. Journal of Neuroendocrinology. 1990;**2**(6):845-852. DOI: 10.1111/j.1365-2826.1990.tb00650.x

[17] Hoff JD, Quigley ME, Yen SCC. Hormonal dynamics at midcycle: A re-evaluation. The Journal of Clinical Endocrinology and Metabolism. 1983;**57**:792

[18] Irianni F, Hodgen GD. Mechanism of ovulation. Endocrinology and Metabolism Clinics of North America. 1992;**21**(1):19-38. DOI: 10.1016/S0889-8529(18)30230-5

[19] Jesam C, Salvatierra AM, Schwartz JL, Croxatto HB. Suppression of follicular rupture with meloxicam, a cyclooxygenase-2 inhibitor: Potential for emergency contraception. Human Reproduction. 2010;**25**(2):368-373. DOI: 10.1093/humrep/dep392

[20] Duffy DM. Novel contraceptive targets to inhibit ovulation: The prostaglandin E2 pathway. Human Reproduction Update. 2015;**21**(5):652-670. DOI: 10.1093/humupd/dmv026

[21] Russell DL, Robker RL. Molecular mechanisms of ovulation: Co-ordination through the cumulus complex. Human Reproduction Update. 2007;**13**(3):289-312. DOI: 10.1093/humupd/dml062

[22] Richards JS, Russell DL, Robker RL, Dajee M, Alliston TN. Molecular mechanisms of ovulation and luteinization. Molecular and Cellular Endocrinology. 1998;**145**(1-2):47-54. DOI: 10.1016/S0303-7207(98)00168-3

[23] Devoto L, Henríqucz S, Kohen P, Strauss JF 3rd. The significance of estradiol metabolites in human corpus luteum physiology. Steroids. 2017;**123**:50-54. DOI: 10.1016/j.steroids.2017.05.002

[24] Stocco C, Telleria C, Gibori G. The molecular control of corpus luteum formation, function, and regression. Endocrine Reviews. 2007;**28**(1):117-149. DOI: 10.1210/er.2006-0022

[25] Niswender GD. Molecular control of luteal secretion of progesterone. Reproduction. 2002;**123**(3):333-339

[26] Niswender GD, Juengel JL, Silva PJ, Rollyson MK, McIntush EW. Mechanisms controlling the function and life span of the corpus luteum. Physiological Reviews. 2000;**80**(1):1-29. DOI: 10.1152/physrev.2000.80.1.1

[27] Christenson LK, Devoto L. Cholesterol transport and steroidogenesis by the corpus luteum. Reproductive Biology and Endocrinology. 2003;**1**:90. DOI: 10.1186/1477-7827-1-90

[28] Henriet P, Cornet PB, Lemoine P, Galant C, Singer CF, Courtoy PJ, et al. Circulating ovarian steroids and endometrial matrix metalloproteinases (MMPs). Annals of the New York Academy of Sciences. 2002;**955**:119-138. DOI: 10.1111/j.1749-6632.2002.tb02773.x

[29] Munro MG, Critchley HO, Broder MS, Fraser IS, FIGO Working Group on Menstrual Disorders. FIGO classification system (PALM-COEIN) for causes of abnormal uterine bleeding in nongravid women of reproductive age. International Journal of Gynaecology and Obstetrics. 2011;**113**(1):3-13. DOI: 10.1016/j.ijgo.2010.11.011

[30] Hutchens EG, Ramsey KA, Howard LC, Abshire MY, Patrie JT, McCartney CR. Progesterone has rapid positive feedback actions on LH release but fails to reduce LH pulse frequency within 12 h in estradiol-pretreated women. Physiological Reports. 2016;**4**(16). DOI: 10.14814/phy2.12891

[31] Kim SH, Burt Solorzano CM, McCartney CR. Progesterone administration does not acutely alter LH pulse secretion in the mid-follicular phase in women. Physiological Reports. 2018;**6**(8):e13680. DOI: 10.14814/phy2.13680

[32] Skorupskaite K, George JT, Anderson RA. The kisspeptin-GnRH pathway in human reproductive health and disease. Human Reproduction Update. 2014;**20**(4):485-500. DOI: 10.1093/humupd/dmu009

[33] Lehman MN, Coolen LM, Goodman RL. Minireview: Kisspeptin/neurokinin B/dynorphin (KNDy) cells of the arcuate nucleus: A central node in the control of gonadotropin-releasing hormone secretion. Endocrinology. 2010;**151**(8):3479-3489. DOI: 10.1210/en.2010-0022

[34] Bilezikjian LM, Blount AL, Leal AM, Donaldson CJ, Fischer WH, Vale WW. Autocrine/paracrine regulation of pituitary function by activin, inhibin and follistatin. Molecular and Cellular Endocrinology. 2004 Oct 15;**225**(1-2):29-36. DOI: 10.1016/j.mce.2004.02.010

[35] Hale GE, Zhao X, Hughes CL, Burger HG, Robertson DM, Fraser IS. Endocrine features of menstrual cycles in middle and late reproductive age and the menopausal transition classified according to the staging of reproductive aging workshop (STRAW) staging system. The Journal of Clinical Endocrinology and Metabolism. 2007;**92**(8):3060-3067

9

Use of Phytoestrogens for the Treatment of Psychiatric Symptoms Associated with Menopause Transition

Erika Estrada-Camarena, Carolina López-Rubalcava,
Brenda Valdés-Sustaita,
Gabriel Sinhue Azpilcueta-Morales and
Eva María González-Trujano

Abstract

Menopause transition is recognized as a vulnerable period in women life to develop or aggravate symptoms of psychiatric disorders. Several treatments including antidepressants and hormonal restitution with estrogens have been suggested to ameliorate the symptoms. Also, in this period of life is frequent the use of other drugs to treat is also frequent the use of other drugs to treat comorbid pathologies that might even increase the risk of drug-drug interactions. Literature reports that some phytochemicals with estrogenic activity have beneficial effects during menopausal transition without collateral events. This chapter shows evidence about the use of phytoestrogens as an alternative therapy for the treatment of some psychiatric symptoms associated with the menopausal transition. Data derived from preclinical research related to the use of classical phytoestrogens (isoflavones), considering the beneficial effects, as well as adverse events, are discussed. Also, the use of polyphenols and organosulfurate compounds as an alternative for the treatment of anxiety- and depressive-like behavior as well as fibromyalgia is included. A narrative review was conducted using bibliography reporting the use of isoflavones (genistein, daidzein, equol), coumestans or lignans for the reduction of depressive-like or anxiety-like behavior. Furthermore, it is described if the use of this compounds impact in other signs of menopause, i.e. vasomotor and osteoporosis. In addition, due to the high frequency of comorbid pathologies as diabetes mellitus, dyslipidemia or metabolic syndrome with psychiatric disorders, the use of these phytochemicals is discussed.

Keywords: menopause, polyphenols, glycosinolates, phytoestrogens

1. Introduction

With the increase of life expectancy, women potentially spend the last third of their lives in post-menopause. Most of the menopausal women suffer from a variety of symptoms such as hot flashes, night sweats, mood swings, insomnia, vaginal dryness and osteoporosis [1, 2]. Also, the menopause transition could be a vulnerable period to develop some diseases related to mental disorders (i.e., anxiety and depression) and chronic non-degenerative pathologies (metabolic diseases) in addition to menopausal symptoms [3, 4]. This situation implies that women that transit in this period of life could be vulnerable to develop co-morbidities leading to a complex medical management due to the elevated cost and possible pharmacological interactions.

Hormone replacement therapy is considered the first line of treatment for menopause symptoms, mainly vasomotor and night sweats. However, many women refuse it because of their association with increased risk of breast cancer and are considering botanical products or dietary supplements as therapy because they are regarded as safer products [1, 2, 5]. For example, black cohosh is widely employed for hot flashes and mood disorders; others are compounds with estrogenic activity (phytoestrogens) as soy food products, red clover, kudzu, hops, licorice, rhubarb, yam and chasteberry [1].

The use of functional food and nutraceuticals became common to treat menopause symptoms [2]. The term "nutraceutical" combines two words—"nutrient" (a nourishing food component) and "pharmaceutical" (a medical drug). It is defined as "any substance that may be considered a food or part of it that provides medical or health benefits, including the prevention and treatment of diseases." These products include isolated nutrients, dietary supplements and diets genetically engineered "designed" foods, botanical products and processed foods such as cereals, foods and beverages [6]. A nutraceutical is demonstrated to have a physiological benefit or provide protection against chronic disease [6]. On the other hand, functional food according to American Dietetic Association, "functional" implies that the food possesses some identified value leading to health benefits, including reducing the risk of adverse effects for a person consuming it [7].

Nutraceuticals and functional food are classified in several manners taken into account their content of specific food, properties (anti-cancer, positive influence on blood lipid profile, anti-inflammatory, osteogenic or bone protective) or chemical structure [6]. Both nutraceuticals and functional food contain active compounds called phytochemicals that confer their properties. Phytochemicals are products of the secondary metabolism of a plant which are biologically active in humans and other animal species playing a greater beneficial role in health more than only nutritional properties. These products are part of the defense system and plants' protection [8], and in humans, they have activity in several systems such as the digestive, immune, cardiovascular, endocrine and central nervous system [6, 8], among others. Also, phytochemicals confer organoleptic properties to vegetables and fruits [8].

Phytochemicals are classified into four groups according to their impact on health [9, 10]:

1. Terpenoids (i.e., carotenoids and phytosterols)
2. Phenols (i.e., flavonoids, phenolic acids, tannins, stilbens and curcuminoids)

3. Organosulfurate compounds (i.e., glycosinolates and isothiocyanates)
4. Nitrogen compounds (i.e., alkaloids, betalainas, indol-glycosinolates)

The distribution of phytochemicals' sources could be at the same time diffuse and copious as well as specific depending on the product, for example, carotenoids are frequently found in several products (carrots, tomato, orange, mango, pumpkin, guava), whereeas glycosinolates are found only in cruciferous (broccoli, brussel sprout, cabbage, horseradish, rutabaga) [8]. The concentration of the phytochemical could vary depending on the morphological factors: skin, seed, pulp, peel, leaves, also on agronomic factors: weather, agricultural soil, technical procedure, physiological stress; and postharvest: maturity, processing and storage, among the others [8].

2. Phytochemicals: polyphenols

Polyphenols can be found in a large variety of food mainly of vegetable origin. They constitute the major group of natural compounds known (around 8000 identified) in the plant kingdom [11]. These compounds result of the secondary metabolism of carbon by the acetate-malonate and shikimate pathways. They are characterized by the presence of phenolic structures with a potent antioxidant activity that confers protection to plants against oxidative stress, ultraviolet radiation and other harmful factors of the environment such as pollutants and pathogens [12]. There are a wide variety of polyphenols but, in general, they have been classified into two groups according to their chemicals properties: flavonoids and non-flavonoids (**Figure 1**).

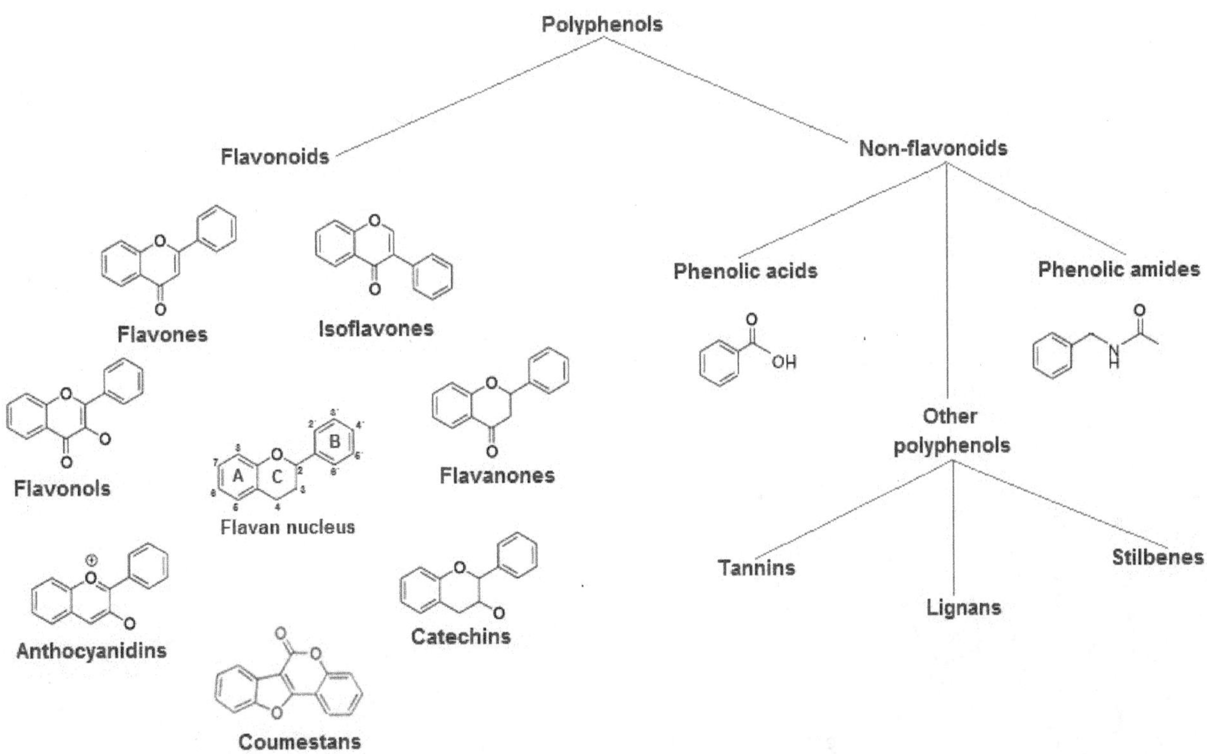

Figure 1. The scheme illustrates the main polyphenols and their division. Phytoestrogens are products of the metabolism of polyphenols: isoflavones and coumenstans are flavonoids, whereas lignans and stilbens are non-flavonoids.

The flavonoid group includes compounds whose structure contains the flavan nucleus (diphenyl propane; C:15: C3, C6, C3), such as anthocyanidins, proanthocyanidins, catechins, flavones, flavonols, flavanones, isoflavones and coumestans (**Figure 1**). The non-flavonoids group includes phenolic acids, phenolic amides and other polyphenols, such as tannins, lignans and stilbene compounds (**Figure 1**). Polyphenols, flavonoids and nonflavonoids have biological importance and are considered as nutraceuticals, not only for their antioxidant effect but also for their beneficial effects on health such as cardiovascular, diabetes and neurodegenerative protection, cancer prevention and anti-infection effect [11].

Recently, it has been determined that some polyphenols, especially isoflavones, flavonols, anthocyanidins, lignans, stilbenes and coumestans, have estrogenic activities, for which they have been denominated as phytoestrogens.

3. Phytoestrogens

Phytoestrogens are non-steroidal compounds that have a unique similarity in molecular weight and the arrangement of aromatic rings with hydroxyl groups to the cyclopentanoperhydrophenanthrene of 17β-estradiol (the most important endogenous estrogen; **Figure 2**).

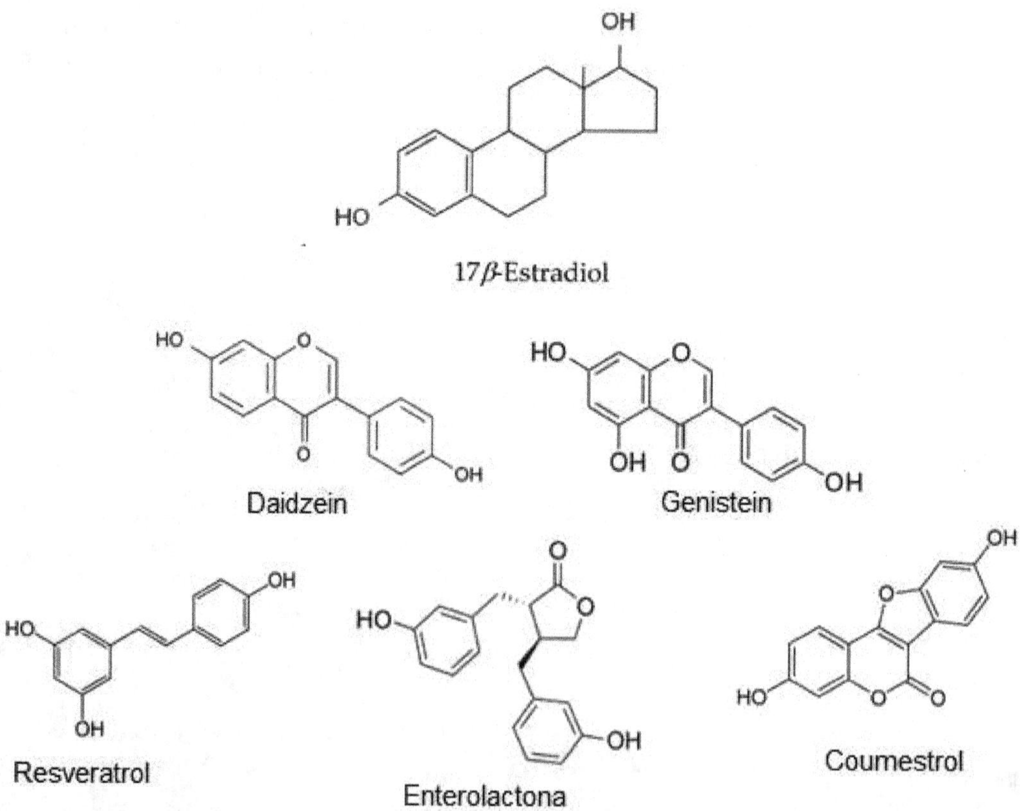

Figure 2. Phytoestrogens. The figure illustrates comparatively the chemical structure of 17β-estradiol and some phytoestrogens. Phytoestrogens are non-steroidal compounds that have a unique similarity in molecular weight and the arrangement of aromatic rings with hydroxyl groups to the cyclopentanoperhydrophenanthrene of 17β-estradiol.

The types of phytoestrogens are isoflavones, lignans, coumestans, ellagitannins and stilbens [13–15]. **Figure 3** shows the main sources of phytoestrogens and the phytochemicals with estrogenic properties. The primary sources of lignans are flaxseed, whole grain cereal and some beverages, such as coffee, tea and wine [15]. For isoflavones are legumens such as soybeans and peanuts, chickpeas and kudzu, lupine, fava, alfalfa, peanuts and chickpeas [15]. In the case of clover alfalfa and soybean sprouts, these are sources of coumestans [13]. Ellagitannins are abundant in fruits, nuts and seeds such as pomegranate, black raspberries, strawberries, walnuts and almonds [16]. The main source of stilbens such as revestratrol is the red wine and peanuts [15].

It is important to note that the beneficial actions of phytoestrogens are mostly given by the estrogenic/anti-estrogenic effect dependent on the resultant concentration of the metabolism

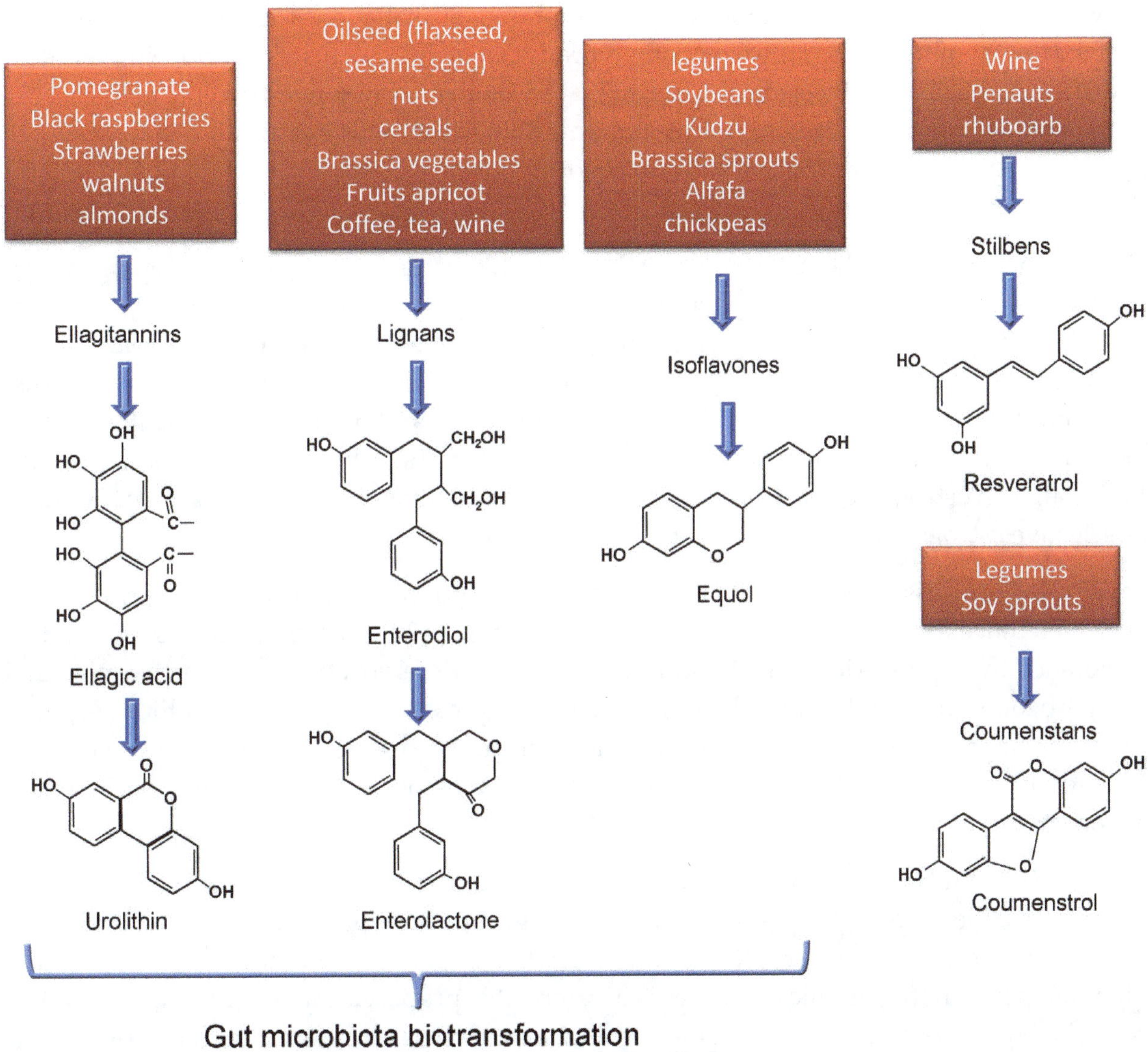

Figure 3. Phytoestrogens and their main food or beverage source. Ellagitannins, lignans and isoflavones require of microbiota biotransformation to release an active compound (urolithins A and B, enteronolactone or Equol, respectively) that produces their estrogen-like effects on different tissues. In contrast, stilbens and coumestans production appears to be independent of microbiota.

of phytoestrogens. It is known that phytoestrogens are mostly as glycosides and that only the aglycone fraction is bio-available to produce biological effects [17]. Some phytoestrogens, such as isoflavones, ellagitannins and lignans, require the action of gut bacterial enzymes to produce equol, urolithins and enterolignans, respectively [16, 18, 19]. These subproducts have more bioavailability and have more estrogenic/anti-estrogenic and anti-oxidant, anti-inflammatory and anti-proliferative activity than their precursors [20]. Furthermore, it is proposed that the biotransformation of isoflavones, ellagitannins and lignans by intestinal microbiota is essential in protection against menopausal symptoms. Also against certain chronic diseases, such as cancer, cardiovascular disease and osteoporosis [15], suggesting that the main discrepancies between a successful treatment versus lack of effect could be explained by the low bioavailability of phytoestrogens [21].

In this line, several reports indicate that coumestans—coumestrol and methoxycoumestrol—show estrogenic activity; the most active compound of isoflavones is daidzein intestinal-derived metabolite equol. However, other products such as genistein, daidzein, glycitein and their respective β-glycosides of genistein and daidzein possess estrogenic activity [13]. Ellagitannins are metabolized to urolithin A and B which showed estrogenic activity [15, 22]. Also, lignans are metabolized in the gut to produce the most estrogenic enterolignans, enterodiol and enterolactone [18].

On the other hand, the chemical similarity between 17β-estradiol and phytoestrogens confers the capability to interact with estrogen receptors (ERs). They produce effects through genomic actions with ERs alpha and beta (α, β) or non-genomic actions via membrane G-protein receptors (GPER) such as GPR30 and mERα and mERβ [23]. These receptors differ in tissue distribution, ligand selectivity and transcriptional processes and, therefore, also differ in their physiological effects on its activation [24–26]. These interactions between phytoestrogens and ERs results on estrogenic and/or anti-estrogenic effects, so that phytoestrogens are considered as selective estrogen receptor modulators (SERMs) [27–29].

Several in vitro assays suggest that phytoestrogens, especially isoflavones, have a significant preference for ERβ rather than for ERα (8- to 40-fold) [30–33]. Some authors explain this preference through steric interaction and through the difference in the attractive potential of hydrogen bonds between the ERs and phytoestrogens, which is higher in ERβ [34]. It is thought, that in some way the beneficial actions of the estrogenic compounds are related to the ERβ, in part because the activation of ERβ has been associated with the anti-proliferative actions of phytoestrogens [35–37].

GPER activation by phytoestrogens has been relatedto cardiovascular, liver enzymatic and neuroprotective actions [35, 38–40]. Some research groups have proposed that the GPR30 also take part in the endocrine disrupting action of phytoestrogens [41]. Phytoestrogens also show high potency in non-genomic responses. Therefore, it is proposed that their binding affinities could be higher for mERs [42] albeit the involvement of these receptors in the phytoestrogens actions is less explored.

As it can be seen phytoestrogens also possess a complex mechanism of actions to exert their properties, for example, the rapid neuroprotective activity of resveratrol against cerebral ischemia is mediated by ERα and ERβ, and it is blocked by the estrogen receptor antagonist ICI 182 780 [36]. In contrast, Daidzein protects from excitotoxicity induced by glutamate via ERβ and GPR30 [35].

4. Alternative to the hormone replacement therapy on menopause

4.1. Clinical studies

During menopause, symptoms such as body weight changes, vaginal dryness, hot flushes, sweating, sleep disturbances and loss of bone density may occur, also cognitive disturbance, mood changes and depression episodes that lead women to a poor quality of life [43]. Symptoms could vary in intensity and in some women, they could be debilitating, particularly for those women who have a previous experience of depression and anxiety in addition to vasomotor, insomnia, weight gain and stressful life events [44].

Hormone replacement therapy (HRT) is the first line of treatment followed by the treatment with selective serotonergic reuptake inhibitors antidepressants [2, 45]. Despite their benefits and efficacy for reducing most of the discomforts of menopausal women, the long-term use of HRT has been extremely controversial because of the adverse events associated. These include an increase in the risk of stroke and venous thromboembolism, an increase in endometrial, ovarian and breast cancer, in addition to the regular side effects of HRT such as headaches, weight changes, nausea and pruritus, among others. On the other hand, it has been reported that the adverse effects depend on several factors. Randomized trials have shown that the risk of presenting adverse effects is mainly given in women older than 60 years old, women during postmenopausal and after 5 years of the continued usage of the HRT.

Other therapies including non-pharmacological interventions have been recommended such as psychotherapy to address the psychological symptoms, acupuncture, physical exercise, nutritional interventions, botanical products and folk medicine, among others [44, 46].

Nevertheless, it is increasingly common for women to prefer an alternative therapy based on the intake of therapeutic compounds of natural origin instead. The alternative therapy can be based either on the consumption of food that may provide health benefits beyond nutrition (functional food) or on the administration of compounds isolated from food (nutraceuticals) with the same purpose. In this sense, phytochemicals as phytoestrogens have received much attention because of their particular health benefits which have allowed the emergence of an alternative to HRT.

Most of the therapies used to treat menopausal symptoms have been focusedon alleviating vasomotor and night sweat complaints. One of the most popular therapies is based in the use of black cohosh [33], Valerian and St John's wort [33, 46] due to the lack of estrogenic effects.

Briefly, black cohosh (*Cimicifuga racemosa L. Synonym Actearacemosa L.*) has been used for centuries by native Americans for a variety of women's health issues [33]. It is agreed that black cohosh is not estrogenic and its mechanism of action may involve modulation of the serotonergic system in a similar manner than antidepressants [1]. This botanical product has been tested in several trials given contradictory results. Indeed, the main effects appear to be related to vasomotor and emotional symptoms [33, 47]. For example, in a multicenter randomized, double-blind, placebo-controlled, parallel group trial, the effect of several doses of black cohosh was tested taking into consideration as a primary outcome the difference in menopausal symptoms (vasomotor, psychological and somatic), assessed by the Kupperman Menopausal Index between baseline and week 12. Secondary efficacy variables were patients' self-assessments of General Quality of Life (QoL), responder rates and safety. Compared to placebo, patients receiving black cohosh showed a significant reduction in the severity of vasomotor and psychological symptoms and improved general QoL in a dose-dependent manner from baseline to endpoint [47]. In contrast, recent clinical trials have reported adverse effects of black cohosh with no significant difference from placebo for relief of hot flashes or improving QoL in Thai women [48].

The phytoestrogens mostly used with documented effects are isoflavones. These compounds obtained from different sources have been used primarily to alleviate vasomotor symptoms, but the results appear not to be consistent on mood complaints. For example, in a metaanalysis (43 randomised controlled trials with 4364 participants) that evaluate the effect of isoflavones from soy and red clover in the treatment of hot flushes and insomnia associated with menopause, no significant difference overall was reported in the incidence of hot flushes between participants taking Promensil (a red clover extract that contains isoflavone biochanin A and formononetin) and those given placebo. In this review, four trials suggested that extracts with high levels (>30 mg/d) of genistein consistently reduced the frequency of hot flushes. Some of these trials found that phytoestrogen treatments alleviated the frequency and severity of hot flushes and night sweats when compared with placebo, but many trials were small and were determined to be at high risk of bias. A strong placebo effect was noted in most trials, with a reduction in frequency ranging from 1 to 59% with placebo. Discrepant results could be related to the amount of isoflavone in the active treatment arm, the severity of vasomotor symptoms or trial quality factors [49].

Other studies tested the effect of red clover and also found controversial results. For example, a trial of 72 women randomly divided between placebo and 40 mg dried red clover daily for 12 weeks showed a significant reduction in menopausal symptoms as measured by the Menopause Rating Scale [50]. In contrast, other clinical trials have not shown a significant difference from placebo, particularly for hot flashes relief [5]. Interestingly, red clover has proestrogens, biochannin A and formonetin, which are metabolized by CYP 450 in the gut and liver in genistein and daidzein [51], suggesting more bioavailability compared with soy products. This could be a reason why the use of red clover appears to be more effective than soy in the clinical trials [52].

Kudzu (*Pueraria lobata* Willd.) Ohwi (Fabaceae) is a traditional Chinese medicine for the treatment of the symptoms of menopause [1]; the major isoflavone in kudzu is puerarin, which is metabolized to daidzein by gut microbiota. Clinical trials with kudzu reported no significant changes in the menopausal complaints compared with control group [53].

Other compounds with estrogenic activity that differ from isoflavones have been tested, for example Hop (*Humulus lupulus* L.) (Cannabaceae). Hop extracts are in some dietary supplements used for managing menopausal symptoms [54]. The most potent phytoestrogen in hops is the ERα-selective agonist 8-prenylnaringenin (8-PN), which is 100-fold more potent than the ERβ-selective isoflavones genistein and daidzein [33]. Clinical trials suggest positive results of 8-PN in reducing the symptoms of menopause [54] however due to their high affinity to ERα; it is important to evaluate the safety on the endometrium and other hormone-sensitive tissues [33].

Rhubard (*Rheum rhaponticum* L.) (Polygonaceae). Rhubard is a plant used for menopausal symptoms relief in Germany [54]. The extract from roots of rhubard mainly consists of rhaponticin and desoxyrhaponticin, which are converted to the resveratrol-like aglycones rhapontigenin and desoxyrhapontigenin by the microbiome. Rhapontigenin is more active than desoxyrhapontigenin, and it is suggested that P_{450}-catalyzed O-demethylation giving the resveratrol-catechol piceatannol might be responsible for its estrogenic activity [14, 55]. Clinical trials show that the rhubarb extract was effective and successfully decreased the Menopause Rating Scale and increased QoL [56–58].

Flaxseed (*Linum usitatissimum* L.) (Linaceae). Flaxseed is a primary source of lignans that are metabolized by the microbiota into the phytoestrogens, enterolactone and enterodiol [18]. In a randomized placebo-controlled clinical trial (90 women, 1 g/day flaxseed extract), modest but significant effects were observed in self-reporting relief of menopausal symptoms [59]. Nevertheless, a meta-analysis that included randomized clinical trials examining the efficacy of flaxseed for menopausal symptoms, concluded that there is little evidence to support the use of this dietary supplement for menopause or bone health [60].

Another product most employed in South America is maca (*Lepidium meyenii* Walp.) (Brassicaceae), it is used for hormonal balance, especially for menopausal symptoms [54]. Albeit the active phytoestrogen has not been detected, the extract of maca showed estrogenic effect increasing proliferation in MCF-7 cells. A systematic review of clinical trials concluded that evidence of the effectiveness of maca for the relief of menopausal symptoms was limited. However, because of the sample size, the number of trials and the quality of the trials, it is not pertinent to establish definite conclusions about the efficacy and safety [61].

Recently, in a placebo-controlled trial, the efficacy of resveratrol and equol supplementation was tested on menopausal women aged 50–55 years who received 200 mg of fermented soy containing 10 mg of equol and 25 mg of resveratrol (1 tablet/day) during 12 weeks. The primary outcome was the change in score on the Menopause Rating Scale, used to evaluate the severity of age-/menopause-related complaints. Additional outcomes included the Hamilton Rating Scale for Depression (HAM-D) and Nottingham Health Profile (NHP), which were used specifically to assess sleep quality. Treatment was effective to reduce Menopause Rating Scale and HAM-D scores, importantly on work and activity items and with a slight effect on anxiety-related items [62].

According to the results of meta-analyses, there is no enough clinical evidence that supports the use of phytoestrogens as HRT to alleviate all symptoms of menopause. Albeit an improvement in the quality of life is reported. An important issue to consider is the use of standardized phytoestrogens and ethnicity of the women included in the studies since these factors could be crucial to obtain a positive result for those phytoestrogens that require specific microbiota biotransformation. Promising results are derived from isoflavones and their precursor because of non-adverse effects reported. However, in all cases, more controlled-clinical trials using large samples with women of different ethnicities are required.

4.2. Preclinical studies

In contrast to the clinical studies where the phytoestrogens were evaluated mainly to prevent or alleviate the vasomotor symptoms, in preclinical data, studies were focused on the evaluation of anxious and depressive-like behaviors. Some of the phytoestrogens are considered selective estrogens receptors modulators and are derived from the metabolism of isoflavones. Importantly, most of them showed an affinity for ERβ, characteristic that may explain their effect partially as an antidepressant [63]. However, others showed an affinity for ERα or membrane receptors, making the study of their mechanism of action complex.

Early studies evaluated the effect of dietary phytoestrogens as anxiolytic-like agents [64]. The authors tested the effect of phytoestrogens in the offspring of mothers fed with a dietary soy derived phytoestrogens (600 μg/g) and found a reduction in the anxiety behavior in those animals that were maintained with soy diet when adulthood. Rodents fed with soy also showed less body weight [64]. Unfortunately, in this paper, the authors did not indicate the phytoestrogens bounded with the behavioral effect but reported high levels of equol in plasma, the more active metabolite of isoflavones found in the soy [14].

After that, several doses of a diet rich in phytoestrogens (200 or 600 ppm of phytoestrogens in diet) and equol injections (5 mg/kg) were evaluated in the forced swimming test in rats under different endocrine conditions: intact, ovariectomized and aged rats with natural ovarian failure [65]. Interestingly, the latter group resembles an animal model of "natural menopause" because rats are acyclic, and it is the only report, as far as we know, that evaluate the effect of the isoflavones under this condition. Authors showed that soy diet rich in phytoestrogens and equol produced antidepressant-like effects at the same time that induces a reduction of body weight and white adipose tissue in all endocrine conditions. After the soy-rich diet, high plasmatic levels of genistein, daidzein and equol were detected in those animals that received the highest dose [65]. Unfortunately, the authors did not evaluate anxiety-like behaviors.

In contrast, no effect or anxiogenic effect was reported after a rich isoflavone diet administration [66, 67]. It is important to mention that these data were generated in male rats instead of female rats where more information is needed. Briefly, when a soy-rich diet containing 150 μg/g total isoflavones (daidzein and genistein) was dispensed to young male Lister rats, an anxiogenic effect was reported in the elevated plus-maze and social interaction test. Diet neither affected water intake nor the weight of rats but enhanced the corticosterone and vasopressin stress-response [66], suggesting an increase in sensitivity to stress. The authors explained the apparent discrepancy between results, i.e. Lund and Lephard [64] versus Hartley et al. [66] considering timing and dose used (150 μg/g versus 600 μg/g). Other difference that could be noted is the strain of rats, Long-Evans [64] versus Lister rats [66] and the sex of the rats. The latter is an important issue since Harley et al. [66] used intact male rats, and Lund and Lephard [64] used intact male and female rats finding positive results in anxiety in females but impaired the anxious-like state in males. Further, Patisaul et al. [67]

showed that the administration of a soy-rich (600 μg/g) diet to gonadally intact male rats produced anxiogenic effects. Furthermore, authors tested high (20 mg/kg) and low (3 mg/kg) doses of equol and resveratrol (3 and 20 mg/kg) in two animal models of anxiety in intact male rats. The authors reported that these compounds did not produce any effect after 3 days of treatment and discussed the possibility that the endocrine condition that prevails in males could be a factor to explain the lack of effect [67].

Following this idea, recently it was hypothesized that the role of isoflavones in the regulation of anxiety and depressive-like behavior depends on the endocrine status [68]. To test this hypothesis, the authors evaluated the anxiolytic- and antidepressant-like effect of isoflavone-rich diet (199.4 μg/g) in ovariectomized rats exposed, or not exposed, to estradiol replacement. Data showed that anxiolytic and antidepressant-like effects depend on the endocrine state that prevails during the treatment with isoflavones. In this case, an isoflavone diet combined with estradiol restitution promotes anxiety; in contrast, the same combination promoted an antidepressant-like effect [68]. Unfortunately, authors did not show evidence about the phytoestrogens that could be responsible for the observed effect.

The isoflavone genistein has been evaluated as an antidepressant and anxiolytic compound. This phytoestrogen also showed more affinity for ERβ than ERα [69], and recent reports also suggested that it binds to ERm. Rodríguez-Landa et al. [70]) assayed several doses of this compound (0.25, 0.5 and 1.0 mg/kg, i.p.) after 4 days of administration in Wistar rats with 12-weeks after the elimination of ovaries. This model resembled a long-term period of menopause and was used to evaluate if genistein was able to induce anxiolytic-like effects as hormone replacement therapy after a long-term ovariectomy. In this study, authors showed that genistein was effective in reducing anxiety-like behavior in the black and white model after a long-term postovariectomy. Interestingly, it has been reported that E_2 is ineffective to produce behavioral effects after a long-term ovaries removal [71–73]. Therefore, the results obtained with genistein open the opportunity to use this compound as a restitution therapy. Furthermore, clinical and preclinical studies reported that genistein lacks stimulatory effects in breast and uterus [33]. Genistein also showed antidepressant-like effects in rats subjected to the forced swimming test. In this case, genistein (10 mg/kg) was administered during 14 days to ovariectomized rats and reduction of immobility behavior was observed. Data also indicated that genistein increased dopamine and restored the serotonin levels in the hippocampus at a dose of 10 mg/kg [74]. Interestingly, the effect of this compound was also tested after a subacute administration (i.e., three injections in 24 hours) and no effect was observed. This result suggested a genomic mechanism of action [74].

Another compound with estrogenic properties that has been tested is coumestrol (7,12-dihydrocoumenstan), which is considered a SERM that shows an affinity for the ERβ [69]. This compound was assayed in the forced swimming test and several models of anxiety after systemic (10 μg/kg) and intracerebral administrations (2 μg/μl/slide) to ovariectomized rats. A reduction of depressive-like and anxiety-like behavior was reported after both routes of administration [63]. As it can be noted, coumestrol is effective as an anxiolytic or antidepressant compound in ovariectomized rats; however, it is necessary to evaluate its effect in young intact and acyclic female rats to establish whether the effect of this compound remains even in the presence of ovarian secretion.

Also, secoisolariciresinol (SECO) is a lignan type phytoestrogen mainly found in flaxseed that can be metabolized to enterodiol and enterolactone. This compound was administered (5, 10 and 20 mg/kg, intragastric) during 14 days to ovariectomized mice and tested in two animal models for the screening of antidepressant drugs, the tail suspension test and the forced swimming test. The authors reported an antidepressant-like effect of SECO in both behavioral tests. Furthermore, this compound restored noradrenaline brain levels and increased dopamine and serotonin concentrations without promoting a stimulatory effect on the uterus [75]. An important difference in comparison to other protocols presented here is that SECO was administered immediately after the ovariectomy. Therefore, the restitution started before a real drop in endogenous estrogen levels, suggesting a model of perimenopause rather than a menopause model.

Phytoestrogens appear to promote anxiolytic and antidepressant-like actions in animal models. However, it can be noted that the time, the dose and endocrine state are factors that may condition the effect of these estrogenic compounds. In general, acute interventions are ineffective; most of the reports indicate that more than 3 days are necessary to observe an anxiolytic or antidepressant-like effect. For isoflavones, their effect appears to depend on the time of restitution and the endocrine state of rats. In this line, the fact that their anxiolytic-like effect is observed in ovariectomized or acyclic females but not in intact rats suggests that isoflavones are working as a restitution therapy and the levels of phytoestrogens that are bioavailable after diet administration are enough to induce changes in the respective receptors like a natural estrogen.

5. Alternative sources of phytoestrogens

5.1. *Punica granatum* L. (Lythraceae)

Pomegranate is a fruit native of Western Asia and North Africa. However, it is now cultivated in most of the Mediterranean and North America region [76]. **Table 1** shows the main phytochemicals reported for pomegranate.

Over the last decades, pomegranate and pomegranate extracts have demonstrated to possess several beneficial health effects for which it is considered a functional food. Clinical and preclinical studies have shown that pomegranate has anti-oxidant [77], anti-inflammatory, antitumorigenic, anti-microbial [78], anti-obesity [79], anti-nociceptive [80], neuroprotective [81] and antidepressant-like properties [82–84]. Interestingly, most of the health benefits of pomegranate are attributed to its high content of polyphenols, which represents the 26–30% of the total weight of the fruit [85]. The main polyphenols present in the pomegranate are ellagitannins, such as punicalagin (α and β), and flavonoids such as anthocyanidins, catechins, flavonols and isoflavones [80, 86–88]. Ellagitannins are a type of hydrolyzable tannins with several hexahydroxydiphenoyl (HHDP) groups esterified to sugar moieties. When consumed, ellagitannins are easily hydrolyzed to ellagic acid in the acidic conditions of the gastric juice because of its hydrophilic nature. Therefore, on different portions of the small and large intestine, ellagitannins are transformed by bacterial metabolism to dibenzopyranone compounds called urolithins. These compounds have recently demonstrated to possess estrogenic activity on *in-vitro* assays; this particularity makes pomegranate an excellent source of phytoestrogens [16, 22, 78, 89]. Under this premise, some

Part of the pomegranate	Phytochemicals
Whole	Ellagitannins
	Anthocyanins
	Anthocyanidins
	Catechin
	Proanthocyanidins
Seed and oil	Acid derivates
	Fatty acids
	Triglycerides
	Sterols
	Terpenoids
Peel and pericarp	Ellagitannins
	Gallotannins
	Hydroxybenzoic acids
	Proanthocyanidins
	Flavonols
Leaves	Ellagitannins
	Flavones
	Flavonols
	Flavone glycosides
	Alkaloids
	Acid hydroxybenzoic
	Triterpenoids
	Flavones

Phytochemicals found in several parts of pomegranate [79, 80, 86, 87].

Table 1. Phytochemicals found in *Punica granatum* L.

research groups have sought its therapeutic potential for the treatment of symptoms in menopause. In 2012, the therapeutic effect of a 12-week schedule of pomegranate seed oil (PGS) on menopausal symptoms was investigated with a neutral response, i.e., PGS reduced menopausal symptoms, but with no significance, authors remarked the importance of evaluating the PGS for a longer period [90]. Furthermore, a systematic review reported the effect of pomegranate juice in osteoporosis, osteoarthritis, or rheumatoid arthritis. All the studies reported positive effects of pomegranate extract or juice on osteoporosis, osteoarthritis and rheumatoid arthritis [91].

Preclinical studies have reported that the juice of pomegranate reduced menopausal symptoms in animal models by inducing antidepressant-like effects and decreasing bone loss [92].

In our laboratory, an extract of pomegranate in the elevated plus-maze for the screening of anxiolytic action and the forced swimming test for an antidepressant-like effect (unpublished results) was evaluated. This extract has a high content of ellagitannins and previously showed anti-inflammatory and antinociceptive properties [80] After 7 days of intraperitoneal administration, a reduction of anxiety-like behavior was detected and a lack of effect in the forced swimming test. The decrease of anxiety was detected at 1.0 mg/kg (see **Figure 4**). Importantly,

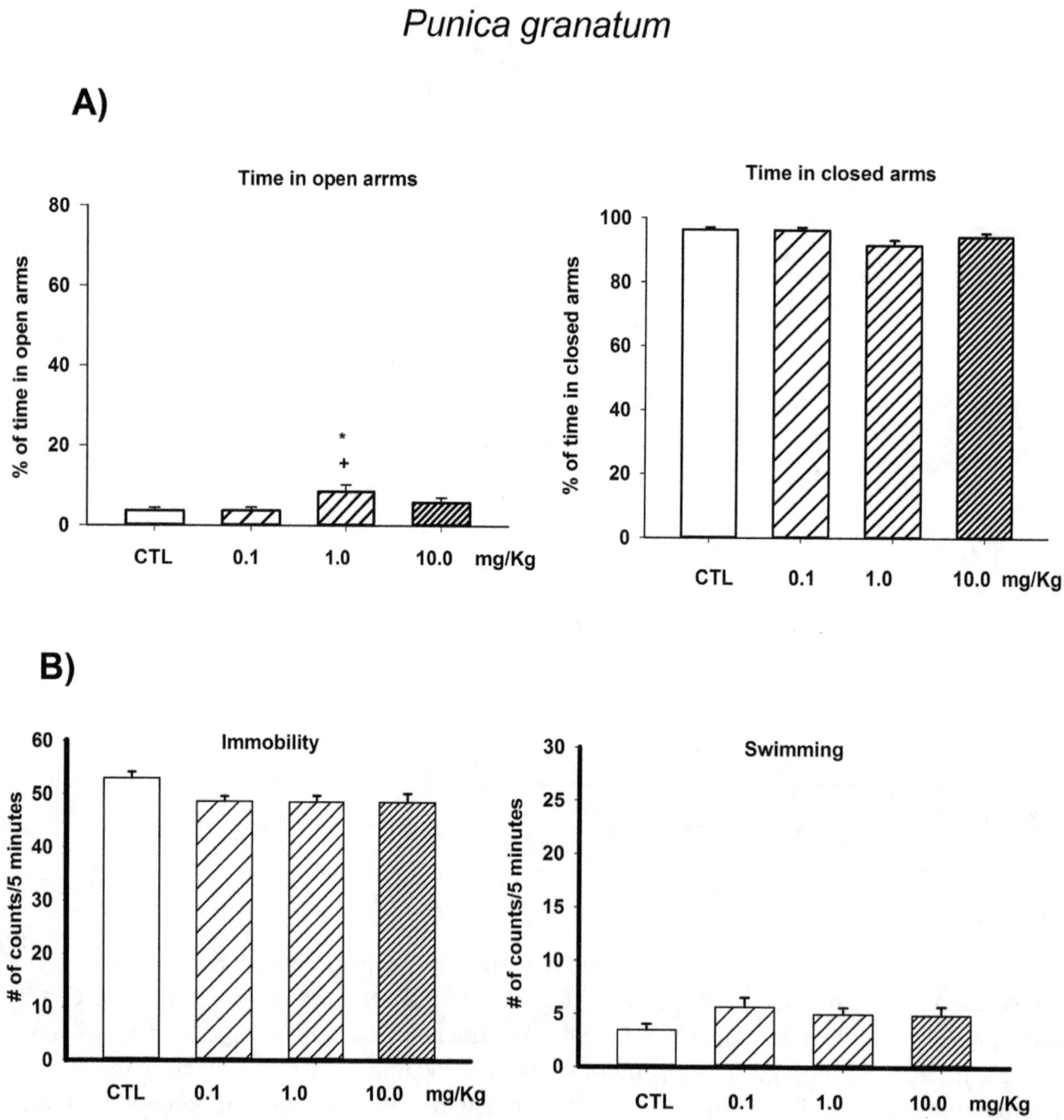

Figure 4. Effect of several doses (0.1, 1.0, 10 mg/kg, i.p) of aqueous extract of pomegranate (*Punica granatum* L.) in the elevated plus-maze (A) and the forced swimming test (panel B) after 7 days of treatment. Pomegranate extract reduced the anxiety-like behavior (panel A) but lacks antidepressant-like effect (B). Data are presented as mean ± SE of 10–12 ovariectomized rats per group. **p* < 0.05 versus control group; +*p* < 0.05 versus 0.1 mg/kg, One-way-ANOVA followed by Student-Newman Keuls test. Unpublished results.

the fact that the administration route was intraperitoneal suggests that other phytochemicals more than ellagitannins, which require of microbiota transformation, could be present in the extract. Future experiments may contribute to elucidate the phytochemical bounded in the anxiolytic effect of pomegranate.

5.2. *Brassica oleraceae* var. *italica*

Broccoli (*Brassica oleracea* var. *italica* Plenck) belongs to the Brassicaceae of cruciferous family where cabbage, brussels sprouts and radish can also be found [93]. It is native to the Anatolian peninsula and now is widely cultivated in other parts of the world. The phytochemical content of broccoli is shown in **Table 2**. As it can be seen, broccoli is also a source of important polyphenols, and consequently, phytoestrogens since in its composition, it can be detected quercetin, kaempferol, daidzein, antocyanins [93, 94], coumestans and lignans [45, 95].

Phytochemicals	Unity	Broccoli
β-Carotene	UI	318.56
Zeaxanthin	UI	22
Lutein	μg	1123.76
β-Cryptoxanthin	UI	0.88
Quercetin	mg	2.2
Kaempferol	mg	0.008
Myricetin	mg	3.5288
Daidzein	mg	0.0352
Anthocyanin	μg	0.01
Lignans	μg	0.528
Glucoiberin	μmol	145.2
Glucoraphanin	μmol	646.8
Progoitrin	μmol	80.15
Glucoalyssin	μmol	69.78
Gluconapin	μmol	22.88
Glucobrassicanapin	μmol	23.707
Gluconasturtiin	μmol	9.52
Glucobrassicin	μmol	308
Neo-glucobrassicin	μmol	84.48
Chlorophyll (A)	mg	0.88
Chlorophyll (B)	mg	0.748

Phytochemicals of Broccoli. Data are expressed as UI, mg, μg or μmol per 98 g of dried sample [96–117].

Table 2. Phytochemicals in different parts of *Brassica oleraceae*.

Broccoli is also a source of a potent anti-oxidant and anti-inflammatory compound called sulforaphane (1-isothiocyanato-4-methylsulfinylbutane) which is an organosulfur compound [118]. Several reports indicated that this compound might prevent depressive-like behavior induced by the inflammatory process. For example, acute sulforaphane at 3–30 mg/kg and glucorophanin (glucosinolate precursor of sulforaphane) in the diet were tested in male C57BL/6 mice. In this case, it was to determine whether these compounds were able to prevent the onset of depression-like behavior after an induction of inflammation by lipopolysaccharide administration [118]. In this chapter, authors also evaluate the effect of sulforaphane on brain-derived neurotrophic factor (BDNF) levels, synaptogenesis protein and dendritic spine density in the brain. The results showed that sulforaphane prevents the increase of TNF-α, IL-10 and microglia activation blocking the inflammation process at the same time that decreased the depressive-like behavior evaluated by two behavioral test. Interestingly, sulforaphane also reverses the reduction of BDNF expression and dendritic spines induced by inflammation process [118].

In another study, the effect of sulporaphane and glucorophaninwas tested on depressive-like behavior after repeated social defeat stress using Nrf2 knock-out mice. Nrf2 is a transcription factor keap-1 system that plays a role in the inflammation and evidence has shown that both peripheral and central inflammation plays a crucial role in the pathophysiology of depression [119]. The administration of diet rich in sulforaphane and glucorophanin prevented the depressive-like behavior during adulthood; further authors showed that dietary intake of SFN-rich food during juvenile stages and adolescence could confer stress resilience in adulthood [119].

Contrasting results have also been reported, for example, Balb/c mice received sulforaphane (50 mg/kg) previous to the injection of lipopolysaccharide afterward sickness behavior (an animal model of depression), and the proinflammatory response was evaluated in the hippocampus. The authors reported that sulforaphane administration prevented the induction of pro-inflammatory mediators (IL-b; IL-6, Cybb, INOS) but did not improve sickness behavior [120, 121]. Therefore, the use of sulforaphane to prevent depression-like behavior is inconclusive.

As far as we know, there is no information about the use of sulforaphane or glucorophanin in animal models of menopause. However, it has been suggested that the advantage of broccoli consumption is that some phytochemicals promote the conversion of 16-a-hydroxyestrone to 2-hydroxyestrone, the first is a carcinogenic metabolite that has been linked to breast cancer risk whereas the latter product does not exhibit estrogenic properties in breast tissue. Apparently, the ingestion of broccoli sprouts could be a good strategy for the treatment of menopause symptoms [2, 122, 123].

In our laboratory, several doses (0.1, 1.0, 10 mg/kg, i.p) of an extract of broccoli were evaluated for its anxiolytic and antidepressant-like effects after 7 days of administration to 3-week post-ovariectomized rats. The results indicated an anxiolytic—but not antidepressant-like effect (**Figure 5**, unpublished results). The phytochemical involved in this action is unknown and studies to reveal it are running.

The fact that sulforaphane exerts anti-inflammatory properties and that according to the aetiology of depression, the inflammatory process plays a major role in its aetiology, the consumption of food or nutraceuticals with sulforaphane could be suitable.

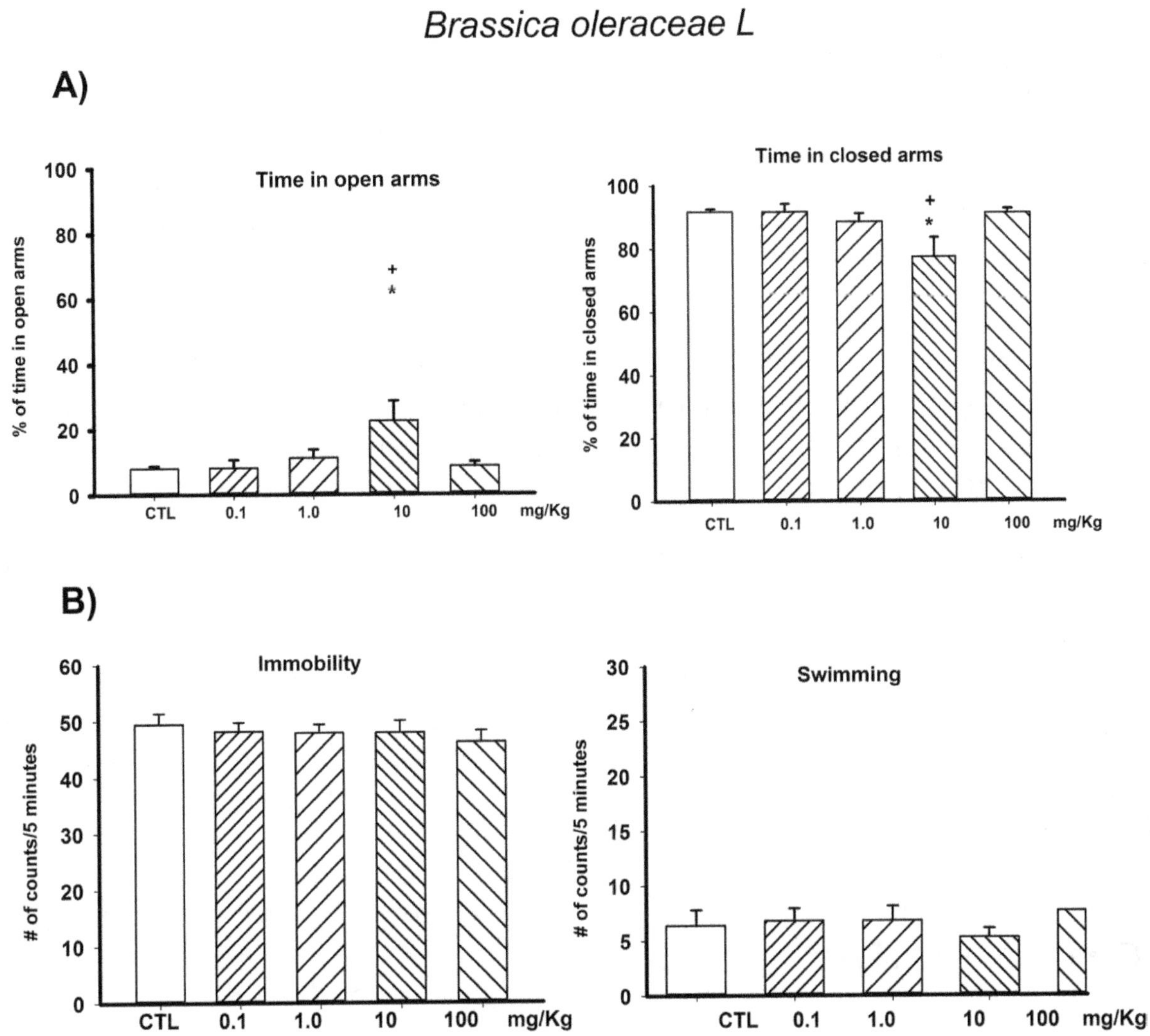

Figure 5. Effect of several doses (0.1, 1.0, 10 and 100 mg/kg, i.p) of aqueous extract of broccoli (*Brassica oleraceae* L) in the elevated plus-maze (A) and the forced swimming test (B) after 7 days of treatment. Broccoli extract reduced the anxiety-like behavior (A) but lacks antidepressant-like effect (B). Data are presented as mean ± SE of 10–12 ovariectomized rats per group. *$p < 0.05$ versus control group; +$p < 0.05$ versus 0.1 mg/kg, One way-ANOVA followed by Student-Newman Keuls test. Unpublished results.

6. Comorbidity in menopause and alternative medicine

Fibromyalgia (FM) is a chronic, generalized pain syndrome that affects the musculoskeletal system [124]. It is characterized not only by a widespread pain observed due to the presence of multiple tender points but also by depressive behavior, fatigue and sleep disturbances without any structural or inflammatory cause [125, 126]. Studies have consistently demonstrated a female predominance of this disease [127] with a major frequency in pre- and post-menopause condition supporting that an abrupt decline or a reduced time of exposure to ovarian hormones may contribute to FM [128].

Although FM is not an inflammatory disease, it is known that a neuroinflammation process can occur, which is described as an increase in the production of interleukins at the central nervous system level, such as IL-1β, IL-6, IL-8, IL-10 and TNF-α, and not at the peripheral level [129]. To date, it has not been possible to establish whether their elevated levels are associated with the painful process in FM since these have also been observed in patients with depression and sleep disorders [130]. The neuroendocrine alterations observed are usually at the level of the hypothalamic-pituitary-adrenal axis where there is hyperactivation, and it has been related to deficient levels of hormones [131] that could be part of the reasons of a major frequency in menopause [128].

As it was mentioned, anthocyanidins belong to the flavonoid group of plant-derived chemicals, which have been commonly used for the treatment of chronic diseases. One randomized clinic test was done to evaluate the efficacy of this compounds (40, 80 and 120 mg/day) in the treatment of FM compared with a placebo group. The evaluation had duration of 52 weeks with each treatment given for 12 weeks, preceded by a 4-week baseline period. Authors conclude that anthocyanidins showed small but significant benefits at a dosage of 80 mg/day in the treatment of primary FM, mainly in the sleep disturbance in the presence of minor adverse effects like indigestion or nausea [132].

Chronic fatigue syndrome is also comorbid linked to early menopause and FM since it involves the muscular, nervous, hormonal and immune systems; it is often misdiagnosed as depression [133]. Isoflavones (daidzein and genistein) were capable of reversing alterations like chronic fatigue syndrome in an experimental model in mice suggesting their protective effect in this neuroimmune-endocrine disease [134].

7. Concluding remarks

1. Clinical reports show inconsistent results about the use of phytoestrogens effectiveness to treat vasomotor and psychiatric disorders associated with menopause. The biotransformation by microbiota to deliver the main active compounds appears to be fundamental to observe positive effects.
2. Preclinical data show that the effect of phytoestrogens depends on the time of administration as well as the endocrine state of rats, suggesting that these factors could also contribute to explain the inconsistency between results observed in humans.
3. More studies are necessary to evaluate if the same phytoestrogen can induce both anxiolytic- and antidepressant-like action and if their effect depends on the endocrine state.
4. Clinical and preclinical studies indicated that the use of phytoestrogens is safe due to the high antioxidant activity. However, meta-analysis studies are inconclusive. Therefore, phytoestrogens as restitution therapy should be monitored.
5. Functional food and nutraceuticals are an important source of a wide variety of phytoestrogens.

Author details

Erika Estrada-Camarena[1*], Carolina López-Rubalcava[2], Brenda Valdés-Sustaita[2], Gabriel Sinhue Azpilcueta-Morales[1] and Eva María González-Trujano[3]

*Address all correspondence to: estrada@imp.edu.mx

1 Laboratory of Neuropsychopharmacology, Neuroscience Division, National Institute of Psychiatry "Ramón de la Fuente", Mexico, Mexico

2 Departamento de Farmacobiología, Centro de Investigación y de Estudios Avanzados del IPN, Mexico, Mexico

3 Laboratory of Neuropharmacology of Natural Products, Neuroscience Division. National Institute of Psychiatry "Ramón de la Fuente", Mexico, Mexico

References

[1] Hajirahimkhan A, Dietz BM, Bolton JL. Botanical modulation of menopausal symptoms: mechanisms of action? Planta Medica. 2013;**79**:538-553

[2] Comhaire FH, Depypere HT. Hormones, herbal preparation and nutraceuticals for better life after the menopause: Part II. Climateric. 2015;**18**:364-371

[3] Parry BL. Perimenopausal depression. The American Journal of Psychiatry. 2008;**165**: 23-27

[4] Rocca WA, Grossardt BR, Shuster LT. Oophorectomy, menopause, estrogen, and cognitive aging: The timing hypothesis. Neurodegener Ative Diseases. 2009;**7**:163-166

[5] Geller SE, Studee L. Botanical and dietary supplements for menopausal symptoms: What works, what does not. Journal of Women's Health. 2005;**14**:634-649

[6] Wildman R, Kelley M. Nutraceuticals and functional foods. In: Wildman R, editor. Handbook of Nutraceutical and Functional Foods. 2nd ed. New York: CRC Press, Taylor & Francis Group; 2006. Chapter 1

[7] American Dietetics Association. Position of the American Dietetic Association: Functional foods position statement. Journal of the American Dietetic Assocciation. 2004; **104**:814-826

[8] Gonzalez-Laredo R, Rocha-Guzmán E, Gallegos Infante JA. Fitoquímicos en los alimentos. In: Álvarez E, editor. Antioxidantes en alimentos y salud. México D.F.: Clave; 2012. pp. 133-154. Cap. 6

[9] Rodríguez EB, Flavier ME, Rodríguez-Amaya DB, Amaya-Farfán J. Phytochemicals and funcrional foods. Currem Situation and prospect for developing countries. Seguridad Alimentaria en Nutrició, Campinas. 2006;**13**:1-22

[10] Crozier AM, Clifford N, Ashihara H. Plant Secundary Metabolites. Occurrence, Structure and Role in the Human Diet. Oxford, RU: Blackwell; 2006

[11] Tsao R. Chemistry and biochemistry of dietary polyphenols. Nutrients. 2010;**2**:1231-1246

[12] Duda-Chodak A, Tarko T, Satora, P, Sroka P. Interaction of dietary compounds, especially polyphenols, with the intestinal microbiota: A review. European Journal of Nutrition. 2015;**54**:325-341

[13] Philp HA. Hot flashes—a review of the literature on alternative and complementary treatment approaches. Alternative Medicine Review. 2003;**8**:284-302

[14] Gaya P, Medina M, Sánchez-Jiménez A, Landete JM. Phytoestrogen metabolism by adult human gut microbiota. Molecules. 2016;**21**:1034. DOI: 10.339.

[15] Landete JM, Arqués J, Medina M, Gaya P, de Las Rivas B, Muñoz R. Bioactivation of phytoestrogens: Intestinal bacteria and health. Critical Review in Food Science and Nutrition. 2016;**56**:1826-1843

[16] Landete JM. Ellagitannins, ellagic acid and their derived metabolites: A review about source, metabolism, functions and health. Food Research International. 2011;**44**(5): 1150-1160

[17] Cederroth CR, Nef S. Soy, phytoestrogens and metabolism: A review. Molecular and Cellular Endocrinology. 2009;**304**:30-42

[18] Landete JM. Plant and mammalian lignans: A review of source, intake, metabolism, intestinal bacteria and health. Food Research International. 2012;**46**:410-424

[19] Setchell KDR, Brown NM, Desai PB, Zimmer-Nechimias L, Wolfe B, Jakate AS, Heubi JE. Bioavailability, disposition, and dose-response effects of soy isoflavones when consumed by healthy women at physiologically typical dietary intakes. The Journal of Nutrition. 2003;**133**(4):1027-1035

[20] Seeram NP, Aronson WJ, Zhang Y, Henning SM, Moro A, Lee RP, Sartippour M, Harris DM, Rettig M, Suchard MA, Pantuck AJ, Belldegrun A, Heber D. Pomegranate ellagitannin-derived metabolites inhibit prostate cancer growth and localize to the mouse prostate gland. Journal Agricultural and Food Chemestry. 2007;**55**:7732-7737

[21] Landete JM, Arqués J, Medina M, Gaya P, de Las Rivas B, Muñoz R. Bioactivation of phytoestrogens: Intestinal bacteria and health. Critical Reviewsin Food Scienceand Nutrition. 2015;**56**:1826-1843

[22] Larrosa M, González-Sarrías A, García-Conesa MT, Tomás-Barberán F, Espín JC. Urolithins, ellagic acid-derived metabolites produced by human colonic microflora, exhibit

estrogenic and antiestrogenic activities. Journal of Agricultural and Food Chemistry. 2006;**54**:1611-1620

[23] Watson CS, Bulayeva NN, Wozniak AL, Finnerty CC. Signaling from the membrane via membrane estrogen receptor-alpha: Estrogens, xenoestrogens, and phytoestrogens. Steroids. 2005;**70**(5-7 SPEC. ISS.):364-371

[24] Paterni I, Granchi C, Katzenellenbogen J, Minutolo F. Estrogen receptors alpha (ERα) and beta (ERβ): Subtype-selective ligands and clinical potential. Steroids. 2014;**90**:13-29

[25] Prossnitz ER, Barton M. The G-protein-coupled estrogen receptor GPER in health and disease. Nature Reviews Endocrinology. 2011;**7**:715-726

[26] Jeng YJ, Kochukov MY, Watson CS. Membrane estrogen receptor-alpha-mediated non-genomic actions of phytoestrogens in GH3/B6/F10 pituitary tumor cells. Journal of Molecular Signaling. 2009;**4**:2

[27] Díaz-Yamal I, Munévar-Vega L. Fitoestrógenos: Revisión de tema Phytoestrogens : Atopicreview. Rev. Colombiana de Obstetricia y Ginecología. 2009;**60**(3):274-281

[28] Moreira AC, Silva AM, Santos MS, Sardão VA. Phytoestrogens as alternative hormone replacement therapy in menopause: What is real, what is unknown. Journal of Steroid Biochemistry and Molecular Biology. 2014;**143**:61-71

[29] Patisau HB, Jefferson W. The pros and cons of phytoestrogens. Frontiers in Neuro-endocrinology. 2010;**31**(4):400-419. DOI: 10.1016/j.yfrne.2010.03.003.

[30] Nikov GN, Hopkins NE, Boue S, Alworth WL. Interactions of dietary estrogens with human estrogen receptors and the effect on estrogen receptor-estrogen response element complex formation. Environmental Health Perspectives. 2000;**108**(9):867-872. DOI: 10.1289/ehp.00108867

[31] Zand RS, Jenkins DJ, Diamandis EP. Steroid hormone activity of flavonoids and related compounds. Breast Cancer Research and Treatment. 2000;**62**:35-49

[32] Zava DT, Blen M, Duwe G. Estrogenic activity of natural and synthetic estrogens in human breast cancer cells in culture. Environmental Health Perspectives. 1997;**105**(Suppl):637-645. DOI: 10.1289/ehp.97105s3637

[33] Dietz BM, Hajirahimkhan A, Dunlap TL, Bolton JL. Botanicals and their bioactive phyto-chemicals for women's health. Pharmaceuticals Reviews. 2016;**68**:1026-1073

[34] Manas ES, Xu ZB, Unwalla RJ, Somers WS. Understanding the selectivity of genistein for human estrogen receptor-alpha using X-ray crystallography and computational methods. Structure. 2004;**12**:2197-2207. DOI: 10.1016/j.str.2004.09.015

[35] Kajta M, Rzemieniec J, Litwa E, Lason W, Lenartowicz M, Krzeptowski W, Wojtowicz AK. The key involvement of estrogen receptor β and G-protein-coupled receptor 30 in the neuroprotective action of daidzein. Neuroscience. 2013;**238**:345-360

[36] Saleh MC, Connell BJ, Saleh TM. Resveratrol induced neuroprotection is mediated via both estrogen receptor subtypes, ER(α) and ER(β). Neuroscience Letters. 2013;**548**:217-221

[37] Vargas KG, Milic J, Zaciragic A, Wen K, Jaspers L, Nano J, Franco OH. The functions of estrogen receptor beta in the female brain: A systematic review. Maturitas. 2016. DOI: 10.1016/j.maturitas.2016.05.014

[38] Lin AHY, Leung GPH, Leung SWS, Vanhoutte PM, Man RYK. Genistein enhances relaxation of the spontaneously hypertensive rat aorta by transactivation of epidermal growth factor receptor following binding to membrane estrogen receptors-alpha and activation of a G protein-coupled, endothelial nitric oxide synthase-dependent pathway. Pharmacological Research. 2011;**63**(3):181-189

[39] Lindsey SH, Chappell MC. Evidence that the G protein-coupled membrane receptor GPR30 contributes to the cardiovascular actions of estrogen. Gender Medicine. 2011; **8**(6):343-354

[40] Pinto Patricia I, Estevao S, Dulce M, Andrade A, Santos, Soraia P, Deborah M. Tissue responsiveness to estradiol and genistein in the sea bass liver and scale. Journal of Steroid Biochemistry and Molecular Biology. 2016;**158**:127-137. ISSN: 1879-1220

[41] Thomas P, Dong J. Binding and activation of the seven-transmembrane estrogen receptor GPR30 by environmental estrogens: A potential novel mechanism of endocrine disruption. Journal of Steroid Biochemistry and Molecular Biology. 2006;**102**(1-5 SPEC. ISS.):175-179

[42] Watson CS, Alyea RA, Cunningham KA, Jeng YJ. Estrogens of multiple classes and their role in mental health disease mechanisms. International Journal Women's Health. 2010;**2**:153-166

[43] Roberts H, Hickey M. Managing the menopause: An update. Maturitas. 2016;**86**:53-58

[44] Brando AR, Shivakumar G, Freeman M. Perimenopausal depression. Hormones, antidepressants, psychotherapy-what would you recommend? Current Psychiatry. 2008; **7**:39-50

[45] Poluzzi E, Piccinni C, Raschi E, Rampa A, Recanatini M, De Ponti F. Phytoestrogens in postmenopause: The state of the art from a chemical, pharmacological and regulatory perspective. Current Medicinal Chemistry. 2014;**21**:417-436

[46] Taylor M. Alternative medicine and the perimenopause an evidence-based review. Obstetrics & Gynecology Clinics of North America. 2002;**29**:555-573

[47] Schellenberg R, Saller R, Hess L, Melzer J, Zimmermann C, Drewe J, Zahner C. Dose-Dependent Effects of the *Cimicifuga racemosa* extract Ze 450 in the treatment of climacteric complaints: A randomized, Placebo-Controlled Study. Evidence-Based Complement Alternative Medicine. 2012;**2012**:260-301

[48] Tanmahasamut P, Vichinsartvichai P, Rattanachaiyanont M, Techatraisak K, Dangrat C, Sardod P. *Cimicifuga racemosa* extract for relieving menopausal symptoms: A randomized controlled trial. Climacteric. 2015;**18**:79-85

[49] Lethaby A, Marjoribanks J, Kronenberg F, Roberts H, Eden J, Brown J. Phytoestrogens for menopausal vasomotor symptoms. Cochrane Database of Systematic Reviews. 2013;**12**(12):CD001395

[50] Shakeri F1, Taavoni S, Goushegir A, Haghani H. Effectiveness of red clover in alleviating menopausal symptoms: A 12-week randomized, controlled trial. Climacteric. 2015; **18**:568-573

[51] Tolleson WH, Doerge DR, Churchwell MI, Marques MM, Roberts DW. Metabolism of biochanin A and formononetin by human liver microsomes in vitro. Journal of Agricultural and Food Chemistry. 2002;**50**:4783-4790

[52] Thomas AJ, Ismail R, Taylor-Swanson L, Cray L, Schnall JG, Mitchell ES, Woods NF. Effects of isoflavones and amino acid therapies for hot flashes and co-occurring symptoms during the menopausal transition and early postmenopause: A systematic review. Maturitas. 2014;78:263-276

[53] Ulbricht C, Bryan JK, Costa D, Culwell S, Giese N, Isaac R, Nummy K, Pham T, Rapp C, Rusie E, Weissner W, Windsor RC, Woods J, Zhou S. An Evidence-Based systematic review of Goji (*Lycium* spp.) by the natural standard research collaboration. Journal of Dietary Supplements. 2015;**12**:184-240

[54] Taylor M. Complementary and alternative approaches to menopause. Endocrinology Metabolism Clinics of North America. 2015;**44**:619-648

[55] Wober J, Möller F, Richter T, Unger C, Weigt C, Jandausch A, Zierau O, Rettenberger R, Kaszkin-Bettag M, Vollmer G. Activation of estrogen receptor-beta by a special extract of *Rheum rhaponticum* (ERr 731), its aglycones and structurally related compounds. Journal of Steroid Biochemistry and Molecular Biology. 2007;**107**:191-201

[56] Heger M, Ventskovskiy BM, Borzenko I, Kneis KC, Rettenberger R, Kaszkin-Bettag M, Heger PW. Efficacy and safety of a special extract of *Rheum rhaponticum* (ERr 731) in perimenopausal women with climacteric complaints: A 12-week randomized, double-blind, placebo-controlled trial. Menopause. 2006;**13**:744-759

[57] Kaszkin-Bettag M, Beck S, Richardson A, Heger PW, Beer AM. Efficacy of the special extractERr 731 from *Rhapontic rhubarb* for menopausal complaints: A 6-month open observational study. Alternative Therapies in Health Medicine. 2008;**14**:32-38

[58] Hasper I, Ventskovskiy BM, Rettenberger R, Heger PW, Riley DS, Kaszkin-Bettag M. Long-term efficacy and safety of the special extract ERr 731 of *Rheum rhaponticum* in perimenopausal women with menopausal symptoms. Menopause. 2009;**16**:117-131

[59] Colli MC, Bracht A, Soares AA, de Oliveira AL, Bôer CG, de Souza CG, Peralta RM. Evaluation of the efficacy of flaxseed meal and flaxseed extract in reducing menopausal symptoms. Journal of Medicine Food. 2012;**15**:840-845

[60] Dew TP, Williamson G. Controlled flax interventions for the improvement of menopausal symptoms and postmenopausal bone health: A systematic review. Menopause. 2013;**20**:1207-1215

[61] Lee MS, Shin BC, Yang EJ, Lim HJ, Ernst E. Maca (Lepidium meyenii) for treatment of menopausal symptoms: A systematic review. Maturitas. 2011;**70**:227-233

[62] Davinelli S, Scapagnini G, Marzatico F, Nobile V, Ferrara N, Corbi G. Influence of equol and resveratrol supplementation on health-related quality of life in menopausal women: A randomized, placebo-controlled study. Maturitas. 2017;**96**:77-83

[63] Walf AA, Rhodes ME, Frye CA. Antidepressant effects of ERbeta-selective estrogen receptor modulators in the forced swim test. Pharmacology Biochemistry and Behavior. 2004;**78**:523-529

[64] Lund TD, Lephart ED. Dietary soy phytoestrogens produce anxiolytic effects in the elevated plus-maze. Behavioural Brain Research. 2001;**913**:180-184

[65] Blake C, Fabick KM, Setchell KD, Lund TD, Lephart ED. Neuromodulation by soy diets or equol: Anti-depressive & anti-obesity-like influences, age- & hormone-dependent effects. BMC Neuroscience. 2011;**16**:12-28

[66] Hartley DE, Edwards JE, Spiller CE, Alom N, Tucci S, Seth P, Forsling ML, File SE. The soy isoflavone content of rat diet can increase anxiety and stress hormone release in the male rat. Psychopharmacology (Berl). 2003;**167**:46-53

[67] Patisaul HB, Burke KT, Hinkle RE, Adewale HB, Shea D. Systemic administration of diarylpropionitrile (DPN) or phytoestrogens does not affect anxiety-related behaviors in gonadally intact male rats. Hormones and Behavior. 2009;**55**:319-328

[68] Russell AL, Grimes JM, Larco DO, Cruthirds DF, Westerfield J, Wooten L, Keil M, Weiser MJ, Landauer MR, Handa RJ, Wu TJ. The interaction of dietary isoflavones and estradiol replacement on behavior and brain-derived neurotrophic factor in the ovariectomized rat. Neuroscience Letters. 2017;**640**:53-59

[69] Kuiper GG, Gustafsson JA. The novel estrogen receptor-beta subtype: Potential role in the cell- and promoter-specific actions of estrogens and anti-estrogens. FEBS Letters. 1997;**410**:87-90

[70] Rodríguez-Landa JF, Hernández-Figueroa JD, Hernández-Calderón BC, Saavedra M. Anxiolytic-like effect of phytoestrogen genistein in rats with long-term absence of ovarian hormones in the black and white model. Progress in Neuropsychopharmacology & Biological Psychiatry. 2009;**33**:367-372

[71] Estrada-Camarena E, Lopez-Rubalcava C, Hernandez-Aragon A, Mejia-Mauries S, Picazo O. Long-term ovariectomy modulates the antidepressant-like action of estrogens, but not of antidepressants. Journal of Psychopharmacology. 2011;**25**:1365-1377

[72] De Chaves G, Moretti M, Castro AA, Dagostin W, et al. Effects of long term ovariectomy on anxiety and behavioral despair in rats. Physiology & Behavior. 2009;**97**:420-425

[73] Walf AA, Frye CA. Administration of estrogen receptor beta-specific selective estrogen receptor modulators to the hippocampus decrease anxiety and depressive behavior of ovariectomized rats. Pharmacology Biochemistry and Behavior. 2007;**86**:407-414

[74] Kageyama A, Sakakibara H, Zhou W, Yoshioka M, Ohsumi M, Shimoi K, Yokogoshi H. Genistein regulated serotonergic activity in the hippocampus of ovariectomized rats under forced swimming stress. Bioscience, Biotechnology, and Biochemistry. 2010; **74**:2005-2010

[75] Wang YF, Xu ZK, Yang DH, Yao HY, Ku BS, Ma XQ, Wang CZ, Liu SL, Cai SQ. The anti-depressant of secoisolariciresinol, a lignan- type phytoestrogen constitutent of flagseed on ovariectomized mice. Journal of Natural Medicines. 2013;**67**:222-227

[76] Bhandari P. Pomegranate (*Punica granatum L*). Ancient seeds for modern cure? Review of potential therapeutic applications. International Journal of Nutrition, Pharmacology, Neurological Disease. 2012;**2**:171-184

[77] Zhang L, Fu Q, Zhang Y. Composition of anthocyanins in pomegranate flowers and their antioxidant activity. Food Chemistry. 2011;**127**(4):1444-1449. DOI: 10.1016/j.foodchem.2011.01.077

[78] Lipińska L, Klewicka E, Sójka M. Structure, occurrence and biological activity of ella-gitannins: A general review. Acta Scientiarum Polonorum, Technologia Alimentaria. 2014;**13**(3):289-299

[79] Al-Muammar MN, Khan F. Obesity: The preventive role of the pomegranate (*Punica granatum*). Nutrition. 2012;**28**(6):595-604

[80] González-Trujano ME, Pellicer F, Mena P, Moreno DA, García-Viguera C. Antinociceptive and anti-inflammatory activities of a pomegranate (*Punica granatum L.*) extract rich in ellagitannins. International Journal of Food Sciences and Nutrition. 2015;**7486**(June 2016):1-5

[81] Yuan T, Ma H, Liu, W, Niesen DB, Shah N, Crews R, Seeram NP. Pomegranate's neuro-protective effects against alzheimer's disease are mediated by urolithins, its Ellagitannin-Gut microbial derived metabolites. ACS Chemical Neuroscience. 2016;**7**:26-33

[82] Naveen S, Siddalingaswamy M, Singsit D, Khanum F. Anti-depressive effect of poly-phenols and omega-3 fatty acid from pomegranate peel and flax seed in mice exposed to chronic mild stress. Psychiatric and Clinical Neurosciences. 2013;**67**:501-508

[83] Abdul RS, Abdul KB, Hidayat BMT, Mohd MMA. Antidepressant-like effect of methanolic extract of *Punica granatum* (pomegranate) in mice model of depression. Journal of Natural Products and Biomedical Research. 2015;**1**:16-20

[84] Shastry R, Sharma A, Sayeli V, Sheetal D. Screening of antidepressant activity of *Punica granatum* in mice. Journal Pharmacognosy. 2017;**9**(1):27-29

[85] Díaz MAG. Calidad nutracéutica de extractos de granada dulce y ácida y bioaccesibilidad de sus compuestos fenólicos en un modelo in vivo. PhD Proposal. 2014;**1**

[86] Choi DW, Kim JY, Choi SH, Jung HS, Kim HJ, Cho SY, Chang SY. Identification of steroid hormones in pomegranate (*Punica granatum*) using HPLC and GC–mass spectrometry. Food Chemistry. 2006;**96**:562-571

[87] Middha SK, Usha T, Pande V. HPLC evaluation of phenolic profile, nutritive content, and antioxidant capacity of extracts obtained from *Punica granatum* fruit peel. Advances in Pharmacological Sciences. 2013;**2013**:296236

[88] Van Elswijk D, Schobel UP, Lansky EP, Irth H, Van der Greef J. Rapid dereplication of estrogenic compounds in pomegranate (*Punica granatum*) using on-line biochemical detection coupled to mass spectrometry. Phytochemistry. 2004;**65**:233-241

[89] Espín JC. Biological significance of the gut microbial ellagic acid-derived metabolites urolithins. JournalHindawi. 2013; **2013**: 1-16

[90] Auerbach L, Rakus J, Bauer C, Gerner C, Ullmann, R, Wilmmer H, Huber J. Pomegranate seed oil in women with menopausal symptoms: A prospective randomized, placebo-controlled, double blinded trial. Menopause. 2012;**19**(4):426-432

[91] Shuid AN, Mohamed IN. Pomegranate use to attenuate bone loss in major musculoskeletal diseases: An evidence-based review. Current Drug Targets. 2013;**14**:1565-1578

[92] Mori-Okamoto J, Otawara-Hamamoto Y, Yamato H, Yoshimura H. Pomegranate extract improves a depressive state and bone properties in menopausal syndrome model ovariectomized mice. Journal of Ethnopharmacology. 2004;**92**:93-101

[93] Rodríguez M. Respuestas fisológicas moleculares y fitoquímicas de variedades *de Brassica oleracea* (grupo itálica) sometidas a estrés abiótico [Tesis recepcional de Doctorado]. España: Universidad de Murcia; 2013

[94] Álvarez PE, de la Rosa LA, González-Aguilar GA, Ayala-Zavala JF. Antioxidantes en alimentos y salud. México: Clave Editorial; 2012. pp. 97-289

[95] Klejin MJ, Van Der YT, Wilson PW, Adlerercreutz H, Mazur W, Grobbe DE, Jacques PF. Intake of dietary phytoestrogens is low postmenopausal women in the United States: The Framingham Study (1-4). Journal of Nutrition. 2001;**131**:1826-1832

[96] Nardini MD' Aquino N, Tomassi G, Gentili V, Di Felice M, Scaccini C. Inhibition of human Low-Density lipoprotein oxidation by Caffeic acid and other hydroxycinnamic acid derivatives. Journal Free Radical Biology & Medicine. 1995;**19**(5):541-552

[97] Rodríguez-Amaya D. Estructuras y características de las Xantofilas comunes en los alimentos. En Carotenoides y preparación de alimentos: Retención de los Carotenoides, Provitamina A en los alimentos preparados, procesados y almacenados. Health and Nutrition. 1999; **1**:3-7

[98] Troxler J. Brócoli. Food and Drug Protection. 2001; **303**: 1-35

[99] Fernández-León MF, Fernández León AM, Lozano M, Ayuso MC, González Gómez D. Identificación y cuantificación de glucosinolatos intactos en dos cultivares de brócoli cultivados en las Vegas Bajas del Guadiana (Extremadura). Actas de Horniticultura. 2012;**60**:767-771

[100] Fernández M. Evolución de los parámetros de calidad físico-química y funcional de distintas Brassicas sometidas a diferentes tratamientos postcosecha. Doctorado. Universidad de Extramadura; 2012

[101] Verkerk R, Dekker M, Wim Jongen MF. Post-harvest increase of indolyl glucosinolates in response to chopping and storage of vegetables. Journal of the Science of Food and Agriculture. 2001;**81**:953-958

[102] Shaban H, Richter C. A2E and blue light in the retina: The paradigm of age-related macular degeneration. The Journal of Biological Chemistry. 2002;**383**(3-4):537-545

[103] Martínez A. Carotenoides distribución y estado natural. Doctorado. Universidad de Antioquia; 2003

[104] Vallejo F, Tomás-Barberán F, García-Viguera C. Health-Promoting Compounds in Broccoli as influenced by refrigerated transport and retail sale period. Journal of Agricultural and-FoodChemistry. 2012; **51**: 3029-3034

[105] Young S, Milner JA. Targets for indole-3carbinol in cancer prevention. Journal of Nutritional Biochemistry. 2005;**16**:65-73

[106] Gallardo C, Jiménez L, García-Conesa MT. Hydroxycinnamic acid composition and in vitro antioxidant activity of selected grain fractions. Journal Food Chemistry. 2006; **99**:455-463

[107] Meléndez-Martínez AJ, Vicario IM. Pigmentos carotenoides: Consideraciones estructurales y fisicoquímicas. Archivos Latinoamericanos de Nutrición. 2007;**57**:112-116

[108] Alquézar B. Caracterización bioquímica y molecular de la carotenogénesis en frutos cítricos. Doctorado. Universidad de Valencia; 2007

[109] Ludueña B. Mastandrea C, Chichizola C, Franconi MC. Isoflavonas en soja, contenido de Daidzeína y Genisteína y su importancia biológica. Red de Revistas Cientificas de América Latina, el Caribe, España y Portugal. 2007;**71**:56-66

[110] Begoña A. Efecto de "nuevos" nutrientes sobre la retina y la función visual. Revista de Nutrición Práctica. 2008;**12**:64-69

[111] Bhagwat S, Haytowitz DB, Holden JM. USDA Database for the Isoflavone content of Selected Foods. Vol. 15. Maryland: US Department of Agriculture; 2008. pp. 43-49

[112] Márques A. Mejora genética en glucosinolatos en semillas de mostaza etíope (*Brassica carinata A. Braun*). Doctorado. Universidad de Córdoba; 2008

[113] Mataíx J. Rodríguez-Navarrete J. Tratado de Nutrición y Alimentación. Alimentos funcionales. 4th ed. Barcelona: OCEANO/ ergon (ed); 2009. Chapter 20

[114] Kim DH, Jung HA, Park SJ, kim JM, Lee S, Choi JS, Cheong JH, Ko KH, Ryu JH. The effects of Daidzin and its aglycon, Daidzein, on the Scopolamine induced Memory Impairment in Male Mice. Archives of Pharmacal Research. 2010;**33**(10):1685-1690

[115] Navarro-Cruz AR, Vera-López O, Muñoz-Bedolla M, Melgoza-Palma N, Lazcano-Hernández M, Gómez CrisostomoMR, Romero Vázquez M. Estudio de la concentración de quercetina en las variedades de manzana (*Malus domestica*) Fuji, red delicius y delicia. Red de Revistas Cientificas de América Latina, el Caribe, España y Portugal. 2010;**25**:901-910

[116] Naso L, Lezama L, Rojo T, González Baró AC, Williams-Patricia AM, Ferrer EG. Efectos antioxidantes del ácido clorogénico y su complejo con el catión oxovanadio. Journal Spectroscopy Letters. 2010;**64**:1-7

[117] Aguilera-Ortíz M, Reza-Vargas MC, CHew-Madinaveitia RG, Meza-Velázquez JA. Propiedades funcionales de las antocianinas. Revista de Ciencias Biológicas y de la Salud. 2011;**12**:16-22

[118] Zhang JC, Yao W, Dong C, Yang C, Ren Q1, Ma M, Han M, Wu J, Ushida Y, Suganuma H, Hashimoto K. Prophylactic effects of sulforaphane on depression-like behavior and dendritic changes in mice after inflammation. The Journal of Nutritional Biochemistry. 2017;**39**:134-144

[119] Yao W, Zhang JC, Ishima T, Dong C, Yang C, Ren Q, Ma M, Han M, Wu J, Suganuma H, Ushida Y, Yamamoto M, Hashimoto K. Role of Keap1-Nrf2 signaling in depression and dietary intake of glucoraphanin confers stress resilience in mice. Scientific Reports. 2016;**6**:306-359

[120] Townsend BE, Johnson RW. Sulforaphane reduces lipopolysaccharide-induced proinflammatory markers in hippocampus and liver but does not improve sickness behavior. Nutritional Neuroscience. 2017;**20**:195-202

[121] Townsend BE, Chen YJ, Jeffery EH, Johnson RW. Dietary broccoli mildly improves neuroinflammation in aged mice but does not reduce lipopolysaccharide-induced sickness behavior. Nutrition Research. 2014;**34**:990-999

[122] Fowke JH, Longcope C, Hebert JR. *Brassica* vegetable consumption shifts estrogen metabolism in healthy postmenopausal women. Cancer Epidemiology, Biomarkers & Prevention. 2000;**9**:773-779

[123] Ambrosone CB, McCann SE, Freudenheim JL, Marshall JR, Zhang Y, Shields PG. Breast cancer risk in premenopausal women is inversely associated with consumption of broccoli, a source of isothiocyanates, but is not modified by GST genotype. Journal of Nutrition. 2004;**134**:1134-1138

[124] Mease P. Fibromyalgia syndrome: Review of clinical presentation, pathogenesis, outcome measures, and treatment. The Journal Rheumatology. 2005;**75**:6-21

[125] Roizenblatt S, Moldofsky H, Benedito-Silva AA, Tufik S. Alpha sleep characteristics in fibromyalgia. Arthritis & Rheumatologym. 2001;**44**:222-230

[126] Arnold LM, Hudson JI, Keck PE, Auchenbach MB, Javaras KN, Hess EV. Comorbidity of fibromyalgia and psychiatric disorders. The Journal of Clinical Psychyatry. 2006; **67**:1219-1225

[127] Clauw DJ. Fibromyalgia: A clinical review. The Journal of the American Medical Association. 2014;**311**:1547-1555

[128] Martínez-Jauand M, Sitges C, Femenia J, Cifre I, González S, Chialvo D, Montoya P. Age-of-onset of menopause is associated with enhanced painful and non-painful sensitivity in fibromyalgia. Jounal of Clinical Rheumatology. 2013;**32**:975-981

[129] Kadetoff D, Lampa J, Westman M , Andersson M, Kosek E. Evidence of central inflammation in fibromyalgia-increased cerebrospinal fluid interleukin-8 levels. Journal of Neuroimmunology. 2012;**242**:33-38

[130] Prados G, Miro E. Fibromyalgia and sleep: A review. Revista De Neurologia. 2012;**54**: 227-240

[131] Cuatrecasas G, Gonzalez MJ, Alegre C, Sesmilo G, Fernandez-Sola J, Casanueva FF, Garcia-Fructuoso F, Poca-Dias V, Izquierdo JP, Puig-Domingo M. High prevalence of growth hormone deficiency in severe fibromyalgia syndromes. The Journal of Clinical Endocrinology & Metabolism. 2010;**95**:4331-4337

[132] Edwards AM, Blackburn L, Christie S, Townsend S, David J. Food supplement in the treatment of primary fibromyalgia: A double blind, cross over trial of anthocyanidins and placebo. Journal of Nutritional & Environmental Medicine. 2000;**10**:189-199

[133] Griffith MP, Zarrouf FA. A systematic review of chronic fatigue syndrome: Don´t assume it´s depression. Primary Care Companion to the Journal of Clinical Psychiatry. 2008;**10**:120-128

[134] Vasiadi M, Newman J, Theoharides TC. Isoflavones inhibit poly(I:C)-induced serum, brain, and skin inflammatory mediators—relevance to chronic fatigue syndrome. Journal of Neuroinflammation. 2014;**11**:1-12

10

Regulation of Ovarian-Menstrual Cycle as a Systemic Problem of Physiology of Humans

Olena Lutsenko

1. Introduction

One of the main manifestations of the vital activity of the female body is the menstrual cycle, which begins during puberty and has a rhythmic (monthly) character.

Endocrine relationships in the hypothalamic-pituitary-ovarian system are formed throughout the period of puberty. This process is regulated by certain neuroendocrine processes, which have different activities depending on age. The determinants of this regulation are the hypothalamus, pituitary gland, gonads, thyroid gland, and adrenal cortex; therefore, a certain interest is the study of the peculiarities of the formation of the hypothalamic-pituitary-ovarian hormonal system.

Back in the late nineteenth century, leading scholars D. O. Ott, S. S. Zikharev, and A. V. Reperov found that menstrual cycle is not a local process, but a wavelike reaction of the organism associated with changes in the system of the hypothalamus-pituitary-ovaries-uterus, which appears from the outside of uterine bleeding. These changes in vital processes in the body of women were called "menstrual wave" [1, 2].

So, the normal menstrual cycle is a finely coordinated cyclic process of stimulating and inhibiting effects that lead to the release of one mature egg. Various factors involved in the regulation of this process, including hormones, paracrine, and autocrine factors, are identified so far [3].

The regulation of the menstrual function passes through a complex neurohumoral path [4–6]. According to modern concepts [7–9], cyclic changes in the body of a woman are related to the implementation menstrual function and occur with the obligatory participation of five levels (or levels) of regulation. Each of them is regulated by the structures located above according to the mechanism of feedback.

The levels (links) of regulating the menstrual (reproductive) function:

1. the cerebral cortex is a cerebral structure;
2. hypothalamus-subcortical centers;
3. pituitary gland-brain application;
4. ovaries-gonads; and
5. uterus-organ-target.

Nowadays, leading scientists insist that the multilateral morphological features are closely related to the functional manifestations of sexual dimorphism [10, 11], which, in its turn, causes the sexual specificity of the processes of adaptation of the organism to external influences and, in particular, to physical activity. For women, the role of estrogen and progestogens is predominant, and for men, androgens. The degree of saturation of the body by sex hormones determines their biological effect [12–16].

Estrogens are an important link in the chain of adaptive-trophic reactions in the body [17, 18]; they have an anabolic effect but are slightly weaker than androgens, determine the degree and nature of the distribution of fatty tissue by female type, increase the growth of pelvic bones, create a female type of body proportions [19, 20], contribute to the closure of epiphyseal bone growth zones, and hinder the development of osteoporosis (resorption of bone tissue). Estrogens suppress erythropoiesis (red blood cells), reduce thrombocytopenia, promote growth of shock and minute volume of the heart, increase cardiac output, increase the volume of circulating blood, and have a positive effect on myocardial tropism and vascular tone [21, 22].

Progesterone, like estrogens, increases systolic and temporal volumes of blood and the frequency of heart contractions. Progesterone has a sodium diuretic effect and reduces the peripheral resistance of the blood vessels, which contributes to lowering blood pressure [23, 24].

Estrogens cause narrowing of the lumen of bronchioles by increasing the release of histamine and serotonin, increasing pulmonary resistance. Its direct effect increases the excitability of the respiratory center; improves the patency of bronchioles by increasing their lumen; decreases the overall pulmonary resistance; as a consequence, increases alveolar ventilation; and decreases the tone of the respiratory muscles [18, 25].

The change in the balance of steroid hormones, in particular the deficiency of progesterone and the excess of estrogens involved in the regulation of water-salt metabolism, increases reabsorption (reabsorption) of sodium in the kidneys while increasing osmotic pressure. As a result, in order to maintain homeostasis, the water is delayed in the body to compensate for the homeostasis, and, as a consequence, the body weight increases in the premenstrual and menstrual phases of the cycle. Scientists have established the influence of sex hormones on the emotional state of women [22, 26]. All of the above suggests that reproductive and exogenital functional systems are closely interrelated, and the reproductive system, in turn, has a different effect on the organs and tissues of other functional systems, which correlates the adaptation, resistance, and reactivity of the female body. In recent years, the distribution and extension theory has intensified, according to which the influence of sex steroids to one degree or another extends to the functional state of all organs and systems [10, 27, 28].

The functional state of the cardiovascular system in women has a number of features due to hormonal changes that accompany the menstrual cycle [29]. In recent years, the study of the role of estrogens and progestogens in the regulation of the function of the cardiovascular system [30].

The increased resistance of women in comparison with men to cardiovascular diseases is associated with the dynamics of cardiodynamics parameters in stressed women [23], which is determined by the sexual characteristics of the nervous and humoral regulation of the cardiovascular system. During stress, more catecholamines are released in the female body [31, 32], and their influence on the heart rhythm becomes more pronounced, but pressor responses are less prolonged than in men, which suggests that the control of the sympathetic adrenal system is more effective in the female body [33]. The factors limiting its activity include the presence of estrogens, which enhance the tone of the parasympathetic nervous system and reduce sympathetic effects on the cardiovascular system. The influence of estrogens on the vegetative level of regulation, along with their peripheral effects on the heart and blood vessels, is the basis of cardioprotective properties of estrogens. Information on the influence of androgens on the cardiovascular system and the mechanisms of its regulation are few and contradictory. Testosterone contributes to the development of hypertension and has an atherogenic effect [34]. At the same time, testosterone improves coronary blood flow in coronary arteries [35] and positively affects the mechanical function of the heart by activating the expression of heavy α chains of myosin [36]. Sexual features in cardiovascular stress reactivity are largely due to differences in the autonomic regulation of the cardiovascular system in the female and male body. Investigation of the mechanisms that determine the differences in the activity of the autonomic nervous system departments convinces in the need to study the role of sex hormones. The scarcity and contradictory nature of research data on the role of autonomic regulation of the cardiovascular system in the female and male organisms, as well as the influence of sex hormones on the autonomic balance, justify the carrying out of complex studies of the revealed phenomenon [37, 38].

Significant are the effective attempts to decipher the mechanism of the influence of sex hormones on the central nervous system that are highlighted in the works of well-known scientists [33]. The beginning of puberty is marked by a significant increase in the threshold of the sexual centers of the central nervous system (gonadostat) to steroids in the feedback system, which was first noticed by Hohlweg and Dohin (1932) and then Donovan and van der Werff Ten Bosch (1965) [38]. Further animal studies and human observation fully confirmed this assumption. The enhancement of the inhibitory effect of sex steroids on the hypothalamus has been linked with a change in the puberty of the spectrum of sex hormones—the shift in the ratio of estrogen to testosterone in favor of the latter, which is allegedly less effective in suppressing the production of gonadotropins. However, this is unlikely.

The scientific assumptions about the importance of changing the metabolism of testosterone and other androgens during puberty have been supported. So, in an experiment in many species of animals, it was discovered and demonstrated that the metabolic activity of the liver and kidneys, aimed at inactivating androgens, increases with age. Small amounts of sex hormones produced by gonads of immature animals give a more pronounced inhibitory effect due to the fact that in adult animals the inactivation of hormones is more pronounced [38]. However, this hypothesis was subjected to devastating criticism, as the androgenic effect on other target organs during puberty does not decrease but increases.

An important role in the onset of puberty may be played by not only inhibiting but also stimulating effects of sex hormones, in particular estrogens. We have convincing evidence of the leading role of estrogens in the formation of systems of the hypothalamic neurons responsible for regulating the gonadotropic function of the pituitary gland. This process begins during the period of sexual differentiation of the hypothalamus, but its final stage falls on the puberty period. It has been experimentally shown that the administration of small doses of sex hormones can cause premature puberty. Although the role of estrogens is particularly significant in the formation of pubertal in girls, however, in boys, estrogens are also an effective stimulator for secretion of gonadotropin and gonadotropins, since central nervous structures do not lose their ability to respond to the stimulating effect of estrogens during sexual differentiation [33].

During the menstrual cycle, there are significant changes in the hypothalamic-pituitary system and in the body as a whole. Cyclical changes in the structures of the hypothalamus and in the anterior lobe of the pituitary gland regulate all processes that ensure the reproductive function of the woman.

Fluctuations in mental processes and functional state during the menstrual cycle have been proven by many researchers, and the association of these oscillations with the nature of secretion of sex hormones is evident. These changes were detected in the attitude of emotional and motivational behavior [39], the electrical activity of the cerebral cortex [23, 40], the autonomic tone [41], the activity of the cerebral hemispheres [42], and the physical and mental performance [80].

However, the clear dependence of the change in the psycho-functional state, depending on the phases of the menstrual cycle, cannot be identified, and the results of the research are mainly controversial (especially concerning the premenstrual and menstrual phases). Thus, the follicular phase is considered by most researchers as a period of high mental and physical working capacity. As for the phase of ovulation, as a period of poor performance, researchers have quite controversial thoughts. At the same time, some scholars tend to believe that the menstrual cycle does not affect the psycho-functional state of the woman [43], and there are those who record a significant deterioration or improvement [26] of mental and physical performance in the premenstrual and menstrual periods.

Investigating the indicators of the functional state of the soccer players in various phases of the ovarian menstrual cycle, Buzzin VR (2009) [44] concluded that the dependence of the level of physical performance in the first phase of CMC depends mainly on the state of central hemodynamics, in stages II and V (from repolarization of the ventricles), in the IV phase (the state of the atrium), and in the III phase (from the general state of the organism). Body mass swims on the studied indicators of the body of soccer players throughout the entire biological cycle. Given that it is an integral indicator of the general state of the organism, the data obtained can be evidenced by the fact that the pursuit of football contributes to the coherence in the activity of the studied systems of the body of athletes. Perhaps, this is due to the individual nature of the body's response to the fluctuations of sex hormones during the menstrual cycle, depending on many variables of psychophysiological factors, mediating the influence of hormones on the central nervous system and higher nervous activity.

The factors that may affect the condition of women in the premenstrual phase include age, type of constitution, level of health, and typological peculiarities of higher nervous activity. Confirmation of the influence of the identified factors can be, in particular, significant differences in the level of sex hormones between people with different typological peculiarities: type of constitution [12], functional asymmetry [23], temperament [45], as well as differences between adolescent and adolescent girls [41].

The study of Naumova [71] illustrates the different effects of the phases of the ovarian-menstrual cycle on the psychomotor quality and properties of the nervous system of women. The author measured these indices during the premenstrual phase (1–3 days before menission), the menstrual phase (1–2 days), and the postmenstrual phase (1–2 days) during the 3-month period. The obtained data were compared with each other and with the background (from the beginning of menstruation on the 10th–12th day). The premenstrual phase is characterized by deterioration of psychomotor performance. Compared with the background (the period between menstruations), muscle strength and maximum frequency of movements decreased much more often than they increased. Endurance in relation to static forces varied slightly during this period and in the direction of increase [47, 48].

The menstrual phase is characterized by an increase in the muscle strength of the majority of the girls studied (but only to the background level) and the maximum frequency of movements (excess of the background level), but the endurance is somewhat reduced. At the same time, the second component of endurance attracts attention—maintaining the effort against the background of increasing fatigue [46–49]. The postmenstrual phase was accompanied by a variety of changes in the studied parameters. The maximum frequency of movements increases even more, and muscle strength and endurance are greatly reduced.

In the premenstrual phase, the mobility of the nervous processes has increased. These changes indicate an increase in the emotional and motor reactivity of women in the premenstrual phase, which corresponds to the findings of the researchers in the literature on increasing the irritability of women before menstruation [50, 51]. It is explained by the fact that thyroid gland swelling is observed in the premenstrual phase of CMC and there are symptoms of thyrotoxicosis, that is, increased production of thyroid hormones [52]. In the postmenstrual phase, the return of the neurodynamics to the background level is observed. Excitement increases, and mobility of nervous processes decreases somewhat.

The strength of the nervous system in various phases of the OMC did not undergo significant and logical changes. Consequently, as can be seen from the data presented, in different phases of the CMC, the psychomotor functions change unevenly and differently, so that the deterioration of performance on one indicator may be accompanied by an improvement in the ability to work after another [53–55]. Thus, the indicators of "external" and "internal" balances in certain phases of CMC vary in a different direction [56]. The effect of phases of the CMC on functional parameters, well-being, and mood should be taken into account in studies related to the female contingent [23, 57, 58].

The revealed neurovegetative and endocrine regularities of regulation of the ovarian-menstrual cycle are realized through individual-typological peculiarities of the hormonal status and morphology of the female body.

1.1 Individual features of central hemodynamics and cardiac rhythm variability in women of reproductive age

The variability of the heart rate (HRV) is a fundamental physiological property of the human body and reflects the state of regulating mechanisms, in particular the autonomic tone of the autonomic nervous system; its study contributes to the development of quality diagnosis, prognostication, and prevention of various diseases [43].

In recent years, the number of studies on the variability in the duration of the interval RR [31, 32, 34, 59, 60], blood pressure [60, 61], shock volume of blood [35, 60], respiratory arrhythmia [31, 32, 40], and communication wave changes in various hemodynamic parameters. This is due to the wide introduction of information technologies to medicine and physiology, as well as to the confirmed or highly diagnostic value of parameters of regulatory rhythms of hemodynamics.

On the adaptive-trophic role of the sympathetic department of the VNS, including in the reproduction, one of the first pointed academician Orbeli [27]. However, until now, the study of the state of the VAS, including heart rate activity, in women during the normal menstrual cycle and in the physiological and complicated pregnancy, remains insufficient. A number of review papers [43, 62] provide data on age and gender changes in some HRV indices. However, they relate mainly to short (2–5 min) records of RR intervals and performed on contingents of persons with different pathologies. At the same time, the characteristics of the wave structure of oscillation of hemodynamic indices in healthy women in different physiological conditions and loads in the ontogenesis process are insufficiently analyzed. Studies by Ketel et al. [12], conducted in randomized tubes for 149 men and 137 middle-aged women, revealed that HRV levels were inversely related to age and heart rate in both sexes. The level of LF in men is significantly higher in women than in women and is negatively related to the level of triglycerides, insulin. The power of the R-R interval for women is higher than that of men.

The widespread introduction of the ECG Holter monitoring method into the clinical practice allowed the evaluation of HRV values in the course of the day and at certain intervals and also used this method for studying the state of autonomic regulation of the cardiac rhythm [64]. Extreme values of total power of the spectrum and power in the range of very low and low frequencies in Holter monitoring of women compared to men were also recorded in Fluckiger et al. [65]. At the same time, the power in the ranges of low and high frequencies was negatively correlated with age. The total power of the spectrum decreased relatively between 20–29 years and 60–69 years by 30%.

The same gender and age characteristics of the wave structure of the cardiac rhythm were also confirmed in measurements of 302 men and 312 women conducted by Bai et al. [36], with 653 persons performed by Aubert et al. [66], and on 276 persons conducted by Barrett et al. [67]. The gender differences of HRV are measured at the sixth decade of a person's life cycle. Changes in the heart rhythm and its spectral components during orthopedic trial at this age did not have sexual differences.

There are significant differences in the reactivity of fluctuations in the duration of the R-R interval and the peripheral pressure of men and women on physical, mental, and cold loads. So in studies OV Peshakova [68] shows that women under these conditions have a greater centralization of mechanisms of regulation of the cardiovascular system, and for men—an increase in the activity of the sympathetic link of the autonomic nervous system.

Many researchers [39, 69] point out that cardiovascular analysis is more appropriate to detect minor fluctuations of the VNS activity during the menstrual cycle than the use of traditional indicators such as heart rate and arterial pressure. However, the results of studies of changes in cardiac rhythm in different phases of the menstrual cycle are still controversial. It should be noted that significant changes in HRF in women of reproductive age, whether alone or in psycho-emotional stresses, may be due to the ovarian cycle [70]. SDNN in young women was highest during the follicular phase of the menstrual cycle [26]. According to Kravchenko and co-authors [71] in women during the luteal phase compared with the follicular showed an increase in the activity of the sympathetic department of the autonomic autonomy of the autonomy according to the HRV indices. However, a group of researchers Grossman et al. [70] insists on the absence of differences in the parameters of the wave structure of blood pressure and heart rate when performing orthopedic and stimulating carotid sinus in women in different phases of the ovarian cycle.

Japanese scientists [39] demonstrate a significant increase in sympathetic and decreased parasympathetic activity in the luteal phase compared to follicular, as evidenced by an increase in LF/HF and LF values, as well as a decrease in HF in the luteal phase. The facts of the increase in the level of LF/HF in the early and middle luteal phase are presented in Hirshoren et al. [72], with the late lutein phase showing a tendency to decrease the level of LF/HF. At the same time, some researchers, Princi et al. [69] and Sato et al. [39], refute this assumption, indicating that there is no significant change. Although some researchers point to an increase in the level of HF in the follicular phase compared with the luteal and menstrual phase, measurements were made only one [15] or twice a week [73] during the cycle. Since hormonal and physiological changes during the menstrual cycle are complex, they cannot be characterized by two measurements, indicating the need for long-term research.

In studies [45], with ten completely healthy women, it was found that spontaneous baroreceptor sensitivity increases during the luteal phase compared to the follicular phase. It was stated that there were certain differences in the logRSA fluctuations during the menstrual cycle, which were related to the average NSC indices.

According to Fleischman [28], there are significant changes in both the wave structure of the cardiac rhythm and its reactivity to the burden on women in the first 20 weeks of pregnancy. So, normally in this period, the power of OT components increases, and often the synchronization of respiratory and baroreflector waves is observed. In pathological development of pregnancy, there is an inversion of such regulatory relations.

The variability of the cardiac rhythm during the physiological course of pregnancy is reduced, which indicates an increase in the activity of the sympathetic department of the autonomic nervous system [12, 13]. In women with gestosis, HRV is more pronounced. Revealed by scientists the facts of changes in HRV with other hypertensive states in pregnant women, as well as in normal and complicated childbirth, are few and controversial. The emphasis is on the prospect of further study of sympathetic activity in relation to the change in HRV in pregnant and childbearing women, as well as on the need for widespread introduction of cardiointervalography in obstetrics.

Many scientists [13, 64, 74] note that in the second and third trimesters of pregnancy, the activity of the VNS is higher (by characteristics of the wave structure of the cardiac rhythm) than in nonpregnant women. The analysis of these works shows that the decrease in HRV during pregnancy is manifested in the reduction of the values of the mathematical expectation, the mod, the mean square deviation, the variational magnitude, the variation coefficient, the power of the OT waves, the normalized power of the OT waves, and the pHN50, as well as in the increase of the amplitude of the mod, index voltage, autonomic equilibrium index, LF wavelengths, normalized LF wavelengths, VLF wavelengths, and LF/HF ratios.

At the same time, it should be noted that until now scientists have not agreed on the change in HRV at the beginning of pregnancy. Thus, Vae et al. [36] investigated that in the first trimester the HRV increases and in the second and third trimesters it decreases. According to other scholars [45, 63], HRV progressively decreases, starting with the first trimester. According to Klinkenberg et al. [75], HRV in the first trimester remains unchanged. The question remains as to the nature of the changes in BCR before delivery: according to some data [64], it increases and it contributes to the normal course of labor, and for the other [1, 13]—does not change.

The reasons for increasing the excitability of VNS during pregnancy are still not studied. Some scientists believe that increased activity occurs under the influence of chronic stress, which is considered pregnancy; others regard it as a compensation in response to systemic vasodilatation, which occurs under the influence of NO, whose production will increase significantly in pregnancy. According to Klinkenberg et al. [75], the increase in VNS activity during pregnancy is the result of a true increase in the activity of higher sympathetic centers under the influence of changes in the production of various hormones during pregnancy, as well as the result of an increase in the effectiveness of b-adrenergic effects on the heart (or a decrease in the effectiveness of M-cholinergic effects). The latter is due to an increase in the content of endogenous b-adrenergic agonists (b-AP) and endogenous b-AP sensitizers or endogenous M-cholinoreceptor blockers (M-HRP) in the blood. Previously, it was shown that in pregnancy, indeed, the content in the blood b-AP increases, while the content of M-HRP does not change. Most likely, in general, the increase in sympathetic activity is a manifestation of adaptation to pregnancy and is aimed at the formation of mechanisms that ensure the growth and development of the fetus, including inhibition of contractile activity of the uterus, increased pumping function of the heart, and gas transport function of the blood.

Studying the health of women during menopause is of great interest, both for practitioners and for theoretical scholars. This is a separate branch of health care that is socially important in all countries of the world, because in connection with the prolongation of life expectancy, the number of women over 50 years old has increased threefold [76, 77], and more than one-third of her life, a woman holds in postmenopausal care [78].

To date, some research on HSR has been devoted to the study of this phenomenon in women engaged in physical exercise and sports. Thus, the specific features of the female body and its response to intensive, often extreme, training and competitive loads, characteristic of certain sports, are rather negligible. It is believed that this circumstance does not allow to accurately formulate the extent of the impact of occupations on various sports and the desire for the highest sports results in the condition of the female body [60, 79]. However, in the HSR studies on women-tongue-men in comparison with the group of men of masters of sports and masters of the international class, it was found that men had more frequencies of HRV, in particular TP, VLF, LF, LF/HF but less HF and HF percentage (%). Thus, we see that the women of single fighters in comparison with men are noticeable strengthening of the sympathetic link of the VNS.

In the study of the variability of the heart rate in the mode of the training day in the gymnasts, it was established that the relationship between the cardiovascular system and the degree of centralization in the management of cardiac rhythm not only is preserved but also varies. At the same time, the dynamics of integral indicators of the functional state of the circulatory system in gymnasiums is rather informative for the assessment of "urgent" training effect [31, 32].

It should be noted that many researchers point out that the athlete's affiliation with a particular sports specialization determines his "vegetative portrait," which is related to the nature of the exercise, which can be offset by gender differences in HRD [78].

Author details

Olena Lutsenko

Address all correspondence to: olena85lutsenko@gmail.com

Department of Theory and Methods of Teaching of Natural Sciences, Hlukhiv National Pedagogical University of Alexander Dovzhenko, Ukraine

References

[1] Bleil ME, Appelhans BM, Adler NE. Pubertal timing, androgens, and obesity phenotypes in women at midlife. Clinics in Endocrinology and Metabolism. 2012;**97**:1948-1952

[2] Lemanska YA. Indicators of cardiac rhythm variability in pregnant women with cardiac arrhythmias according to Holter monitoring. Bulletin of the Institute of Obstetrics and Gynecology. 2007;**3**:15-16

[3] Bazhenova EA, Voronin IM. Evaluation of polysomnographic and hemodynamic indices in healthy girls with daily profile dipper and non dipper. Vesna, Journal of Tambov State University. 2009;**14**(1):33-36

[4] Collins P, Rosano G, Jiang C. Cardiovascular protection by oestrogen-a calcium antagonist effect? The Lancet. 1993;**341**:1264-1265

[5] Collins P. Vascular aspects of oestrogen. Journal of the Climacteric and Postmenopause. 1996;**23**:217-226

[6] Cooke WN. Head rotation during upright tilt increases cardiovagal baroreflex sensitivity. Aviation, Space, and Environmental Medicine. 2007;**78**(5):463-469

[7] Cheng Y, Cohen B, Oréa V. Baroreflex control of renal sympathetic nerve activity and spontaneous rhythms at Mayer wave's frequency in rats. Autonomic Neuroscience. 2004;**111**:80-88

[8] Kovalenko SO, Kudij LI, Lutsenko OI. Peculiarities of male and female heart rate variability. Science and Education a New Dimension. 2013;**1**(2):15

[9] Asso D. Menstruation; Menopause. Chichester, West sussex/New York; 1983. 214 p

[10] Sarafinyuk LA. Features of individual morphofunctional indices in girls with varying degrees of puberty. In: Problems, Achievements and Prospects of Development of Medical-Biological Sciences and Practical Health Care. Vol. 142. 2006. pp. 69-71

[11] Saenko VG, Chekhova VE, Gurmazhenko MO. Anatomical-physiological features of the body of women-united. In: The Repository of Luhansk National University Named after. T.G. Shevchenko. 2012. Available from: http://dspace.luguniv.edu.ua/jspui/handle/123456789/150

[12] Ketel IJ. Microvascular function has no menstrual-cycle-dependent variation in healthy ovulatory women. Microcirculation. 2009;**16**:714-724

[13] Chayka GV, Gunas IV, Mazorchuk BF. Normograms of the levels of hormones in adolescent and adolescent girls in general and different morphotypes in different phases of the menstrual cycle. Biomedical and Biosocial Anthropology. 2010;**15**:185-188

[14] Asso D. Psychological and physiological changes in severe premenstrual syndrome. Biological Psychology. 1992;**33**(2):115-132

[15] Welt CK, DJ MN, Taylor AE, Hall JE. Female reproductive aging is marked by decreased secretion of dimeric inhibin. Clinics in Endocrinology and Metabolism. 1999;**84**:105

[16] Cella F, Giordano G, Cordera R. Serum leptin concentrations during the menstrual cycle in normal-weight women: Effects of an oral triphasic estrogen-progestin medication. European journal of endocrinology. 2000;**142**(2):174-178

[17] Lichkus LG. A brief critical review of the activities of the St. Petersburg obstetric and Gynecological society during the first 25 years of its existence. Journal of Obstetrics and Women's Diseases. 1911;**3**:391-442

[18] Aubert AE, Seps B, Beckers F. Heart rate variability in athletes. Sports Medicine. 2003;**33**(12):889-919

[19] Shaparenko PP. Anthropometric and somatotypological characteristics of practically healthy urban adolescents of both sexes of the Ukrainian ethnic group. Herald Morphology. 2006;**3**(1):339-341

[20] Shepelev AE, Andriychuk VM. Comparative characteristic of somatometric parameters and indicators of harmony of physical development of girls of different medical groups. Biomedical and Biosocial Anthropology. 2012;**18**:C.117-C.120

[21] Scheer FL, Hiltona M, Mantzoros CS. Adverse metabolic and cardiovascular consequences of circadian misalignment. Proceedings of the National Academy of Sciences of the United States of America. 2009;**106**:4453-4458

[22] Wenner MM. Preserved autonomic function in amenorrheic athletes. Journal of Applied Physiology. 2006;**101**(2):590-597

[23] Shutova SV, Chichuk VN, Kopchenkina YM. Biorhythmological features of sensorimotor response in girls. Scientific Records: Series Medicine Pharmacy. 2011;**4**:35-41

[24] Cockerill IM, Cockerill JA, Wormington AM. Menstrual-cycle effects on mood and perceptual-motor performance. Journal of Psychosomatic Research. 1994;**38**(7):763-771

[25] Seebauer MS. Changes of respiratory sinus arrhythmia during the menstrual cycle depend on average heart rate. European journal of applied physiology. 2002;**87**:309-314

[26] Yamamoto M, Tsutsumi Y, Furukawa K. Influence of normal menstrual cycle on autonomic nervous activity and QT dispersion. Bioelectromagnetics. 2003;**23**:152-153

[27] Orbeli LA. Lectures on Physiology of the Nervous System; Leningrad. 1935. 328 p

[28] Tegako LI, Salivon IN. Fundamentals of Modern Anthropology; Minsk. 2010. 68 p

[29] Bosquet L, Gamelin FX, Berthoin S. Is aerobic endurance a determinant of cardiac autonomic regulation? European journal of applied physiology. 2007;**100**(3):363-369

[30] Pankova NB. Analysis of rhythm variability and arterial pressure in various functional tests in women and men. Human Physiology. 2008;**34**(4):64-72

[31] Yabluchansky NI. Fundamentals of Practical Application of Non-Invasive Technology for the Study of Human Regulatory Systems; Kharkiv. 2000. 88 p

[32] Angela R, Gregg P, Pierson A. Ovarian antral folliculogenesis during the human menstrual cycle. Human Reproduction Update. 2012;**18**(1):73-91

[33] Babichev VN. Effect of estrogens on the central nervous system. Bulletin of the Russian Academy of Medical Science. 2005;**6**:45-54

[34] Celeste NT, Mickiewicz AL. The role of the ventral pallidum in psychiatric disorders psychiatric disorders. Neuropsychopharmacology. 2010;**35**(1):337

[35] Brown SJ. The effect a respiratory acidosis on human heart rate variability. Advances in Experimental Medicine and Biology. 2008;**605**:361-365

[36] Baker FC. Circadian rhythms, sleep and the menstrual cycle. Sleep Medicine. 2007;**8**(6):613-622

[37] Barrett CJ, Guild SJ, Maipas SC. Baroreceptor denervation prevents sympathoinhibition during angiotensin II—Induced hypertension. Hypertension. 2005;**46**:168

[38] Elghozi JL. Short-term variability of blood pressure: Physiology and pharmacology. Annales Pharmaceutiques Françaises. 2008;**660**(3):158-168

[39] Siepka SM, Yoo SH, Lee C. Genetics and neurobiology of circadian clocks in mammals. Cold Spring Harbor Symposia on Quantitative Biology. 2007;**72**:251-259

[40] Bolova AA. Forecasting of Peculiarities of Sexual Development of Girls on the Basis of Vegetative Regulation Estimation: Author's Abstract. dis for the Sciences. Degree Candidate Honey. Sciences Moscow; 2009. 20 p

[41] Donovan T, Bosch SS. Physiology of Puberty. London: Edward Arnold Ltd.; 1965

[42] Lutsenko OI. Morphological factors influence on young women arterial pressure levels. Clinical Practice. 2017;**14**(5):334-337

[43] Yabluchansky NI. Variability of the Heart Rate to Assist the Practitioner For True Doctors; Kharkiv. 2010. 131 p

[44] Hinojosa-Laborde C, Chapa I, Haywood JR. Gender differences in sympathetic nervous system regulation. Clinical and Experimental Pharmacology & Physiology. 1999;**26**:122-126

[45] Lewandowski J. Sex hormone modulation of neuropeptide Y and cardiovascular responses to stress in humans. Stress: Molecular Genetic and Neurobiological Advances. 1996;**2**:569-578

[46] Chapuis B, Vidal-Petiot E, Oréa V. Linear modelling analysis of baroreflex control of arterial pressure variability in rats. The Journal of physiology. 2004;**559**:639-649

[47] Bulavenko OV, Levkivska IG. Correlation of echometric parameters of genital organs in different phases of the menstrual cycle with anthroposotometric indices of healthy girls with mesomorphic somatotype. Biomedical and Biosocial Anthropology. 2010;**15**:154-158

[48] Karsch FJ, Dierschke DJ. Sexual differentiation of pituitary function: Apparent difference between primates and rodents. Science. 1973;**179**(2):484-486

[49] Leicht AS, Hirning DA, Allen DA. Heart rate variability and endogenous sex hormones during the menstrual cycle in young women. Experimental Physiology. 2003;**94**(6):441-446

[50] Kravchenko VI. Features of regulation of cardiac rhythm during mental load in women in different phases of the menstrual cycle. Cherkasy University Bulletin: Biological Sciences Series. 2008;**128**:78-87

[51] Hottenrott K. Heart rate variability and physical exercise. Current status. Herz. 2006;**31**(6):544-552

[52] Klinkenberg AV. Heart rate variability changes in pregnant and non-pregnant women during standardized psychosocial stress. Acta obstetricia et gynecologica Scandinavica. 2009;**88**:77-82

[53] McKinley PS. The impact of menstrual cycle phase on cardiac autonomic regulation. Psychophysiology. 2009;**46**:904-1011

[54] To the doctrine of the "monthly" [Text]: diss.—Zhikharev H/SS. Spb: S. Petersburg lips type, 1896. VI, 320 p; il—(Senior doctoral dissertations admitted to protection at the Imperial War) Medical Academy in 1895-1896, No. 60, 63 p

[55] Anokhin PK. The objective reflex as an object of physiological analysis. Magazine of Higher Nervous Activity. 1962;**126**:7-21

[56] Hirshoren N. Menstrual cycle effects on the neurohumoral and autonomic nervous systems regulating the cardiovascular system. Clinics in Endocrinology and Metabolism. 2002;**87**(4):1569-1575

[57] Vasilyeva VV. Mechanisms for the formation and functioning of reproductive dominant in spontaneous and stimulated cycles. Human Physiology. 2010;**3**:55-65

[58] Sato N, Miyake S. Cardiovascular reactivity to mental stress: Relationship with menstrual cycle and gender. Journal of Physiological Anthropology and Applied Human Science. 2004;**23**:215-223

[59] Bouteau N, Tavernier B. Stroke volume variation as an indicator of fluid responsiveness. Anesthesia and Analgesia. 2004;**98**(1):278-279

[60] MacNaughton J, Banah M, McCloud P. Age related changes in follicle stimulating hormone, luteinizing hormone, oestradiol and immunoreactive inhibin in women of reproductive age. Clinical Endocrinology. 2008;**36**:339-345

[61] Fluckiger L. Differential effects of aging on heart rate variability and blood pressure variability. The Journal of Gerontology: Biological Sciences. 1999;**54**(5):219-224

[62] Moroz VM, Gunas IV, Sarafinuk LA. Age and gender characteristics of the indicators of central humor in girls and boys of adolescence. Biomedical and Biosocial Anthropology. 2008;**10**:92-97

[63] Kuczmierczyk AR. Autonomic arousal and pain sensitivity in women with premenstrual syndrome at different phases of the menstrual cycle. Journal of Psychosomatic Research. 1986;**30**(4):421-428

[64] Balgir RS. Morphological and regional variations in body dimensions of the Gujjars of different localities in North-Western India. Anthropologischer Anzeiger. 2003;**61**(3):275-285

[65] Grossman P, Taylor EW. Toward understanding respiratory sinus arrhythmia: Relations to cardiac vagal tone, evolution and biobehavioral functions. Biological Psychology. 2007;**74**(2):263-285

[66] Bai X. Influence of the menstrual cycle on nonlinear properties of heart rate variability in young women. American Journal of Physiology-Heart and Circulatory Physiology. 2009;**297**(2):765-774

[67] Biro FM, Greenspan LC, Galvez MP. Puberty in girls of the 21st century. Pediatric and Adolescent Gynecology. 2012;**25**(5):289-294

[68] Brunt VE. Short-term administration of progesterone and estradiol independently alter carotid-vasomotor, but not carotid-cardiac, baroreflex function in young women. American Journal of Physiology-Heart and Circulatory Physiology. 2013;**305**:1041-1049

[69] Rilling JK. A potential role for oxytocin in the intergenerational transmission of secure attachment. Neuropsychopharmacology. 2009;**34**(13):2621-2622

[70] Budzin VR. Features of the relationship between the indicators of the functional state of the soccer players in different phases of a specific biological cycle. Pedagogics, Psychology, Medical-Biological Problems of Physical Training and Sports. 2009;**5**:29-32

[71] Naumova VA. The influence of the ovarian-menstrual cycle on motor qualities and neurodynamics of female athletes. In: Psychophysiological Issues of Studying the Personality of the Athlete; Lviv. 1976. pp. 124-131

[72] Purdon SE. Menstrual effects on asymmetrical olfactory acuity. Journal of the International Neuropsychological Society. 2001;**7, 6**:703-709

[73] Korkushko OV, Pisaruk AV, Shatilo VB, Lishnevskaya YV, Chebotarev ND, Pogoretsky YN. Analysis of Cardiac Rhythm Variability in Clinical Practice: Age Aspects; Kyiv. 2002. 192 p

[74] Cohen B, Martinelli GP, Raphan T. The vasovagal response of the rat: Its relation to the vestibulosympathetic reflex and to Mayer waves. The FASEB Journal. 2013;**27**(7):2564-2572

[75] Lawrence JE, Ray CA, Carter JR. Vestibulosympathetic reflex during the early follicular and midluteal phases of the menstrual cycle. American Journal of Physiology-Endocrinology and Metabolism. 2008;**20**:1046-1050

[76] Malhotra A. Effects of sex hormones on development of physiological and pathological hypertrophy in male and female rats. American Journal of Physiology. 1990;**259**:866-871

[77] Princi TS. Parametric evaluation of heart rate variability during the menstrual cycle in young women. Biomedical Sciences Instrumentation. 2005;**41**:340-345

[78] Kovalenko SO, Lutsenko OI. Blood pressure and hemodynamics: Mayer waves in different phases of ovarian and menstrual cycle in women. Physiological Research. 2017;**66**:235-240

[79] Lazzaro SC, Rutledge RB, Burghart DR, Glimcher PW. The impact of menstrual cycle phase on economic choice and rationality. PLoS One. 2016;**11**(1):e0144080. DOI: 10.1371/journal.pone.0144080

[80] Veldhuijzen van Zanten JJ. Mental stress-induced haemoconcentration in women: Effects of menstrual cycle phase. Health Psychology. 2009:805-816

11

Secretory Phase and Implantation

Courtney Marsh, Katelyn Schumacher,
Warren B. Nothnick, Robert N. Taylor and
Monique Monard

Abstract

This chapter will explore the latter phase of the menstrual cycle focusing on the secretory phase of the endometrium. In particular, focus will be on the mid-secretory endometrium and appropriate markers and hormonal environment for successful implantation. This will be put in the context of the luteal phase of ovulation and the hormonal support that progesterone provides. We will also review pathologic states, such as endometriosis and related progesterone resistance, which affect mid-secretory phase and implantation. Finally, we will provide a detailed review of the literature on what the current state of knowledge is regarding receptivity and the microenvironment of the mid-secretory endometrium which is essential to implantation.

Keywords: secretory, implantation

1. Introduction

The female reproductive system prepares women for conception and pregnancy through two distinct, but highly integrated, cycles, the ovarian cycle and the endometrial cycle. The human endometrium, under the influence of complex biological signals, undergoes cyclic changes in preparation for implantation and the initiation of pregnancy. An array of molecular activity, still poorly understood, gives rise to relatively consistent morphologic changes of the endometrium during each cycle. In an era of assisted reproductive technologies (ART), there exists an ever-increasing demand to delineate these pathways in order to improve pregnancy rates. Ultimately, success in the field of reproduction and fertility requires an understanding of these complex processes, from molecular to cellular to tissue, in both the healthy patient as well as in the setting of various pathologic states.

This chapter will discuss the endometrial cycle with an emphasis on the secretory phase, including the molecular and biochemical components of endometrial receptivity and implantation. Markers and techniques for assessment of receptivity will be reviewed, as well as pathologic states that alter fertility.

2. The menstrual cycle and the endometrium

The endometrium is comprised of two anatomic layers, the functionalis and the basalis. The functionalis is made up of a compact zone, including stroma underneath the luminal epithelium, and a spongy zone which lies above the basalis layer [1, 2]. It is the functionalis layer that is shed in the monthly menses. The basalis layer lies on the myometrium; it undergoes fewer cyclic changes compared to the functionalis layer and is responsible for regenerating the functionalis after menstruation (**Figure 1**).

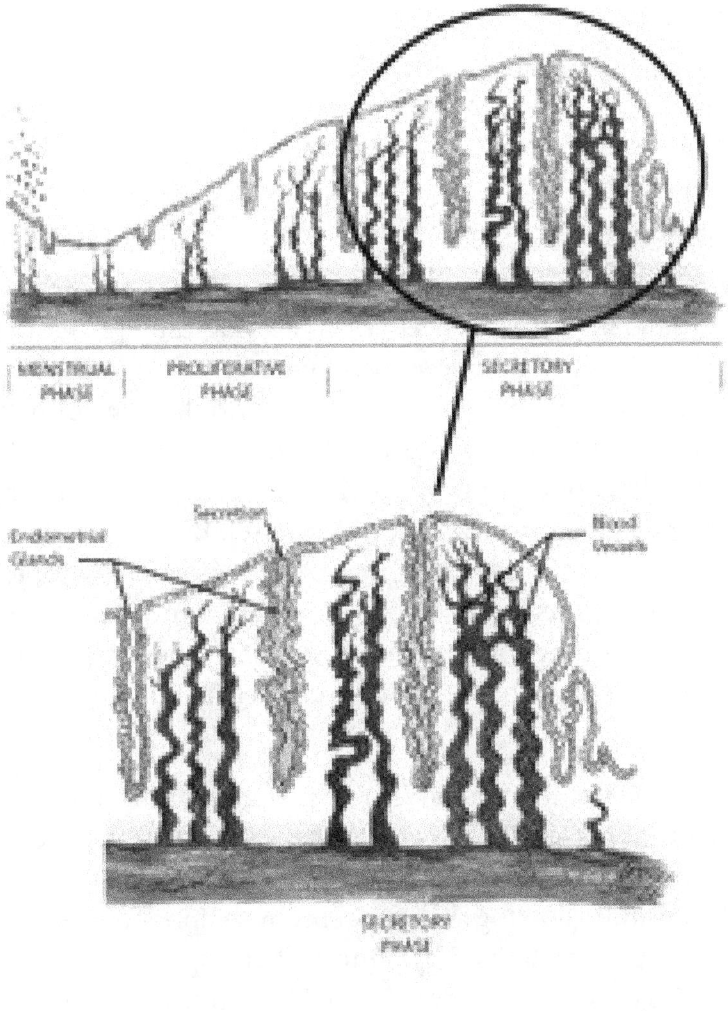

Figure 1. Functional anatomy of the human endometrium during the secretory phase.

The endometrial cycle consists of three sequential phases—the proliferative phase, secretory phase, and menstruation. Each phase is marked by physiologic changes that are controlled by circulating levels of estrogen and progesterone, which are synthesized and secreted from the ovary. The ovarian cycle is characterized by follicular development mediated by FSH (follicular phase), oocyte release mediated by the LH surge (ovulation), and development of the corpus luteum and production of progesterone (luteal phase). In the idealized 28-day cycle, ovulation occurs on day 14. After ovulation, the remnant of the dominant follicle becomes the corpus luteum, a temporary endocrine structure which produces progesterone (**Figure 1**) [1–4]. The corpus luteum becomes atretic on day 28 and menses begins the next day, establishing day 1 of the subsequent cycle.

During the proliferative phase, estradiol derived from the growing follicles drives the restoration of the functionalis layer with re-epithelialization by approximately day 5 of the menstrual cycle. This phase is characterized by hypertrophy and proliferation of glands, increase in stromal matrix, and elongation of terminal arterioles to the endometrial lumen. A gradient of angiogenic factors, particularly VEGF, is released from the endometrial epithelium by estradiol [5]. Estrogen also upregulates the progesterone receptors that orchestrate the environment during the secretory phase, which will be covered in more detail in the next section [2, 4]. In the absence of fertilization, progesterone levels decline due to atresia of the corpus luteum. This leads to vasospasm, ischemia, subsequent tissue death and endometrial shedding, or menses.

3. The secretory phase

For decades, endometrial dating has been assessed histologically [4, 6]. After ovulation, there is an increase in superficial stromal edema that becomes generalized by day 21. Stromal cells near terminal spiral arteries show an increase in cytoplasmic volume and surrounding extracellular matrix, a process termed predecidualization, which eventually encompasses the majority of the superficial endometrium by day 25. This transformation appears to represent a form of mesenchymal-to-epithelial transition (MET) [7]. By day 27, the superficial stromal cells are nearly indistinguishable from decidual cells of pregnancy. The increasing edema during the secretory phase results in the global endometrial thickening that is readily apparent with ultrasonography. Throughout the secretory phase, there are also distinct changes in spiral arteries. They rapidly lengthen, outpacing endometrial thickening, and become increasingly coiled [4, 6, 8, 9].

During the proliferative phase, there is an increase in glandular epithelium mitotic activity and pseudostratification of nuclei. There is a parallel increase in the proliferation of stromal components as well during this phase. After ovulation, this process is replaced by secretory transformation of glands and a slowing of stromal proliferation. At the cellular level, the early-secretory phase glands are characterized by abundant endoplasmic reticulum, accumulation of glycogen-rich vacuoles, and displacement of nuclei centrally. Six days after ovulation, loss of vacuoles from the cytoplasm corresponds with maximal glandular secretory activity [4, 9].

A complex interplay between mesenchymal cells and immune cells highlights the secretory phase of the superficial endometrial stroma. A substantial portion of the uterine leukocyte population is made up of CD56–/CD16+ uterine natural killer (uNK) cells, which are believed to play a tolerizing role in maternal allorecognition of fetal trophoblasts, rather than cytotoxicity. This cell population increases dramatically after ovulation and vanishes before menses in the absence of pregnancy. When conception occurs, the uNK cells are largely found in proximity to spiral arteries and extravillous trophoblasts in early pregnancy. The activity of uNK cells have been shown to be controlled by steroid hormones as well as local chemokines, including those containing the (C-X-C motif) and various interleukins [1, 4].

Macrophages (CD68+ and CD163+) are also found in the superficial endometrium, rapidly accumulating in the stroma after ovulation and declining in the absence of progesterone. T cells are found scattered throughout the endometrium with little to no menstrual-cycle change in concentration, as well as uterine dendritic cells (uDCs) which are most prominent in decidua of pregnancy [4].

The end of the secretory phase and beginning of the premenstrual phase is characterized by degradation of the stromal network, infiltration of the stroma by leukocytes, and cessation of glandular activity in the absence of the appropriate signals, such as hCG from developing trophectoderm. The degradation of the stromal network is catalyzed by matrix metalloproteinases (MMP), which become activated in the setting of falling progesterone levels. Evidence of apoptosis is evident throughout the tissue, and the ultrastructurally electron-dense contents of glandular cells characteristic of secretion vanish. These structures include the well-developed rough endoplasmic reticulum, Golgi apparatus, and glycogen-secreting cytoplasmic projections [1, 4].

4. Microarchitecture and implantation

The implantation of the blastocyst is a highly organized, selective process that, with some variations, is preserved among mammals. In women, nonhuman primates and other hemochorial placental species a narrow "window of implantation" (WOI) exists, during which the endometrium is capable of "receiving" the trophectoderm of the blastocyst. The interaction is orchestrated by a variety of molecules and is overall regulated by steroid hormones [4, 9]. Recent research suggests the WOI only lasts between 12 and 48 h, and is often shifted in patients with infertility [3]. In 1999, Wilcox et al. narrowed the timing of implantation to between 8 and 10 days after ovulation, with increased embryonic losses correlated with later implantation [10].

The process of implantation follows four well-described steps, which is coordinated with endometrial preparation by changes in steroid hormones. The focus here starts with apposition and transient adhesion of syncytial trophoblast cells to the endometrial epithelium, which is followed by firm attachment and finally, trophoblast invasion. As the blastocyst enters the uterine cavity, the zona pellucida is shed allowing for exposure of the trophectoderm [9, 11]. Driven by progesterone, the secretory phase endometrial epithelial cells enter a hypersecretory state, with characteristic features described as the *Arias-Stella reaction*. This hypersecretory state of the tissue provides the necessary histiotrophic nutrition essential for embryo and placental survival, as vascular remodeling occurs later [12, 13].

The molecular basis of blastocyst invasion is of active interest in the field, as failure of these mechanisms is associated with pregnancy loss. Current research suggests that mucin (MUC)1, a large transmembrane mucin and a barrier to implantation is downregulated and/or removed through the action of surface proteases and decreased expression of progesterone receptors. The loss of MUC1 allows for appropriate apposition, adhesion, and attachment of the embryo to the endometrium. Initial transient adhesion is mediated by selectins and galectins. More firm attachment is mediated by integrins, including $\alpha\nu\beta3$ and $\alpha4\beta1$, and CD44 and their shared ligand, osteopontin (OPN). Other attachment-associated molecules include trophinin, HB-EGF, fibronectin, vitronectin, laminin, IGFBP1, and the latency associated peptide linked to TGFβ [2–4, 9, 11].

Specialized surface macromolecules have also been implicated in blastocyst adhesion and invasion. Endometrial epithelium consists of both ciliated and nonciliated, secretory cells, the proportions of which are regulated by estrogen levels. The secretory cells develop transient surface structures in response to progesterone levels, called pinopodes, during the time of maximal receptivity [14]. These structures are involved in pinocytosis and contain various adhesion molecules, including $\alpha\nu\beta3$, glycodelin, and OPN [15]. The development of pinopodes is dependent upon HOXA-10, a homeobox gene whose expression is vital for endometrial receptivity, regulating both endometrial stromal cell proliferation and epithelial cell morphogenesis [16]. Blocking the expression of HOXA-10 results in a significant reduction in the number of pinopodes. Although some evidence points to pinopodes role in adhesion and invasion of the embryo, their precise function and overall importance is still debated [2, 3].

Adhesion via these molecules is static dynamic process. Extracellular contact with appropriate ligands transmits signals, through a variety of pathways, into intracellular cascades that results in gene transcription and protein expression that mediate migration, proliferation, and cytoskeletal remodeling. The overall result is the successful invasion of the embryo into a primed endometrium, where it has the potential for growth and development [2–4].

5. Receptivity markers and clinical applications

The assessment of endometrial receptivity has drastically changed since the establishment of the Noyes' criteria for histologic dating in 1950 [6]. Once the clinical significance of the pathological criteria was questioned, a more detailed understanding of the biochemical pathways influenced by steroid hormones during the menstrual cycle led to new targets to identify endometrial receptivity [17]. Initially, single molecules were analyzed. With the advent of microarray technology and massively parallel, next generation RNA sequencing, vast amounts of molecules can be analyzed at the same time to give a much more complete picture of the endometrial environment [1, 3, 4].

Cytokines are involved in many processes of the ovarian and endometrial cycles and have been shown to play a critical role in implantation. Leukemia inhibitory factor (LIF) is an IL-6 family member and its expression has been demonstrated in the human endometrial epithelium during the mid- to late-secretory phase [16]. In women of proven fertility, endometrial biopsies demonstrated LIF mRNA expression increased from day 18 to 28, with a peak at day 20, and showed a corresponding 2.2-fold increase in LIF protein secretion between the proliferative and secretory phase [18]. IL-6, another cytokine expressed in the endometrium shows a regulated temporal pattern throughout the menstrual cycle with the highest detected levels during the luteal phase. IL-6 mRNA levels increase progressively during the mid- to late-secretory phase and IL-6 protein was strongly expressed in luminal and glandular epithelial cells during the window of implantation. The protein is strongly pronounced. Bone morphogenic protein 2 (BMP2), a member of the TGF-β superfamily, is first detected in the stroma surrounding the site of blastocyst attachment during the mid-secretory phase. BMP2 is considered a critical regulator of decidualization due to its role in regulating proliferation and differentiation, as well as its expression during the implantation period [19, 20].

Amniotic fluid contains very high concentrations (~5 μg/ml) of prolactin (PRL), which is produced by the decidua. It has been determined that endometrial PRL production begins around cycle day 22, and levels rise throughout pregnancy. Similarly, high levels of IGFBP-1 and LEFTY2 are produced by secretory phase endometrium in response to progesterone and expression of these can be recapitulated in vitro. Given their abundance and production during the menstrual cycle, these proteins serve as potential markers for endometrial receptivity, although clinic utility is not yet clear [1–4, 11].

Prostaglandins (PGs) have been shown to play a crucial role for successful embryo implantation due to their vasoactive properties. The generation of PGs from membrane-bound arachidonic acid is achieved by cytosolic phospholipase A_2 (cPLA$_2$) and cyclooxygenase (COX). Studies in female mice lacking cPLA$_2$ or COX-2 enzymes have demonstrated the vital role of PGs in implantation. PGE$_2$ and PGF$_{2\alpha}$ expression was detected in human endometrium throughout all stages of the menstrual cycle but was downregulated during the late-secretory phase [16].

Several integrins have been identified as possible markers of uterine receptivity and have been noted to undergo alterations in the epithelium and decidua during implantation. The co-expression of α1β1, ανβ3, and α4β1 heterodimers marks the period of endometrial receptivity by mediating firm attachment between the embryo and endometrium. The regulated expression of secretory phase integrins suggests that steroid hormones likely play a role in their presence; for example, α1β1/laminin receptor (VLA-1) expression on secretory phase endometrial epithelium is suggestive of progesterone-induced upregulation. The firm attachment mediated by integrins also generates other integrin-associated ligands. OPN, a ligand for ανβ3, is significantly upregulation in endometrial epithelial cells and mediates cellular adhesion and migration during embryo implantation. Calcitonin, a known upregulator of ανβ3, is transiently produced in the uterine epithelia during the period of implantation. It downregulates E-cadherin expression and promotes the outgrowth of trophoblasts into the uterus [16, 21].

Another critical endometrial glycoprotein, MUC1, is a factor that interferes with cellular adhesion. MUC1 is likely the first uterine molecule that the blastocyst encounters during the apposition phase, where it is thought to repel the embryo until the time and place is ideal for firm attachment. This is confirmed by the apparent local downregulation of MUC1 by progesterone before implantation in the receptive endometrium of mice. The reduced expression facilitates embryo-epithelial interactions by unmasking cell adhesion molecules on the endometrial surface [16]. When measured in humans, MUC1 showed increased generalized expression during the peri-implantation period, somewhat contradicting the studies in other species.

Two cytoskeleton-related proteins, stathmin 1 and annexin A2, have opposing regulation in the receptive versus pre-receptive endometrium. Stathmin 1 is a phosphoprotein that regulates microtubule dynamics during cell cycle progression, specifically at the embryo implantation site. In receptive human endometrium, downregulation of stathmin 1 supports decidualization. Annexin A2, an apical surface molecule in receptive human endometrium, is involved in cellular differentiation, regulation of prolactin secretion, and prostaglandin formation. Annexin A2 expression is highest in the mid- to late-secretory phase and decreased in the pre-receptive phase. This pattern of expression, along with in vitro effects on embryo adhesiveness, suggests annexin A2 plays a role in implantation [22].

BCL6, a transcriptional repressor mutated in some lymphomas, is associated with inflammation and significantly elevated values are seen in the secretory phase of patients with endometriosis and otherwise unexplained infertility. Data suggest that BCL6 is associated with progesterone resistance, leading to implantation defects and increased IVF failures [23, 24]. It is being developed as a diagnostic biomarker for endometriosis.

Ion channels and gap junctions in the endometrium have recently demonstrated a role in regulating endometrial receptivity and embryo implantation. The volume of electrolyte-containing fluid in the uterine lumen fluctuates throughout the menstrual cycle under the influence of ovarian hormones and is significantly reduced in the mid-secretory phase, encouraging blastocyst-endometrial apposition. This is suggestive of a net fluid absorption across the endometrium during the receptive phase. Cystic fibrosis transmembrane conductance regulator (CFTR) mediates Cl^- efflux, which is essential for epithelial fluid secretion. The endometrial epithelium is known to contain CFTR, playing an active role in endometrial Cl^- and fluid secretion. Downregulation of CFTR by progesterone during the secretory phase contributes to the decrease in fluid volume, which aids embryo implantation. The epithelial sodium channel (ENaC) also is present in the endometrium establishing a sodium gradient and providing a driving force for water absorption. CFTR has an inhibitory effect on ENaC, so the downregulation of CFTR during the secretory phase enhances the absorptive activity of the endometrial epithelium. ENaC is upregulated by progesterone, furthering the absorptive properties of the endometrial epithelium during the secretory phase. Other ion channels such as K^+ and Ca^{2+} and ion transporters, SLC4 and SLC26, are emerging as important players in regulating certain processes of embryo implantation [19]. Connexin 43 gap junctions also appear to mediate water and small molecule (<1.2 nm Stokes radius) transport and decidual differentiation [7, 25].

Microarray analysis of endometrial tissue allows for assessment of hundreds to thousands of molecules at once. Genomic and proteomic analyses have identified varying levels of genes and proteins implicated in a wide array of activities during decidualization. Receptivity markers are measured in clinical settings to avoid implantation failure and to hopefully provide a more favorable outcome for patients utilizing ART. Although some of the mentioned biomarkers have only recently been discovered as key players in the human receptive endometrium, these discoveries show promise in better understanding the complex interactions throughout the secretory phase and window of implantation.

Aspiration and assessment of secreted uterine fluids, called secretomics, which largely looks at protein and lipid levels, allows for high-throughput analysis of endometrial secretions during the secretory phase without the need for biopsies. Although our understanding of microarray technology as it related to infertility is still evolving, current and future products on the market will likely find clinical utility and are discussed in more detail later in the chapter [3, 26, 27].

6. Pathologic states and the secretory phase

Given the complex nature of endometrial receptivity, it is very vulnerable to perturbation. Local factors that can negatively impact receptivity and implantation can be broadly grouped into mechanical and inflammatory factors. Mechanical abnormalities encompass both congenital anomalies and acquired conditions. Local inflammatory factors include endometriosis, adenomyosis, hydrosalpinges, and endometritis [2, 28, 29].

Mechanical abnormalities of the uterus such as uterine septa, fibroids, polyps, and adhesions result in physical barriers to successful fertilization and implantation. These conditions are linked with recurrent pregnancy loss and infertility and substantial evidence exists that shows surgical correction of these abnormalities can improve outcomes [2, 29].

Given the delicate regulation of the menstrual cycle and the narrow implantation window, inflammatory factors that affect signaling pathways can effectively derail normal physiologic processes. In the setting of local inflammation, progesterone resistance and estrogen receptor dominance can result in impaired implantation. With endometriosis, for instance, there is an increase in inflammatory cytokines including TNFα, INFγ, IL-1, and IL-17. This leads to downstream effects such as phosphorylated STAT3, which in turn leads to an estrogen dominant and progesterone resistant state, shown through microarray analysis [2, 28]. Decreased expression of IL-11 and CCL4, which are associated with embryo receptivity, is found in chronic endometritis and is believed to be related to infertility associated with this condition [30]. Low integrin levels have been associated with inflammatory conditions and reduced $\alpha\nu\beta3$ expression, which can be caused by increased estrogen levels, and have been tied to IVF failure. Conversely, aromatase overexpression is seen in inflammatory states, and is linked with predicting failure in ART cycles. Other chemokines and cytokines, such as interleukins, are similarly linked to inflammation and pregnancy failure [2].

Although there still exist many gaps in our understanding of endometrial receptivity and implantation at the level of the uterus, pregnancy and ART failure cannot be fully explained by local factors. There exist several systemic disorders that can impact the uterine environment and the embryo's ability to implant. These diseases include thyroid dysfunction, vitamin D deficiency, hyperprolactinemia, inflammatory bowel disease, obesity, and smoking. There exists significant evidence relating hypothyroidism and poor fertility/IVF success rates, prompting levothyroxine treatment in patients with TSH < 2.5 mIU/L [2]. Obesity has similarly been linked to infertility, with evidence demonstrating that even modest weight loss improves pregnancy rates [2, 31]. However, our understanding of how these systemic states affect fertility is still limited, and further research is warranted to fully evaluate these relationships.

7. Future directions

Historically, dating of the receptive endometrium was based on morphologic criteria [6]. Shortcomings in the sensitivity and specificity of this method, fueled by significant advances in our molecular understanding of the endometrial cycle, have led to new approaches [17]. Although utilization of single molecular markers has not yielded satisfactory results, high-throughput analysis has been more promising [3]. The recent application of the "-omics" technologies, that utilize high-throughput techniques with sophisticated large data analysis to generate far more detailed patterns of molecular and biochemical processes, has revolutionized our understanding of the receptive endometrium and promises to yield clinically useful tools [3, 4, 26, 27].

The analysis of the endometrial cycle using transcriptomics has been actively investigated for over a decade [3]. Using gene expression microarray techniques, researchers have been able to study the expression of thousands of genes simultaneously during different phases of the endometrial cycle. They have identified unique gene profiles during the window of implantation, which includes important factors previously identified, such as LIF, OPN, CXCL14, glycodelin, IL15, L-selectin ligands, and various antioxidants [3]. One example of a commercially successful diagnostic test based on a transcription signature is the endometrial receptivity array (ERA). In controlled trials, use of this tool identified shifted windows of implantation in women with implantation failure. Using the test to adjust the timing of embryo transfer yielded pregnancy and implantation rates similar to control groups [32].

Although the current transcriptomics method has yielded impressive results, it relies on a tissue biopsy. An alternative matrix that researchers have analyzed since the 1970s is endometrial fluid [16]. More recently, high-throughput analysis of vaginal secretions, coined secretomics, has been utilized [26, 33]. As it focuses on sampling extracellular fluid, the analytes of interest are mainly proteins and lipids, with mass spectroscopy and chromatography used as the analytical methods. Analysis of lipid levels has revealed elevated levels of PGE2 and PGF2α during the WOI. Although preliminary information from endometrial secretions is intriguing, further investigation is required [26, 33].

Our understanding of infertility and endometrial receptivity has come a long way over the past several decades. However, many questions remain unanswered. New molecular and biochemical markers during the endometrial cycle continue to be discovered and they are likely to inform even better diagnostic algorithms. These include potential targets for pharmaceuticals and predictors of therapeutic success. Discoveries in this arena are fueled by advances in research technologies. High-throughput analysis, in particular, has revolutionized the field. Massively parallel sequencing will allow an even more detailed look at the unique genomic and transcriptomic signatures of the receptive endometrium. Translation of this research into clinical trials, and then clinical practice, is expected to have a major impact on the field of reproductive endocrinology and infertility.

Author details

Courtney Marsh[1]*, Katelyn Schumacher[2], Warren B. Nothnick[3,4,5], Robert N. Taylor[6] and Monique Monard[1]

*Address all correspondence to: cmarsh2@kumc.edu

1 Department of Obstetrics and Gynecology, University of Kansas, Kansas City, KS, USA

2 School of Medicine, University of Kansas, Kansas City, KS, USA

3 Department of Molecular and Integrative Physiology, University of Kansas Medical Center, Kansas City, Kansas, USA

4 Department of Obstetrics and Gynecology, University of Kansas Medical Center, Kansas City, Kansas, USA

5 Center for Reproductive Sciences, Institute for Reproduction and Perinatal Research, University of Kansas Medical Center, Kansas City, Kansas, USA

6 Department of Obstetrics and Gynecology, University of Utah, Salt Lake City, UT, USA

References

[1] Critchley HO, Saunders PT. Hormone receptor dynamics in a receptive human endometrium. Reproductive Sciences. 2009;**16**(2):191-199

[2] Fox C, Morin S, Jeong JW, Scott RT Jr, Lessey BA. Local and systemic factors and implantation: What is the evidence? Fertility and Sterility. 2016;**105**(4):873-884

[3] Gómez E, Ruíz-Alonso M, Miravet J, Simón C. Human endometrial transcriptomics: Implications for embryonic implantation. Cold Spring Harbor Perspectives in Medicine. 2015;**5**(7):a022996

[4] Gellersen B, Brosens JJ. Cyclic decidualization of the human endometrium in reproductive health and failure. Endocrine Reviews. 2014;**35**(6):851-905

[5] Taylor RN, Lebovic DI, Hornung D, Mueller MD. Endocrine and paracrine regulation of endometrial angiogenesis. Annals of the New York Academy of Sciences. 2001;**943**: 109-121

[6] Noyes RW, Hertig AT, Rock J. Dating the endometrial biopsy. Fertility and Sterility. 1950;**1**:3-25

[7] Yu J, Berga SL, Johnston-MacAnanny EB, Sidell N, Bagchi IC, Bagchi MK, et al. Endometrial stromal decidualization responds reversibly to hormone stimulation and withdrawal. Endocrinology. 2016;**157**:2432-2446

[8] Rock J, Bartlett MK. Biopsy studies of human endometrium: Criteria of dating and information about amenorrhea, menorrhagia, and time of ovulation. Journal of the American Medical Association. 1937;**108**:2022-2028

[9] Bazer FW, Spencer TE, Johnson GA, Burghardt RC, Wu G. Comparative aspects of implantation. Reproduction. 2009;**138**(2):195-209

[10] Wilcox AJ, Baird DD, Weinberg CR. Time of implantation of the conceptus and loss of pregnancy. The New England Journal of Medicine. 1999;**340**(23):1796-1799

[11] Bazer FW, Wu G, Spencer TE, Johnson GA, Burghardt RC, Bayless K. Novel pathways for implantation and establishment and maintenance of pregnancy in mammals. Molecular Human Reproduction. 2010;**16**(3):135-152

[12] Arias-Stella J. The Arias-Stella reaction: Facts and fancies four decades after. Advances in Anatomic Pathology. 2002;**9**(1):12-23. Review

[13] Burton GJ, Watson AL, Hempstock J, Skepper JN, Jauniaux E. Uterine glands provide histiotrophic nutrition for the human fetus during the first trimester of pregnancy. The Journal of Clinical Endocrinology and Metabolism. 2002;**87**(6):2954-2959

[14] Nikas G, Psychoyos A. Uterine pinopodes in peri-implantation human endometrium. Clinical relevance. Annals of the New York Academy of Sciences. 1997;**816**:129-142. Review

[15] Stavreus-Evers A, Mandelin E, Koistinen R, Aghajanova L, Hovatta O, Seppälä M. Glycodelin is present in pinopodes of receptive-phase human endometrium and is associated with down-regulation of progesterone receptor B. Fertility and Sterility. 2006;**85**(6): 1803-1811

[16] Achache H, Revel A. Endometrial receptivity markers, the journey to successful embryo implantation. Human Reproduction Update. 2006;**12**(6):731-746

[17] Coutifaris C, Myers ER, Guzick DS, Diamond MP, Carson SA, Legro RS, et al. Histological dating of timed endometrial biopsy tissue is not related to fertility status. Fertility and Sterility. 2004;**82**(5):1264-1272

[18] Garrido-Gómez T, Quiñonero A, Antúnez O, Díaz-Gimeno P, Bellver J, Simón C, et al. Deciphering the proteomic signature of human endometrial receptivity. Human Reproduction. 2014;**29**(9):1957-1967

[19] Ruan YC, Chen H, Chan HC. Ion channels in the endometrium: Regulation of endometrial receptivity and embryo implantation. Human Reproduction Update. 2014;**20**(4):517-529

[20] Li Q, Kannan A, Wang W, Demayo FJ, Taylor RN, Bagchi MK, et al. Bone morphogenetic protein 2 functions via a conserved signaling pathway involving Wnt4 to regulate uterine

decidualization in the mouse and the human. The Journal of Biological Chemistry. 2007;**282**(43):31725-31732

[21] Lessey BA. Endometrial integrins and the establishment of uterine receptivity. Human Reproduction. 1998;**13**(Suppl_3):247-258

[22] Dominguez F, Garrido-Gomez T, Lopez JA, Camafeita E, Quinonero A, Pellicer A, et al. Proteomic analysis of the human receptive versus non-receptive endometrium using differential in-gel electrophoresis and MALDI-MS unveils stathmin 1 and annexin A2 as differentially regulated. Human Reproduction. 2009;**24**(10):2607-2617

[23] Evans-Hoeker E, Lessey BA, Jeong JW, Savaris RF, Palomino WA, Yuan L, et al. Endometrial BCL6 overexpression in eutopic endometrium of women with endometriosis. Reproductive Sciences. 2016;**23**(9):1234-1241

[24] Miravet-Valenciano JA, Rincon-Bertolin A, Vilella F, Simon C. Understanding and improving endometrial receptivity. Current Opinion in Obstetrics and Gynecology. 2015;**27**(3): 187-192

[25] Matson BC, Pierce SL, Espenschied ST, Holle E, Sweatt IH, Davis ES, et al. Adrenomedullin improves fertility and promotes pinopodes and cell junctions in the peri-implantation endometrium. Biology of Reproduction. 2017;**97**(3):466-477

[26] Berlanga O, Bradshaw HB, Vilella-Mitjana F, Garrido-Gómez T, Simón C. How endometrial secretomics can help in predicting implantation. Placenta. 2011;**32**(Suppl. 3): S271-S275

[27] Díaz-Gimeno P, Ruíz-Alonso M, Blesa D, Simón C. Transcriptomics of the human endometrium. The International Journal of Developmental Biology. 2014;**58**(2-4):127-137

[28] Ahn SH, Singh V, Tayade C. Biomarkers in endometriosis: Challenges and opportunities. Fertility and Sterility. 2017;**107**(3):523-532

[29] Revel A. Defective endometrial receptivity. Fertility and Sterility. 2012;**97**(5):1028-1032

[30] Kitaya K, Matsubayashi H, Yamaguchi K, Nishiyama R, Takaya Y, Ishikawa T, et al. Chronic endometritis: Potential cause of infertility and obstetric and neonatal complications. American Journal of Reproductive Immunology. 2016;**75**(1):13-22

[31] Marsh CA, Hecker E. Maternal obesity and adverse reproductive outcomes: Reducing the risk. Obstetrical & Gynecological Survey. 2014;**69**(10):622-628

[32] Díaz-Gimeno P, Horcajadas JA, Martínez-Conejero JA, Esteban FJ, Alamá P, Pellicer A, et al. A genomic diagnostic tool for human endometrial receptivity based on the transcriptomic signature. Fertility and Sterility. 2011;**95**(1):50-60. 60.e1-15

[33] Cheong Y, Boomsma C, Heijnen C, Macklon N. Uterine secretomics: A window on the maternal-embryo interface. Fertility and Sterility. 2013;**99**(4):1093-1099

12

Menopause Female Reproductive Senescence from the Viewpoint of Evolutionary Anthropology

Sylvia Kirchengast

Abstract

Female reproductive senescence is characterized by the so-called menopausal transition taking place between the ages of 40 and 60 years. The major event of menopausal transition is menopause itself, which is biomedically defined as the cessation of menstrual function and the irreversible termination of female reproductive capability. Recent human females experience a postreproductive period from about 30 years. Such a long postreproductive period is absolutely uncommon among animals. Consequently, human menopause is still an evolutionary puzzle and several theories to explain the evolutionary basis of menopause have been presented. Menopausal transition, however, is also seen as a period of increased somatic and psychic symptoms which make this phase of life quite uncomfortable for affected women. In the present study, menopause and climacteric complaints are discussed from the viewpoint of evolutionary anthropology.

Keywords: menopause, human evolution, climacteric symptoms, reproductive senescence

1. Introduction

Recent *Homo sapiens* has the longest lifespan of all terrestrial mammals, however, human females stop to reproduce in the middle of it [1, 2]. Every woman who lives until about 50 years and beyond experiences the irreversible cessation of reproductive function, i.e., menopause. The World Health Organization (WHO) has defined menopause as the last spontaneous menstrual bleeding or the permanent cessation of menstruation resulting from loss of ovarian follicular activity [3]. Menopause is preceded by a phase of irregular cycles and starting hormonal changes, which is commonly called perimenopause. Perimenopause continued until 12 months after the last spontaneous menstrual bleeding, because no human female knows exactly that the actual bleeding is really the last one [4]. Therefore, the phase of postmenopause is reached when a woman had no menstrual periods over 12 months. Menopause is a universal, one-time life event, which marks the transition from reproductive to postreproductive life in females [5]. Consequently, menopause is a marker of reproductive ageing patterns typical of the female *Homo sapiens* [6]. Menopause occurs usually between 45 and 55 years, recent human females, however, routinely live for about 30 years after the cessation of reproductive function [2]. Furthermore, reproductive senescence is markedly accelerated relative to general somatic aging among female *Homo sapiens* [7]. Even in traditional foragers societies such as the Ache, Hadza, or !Kung San, that do not enjoy the benefits of modern medicine women can expect 20 and more years of active life following menopause [8–10]. From the viewpoint of evolutionary biology, this extraordinary long postreproductive phase among human females is in strict contradiction to the biogenetic imperative and the paradigm that natural selection forces organisms to maximize reproductive success [11]. According to these assumptions, reproductive senescence and in particular menopause followed by a long postreproductive period should be rare in nature. In the present review, the phenomenon of menopause and extended postreproductive life span is focused on from the viewpoint of evolutionary anthropology, in particular, human life history theory. For an appropriate analysis of menopausal transition, we have to consider two different levels of causality in biology, i.e., proximate and ultimate explanations of biological phenomena [11]. Proximate causes are immediate mechanisms, such as physiological or ontogenetic factors, whereas ultimate explanations, in contrast, tried to interpret biological phenomena in an evolutionary sense [11]. Therefore, proximate as well as ultimate causes of menopause are discussed.

2. Human life history theory

As pointed out above, according to the biogenetic imperative and natural selection theory, menopause should be rare in nature. Among *Homo sapiens*, however, menopause is an obligatory part of female life history. Before we discuss menopause from the viewpoint of evolutionary anthropology, we have considered life history theory.

Every species has evolved its own patterns of ontogeny of the individual organism from conception to death. This species typical process contains somatic growth, development, maturation, reproduction, and senescence—all of them are energetically costly events [12]. Life history theory tries to explain the evolution of these patterns of growth and reproduction by identifying trade-offs [13]. An important trade-off is between somatic growth and the maintenance on the one hand and successful reproduction on the other. For most organisms, it is not possible to provide enough energy to grow and to reproduce simultaneously. Therefore many organisms have evolved a timely separation between growth and reproduction. A period where energy is provided for growth and development is followed by a period where energy is used for successful reproduction. Human life history differs from that of other social mammals in several puzzling details. Even our next living relatives, the nonhuman primates, exhibit marked differences in certain features of life history [14]. In detail, human infants are weaned relatively early, on average by age 36 months, but after weaning human children depend on their mothers or other older group members for food and protection much longer than do the offspring of any other mammal, usually until they age about 7 years [12, 13]. From the viewpoint of evolutionary anthropology and human life history theory, the period between weaning and age of 7 years is defined as childhood stage, which is characterized by a set of biological and behavioral traits. This life history definition of childhood differs from the commonly used term childhood which refers to any time between birth and sexual maturation. It is assumed that the life history stage of childhood evolved about 2 million years ago among *Homo erectus*. The stage of childhood is not found among nonhuman primates [15]. Furthermore, humans reach puberty, i.e., sexual maturation, later than nonhuman primates and the short-term event of puberty is followed by an extended period of adolescence [15]. Adolescence is assumed to be a quite young stage of human life history occurring among *Homo sapiens* only. Since reproduction during early adolescence is rare, the interval between sexual maturation and first reproduction is much longer among humans than among nonhuman primates. Consequently, the age at first reproduction is much older than that of nonhuman primates; nevertheless human fertility may be higher than that among our nonhuman relatives. Modern humans however differ not only in the subadult stages of life history and reproductive success markedly from nonhuman primates and all other social mammals, the most distinct features are the extraordinary long life span and the prolonged period of female reproductive senescence, i.e., a long postmenopause [16]. During the fifth decade of life, fertility declines to essentially zero in human females; although one can expect to live for about further 30 years. This marked discrepancy between ovarian ageing and general ageing is a typical feature of female *Homo sapiens*. A prolonged postreproductive phase is not found among other animals, even among great social mammals with the exception of some toothed whale species.

3. Reproductive senescence among animals

As pointed out above, human females experience the cessation of reproductive function long before they die. Some signs of reproductive ageing are found among invertebrates in particular tephritid fruit flies [17] and the nematode *Caenorhabditis elegans* [18]. A kind of reproductive ageing characterized by a decline of sex steroid levels and a reduced probability of successful reproduction is found among several free living social mammals such as toothed whales, elephants, lions, or first of all primates [19–25]. An obligatory postreproductive life stage of 30 years and more, however, is exclusively found among human females [23]. Long postreproductive periods are uncommon among animals, even among large social mammals such as nonhuman primates and elephants. Only two Cetacean species such as short-finned pilot whales (*Globicephala macrorhynchus*) and killer whales (*Orcinus orca*) exhibit postreproductive life spans comparable to those of female *Homo sapiens* [22, 26]. Female short finned pilot whales stop to reproduce by about 36 years of age but they can live up to 65 years [22]. Female killer whales stop breeding by 48 years but they can live up to 90 years [22]. Baleen whales in contrast continue to reproduce into their nineties. Among large terrestrial mammals, elephants continue to reproduce into their sixties [27]. Quite difficult is the situation among our next living relatives, the nonhuman primates, because only few studies on reproductive ageing patterns among wild living as well as captive primates exist. Some studies suggest that with increasing age a period of reproductive instability is quite common among female primates [28]. Data from *lemurs* and *callitriche* plead for age-related decline in reproduction in some species [28]. Furthermore, hormonal changes—comparable to menopausal hormonal transition among human females—have been noted in many primate species [24]. An increasing cycle length with increasing age was reported for captive chimpanzees but not for the wild chimpanzees [24]. The main problem is that nearly all studies of chimpanzees are based on very small samples and these studies have not provided clear conclusions. According to Thompson et al., there is no evidence that menopause is an obligatory characteristic of chimpanzee life history [29]. Data concerning Orangutan and Gorilla are still rare. Some evidence for an extended postreproductive phase exists for rhesus monkeys (*Macaca mulatta*) [24]. We can summarize that menopause and a long postreproductive phase is found exclusively among humans and some toothed whales. Consequently, menopause seems to be a typical feature of *Homo sapiens* and therefore we have to ask, why do human females loose the capability of reproduction much earlier than their next living relatives and most other social mammals?

4. Physiology of menopause: proximate approach

In the first step, we have to analyze the proximate or physiological basis of female reproductive senescence. From a proximate viewpoint, menopause results from follicular atresia that starts extremely early in female ontogeny, i.e., during intrauterine phase and continues until menopause [23, 30]. In the female embryo, primordial germ cells originating from the yolk sac develop into oogonia, immature sex cells. Germ cell numbers peak at approximately 3×10^5–7×10^6 by the fifth month of fetal development [31]. Oogonia develop to oocytes. Oocyte formation, however, ceases by the time a female fetus is 5 months old. Consequently, human females are unable to continue to produce oocytes past their fifth month in utero. At this time process of follicular degeneration and resorption from 3.4 to 7 million germ cells to less than 1000 remaining follicles at the time of menopausal transition, starts. The exorbitantly high number of 7 million oogonia declines to about 2 million oocytes at the time of birth and to about 400000 at pubertal onset. Oocytes are embedded in follicular cells. The vast majority of follicles are nonproliferating, produces steroids and succumb to atresia by apoptosis [23]. Only few follicles develop to preovulatory follicles with a thick layer of granulosa and theca cells, consequently only few oocytes undergo ovulation. The majority of follicles and oocytes, which are developmental units, degenerates before ovulation. Fertility declines in human females before total depletion of oocytes. A gradual decline in fertility is observable between the ages 35 and 40 years, after this period the decline accelerates. This reduced fertility from about 35 years onward is mainly due to defects in oocytes [31]. Oocyte or follicular depletion accelerates as menopause got closer. At the time of menopause, the activity of the few remaining follicles declines drastically [23].

The follicular decline results in marked hormonal disturbances typical of perimenopause and postmenopause [4]. The main feature of menopausal transition is the dramatic decline in estrogen levels [32, 33]. These hormonal disturbances are caused by the depletion of follicular cells. The theca and the granulosa cells of the follicle, however, are essential for estrogen synthesis in the ovary. Consequently, estrogens are no longer converted from androgen in the granulosa cells during menopausal transition [23]. The decrease of estrogen secretion resulted in consecutive disturbances of the hypothalamus-pituitary-gonad axis (HPO-axis). During reproductive phase, menstrual cycle patterns are regulated by this hormonal axis. The hypothalamus secretes gonadotropin releasing hormone (GnRh) directly to the anterior pituitary. The secretion patterns of GnRh are modified by neurotransmitters such as dopamine, serotonin, epinephrine, or endorphin. Receptors in the anterior pituitary sense the pulse frequency and amplitude of GnRh and direct the production of the gonadotropins, follicle stimulating hormone (FSH), and lutenizing hormone (LH), which are essential for reproduction. FSH stimulates follicle development, LH the estrogen synthesis in the ovaries. Both stimulate ovulation and LH induces corpus luteum development and in this way progesterone synthesis. FSH binds to specific hormone receptors on the membrane of the granulosa cells, whereas LH binds to receptors of the granulose and theca cells. Androgens are secreted under LH stimulation from the theca cells, in the granulosa cells these androgens are converted into estradiol. The hormone secretion of the HPO-axis is regulated by a negative feedback mechanism. During reproductive phase, female sex hormone secretion underlies dramatic cyclic fluctuations [32, 33].

Menopausal transition is characterized by marked endocrine changes which are mainly induced by changes within the ovary but also central neuroendocrine changes. The reduction of ovarian follicles during perimenopause results in declining levels of inhibin B, a dimeric protein, and a rise of follicle stimulating hormone (FSH) and lutenizing hormone (LH) levels. During perimenopause, estradiol levels remain relatively unchanged presumably in response to the elevated FSH levels [32, 33]. As the follicular supply is exhausted, estradiol (E_2) and estrone (E) decrease dramatically; FSH and LH, however, remain elevated. Estradiol, the most physiologically active estrogen, declines most markedly, whereas estrone continues to be produced through the conversion of androstenedione to estrone in muscle, adipose, and other tissues. Consequently, the hypothalamus-pituitary gonad axis (HPG-axis) is irreversible disturbed. Beside the decline in estrogens and progesterone (P), a decrease of testosterone (T), androstenedione (A), dehydroepiandrosterone (DHEA), dehydroepiandrosterone sulfate (DHEA-S), and sex hormone binding globulin (SHBG) levels after menopausal transition was observed [32, 33]. Additionally, thyroxine (t_4) and triiodothyronine (t_3) levels as well as growth hormone (GH) decrease as a result of the general ageing process. This dramatic hormonal transition is often associated with weight gain and changes in body composition, in particular fat distribution patterns [34–41]. We can summarize from a proximate viewpoint that menopausal transition is caused by the final depletion of germ cells and it is characterized by marked hormonal disturbances which are associated with significant changes in body composition and fat patterning.

5. Evolutionary explanations of menopause: ultimate approach

According to Theodosius Dobzhansky, "nothing in biology makes sense except in the light of evolution" [42]. Consequently, we have to analyze menopausal transition from an ultimate or evolutionary viewpoint. There is no doubt that menopause is clearly a biological phenomenon and consequently, we can assume that menopause has an evolutionary origin [43–45]. The majority of women in First world countries experience menopause usually between 47 and 55 years of life [46]. Considering an average life expectancy of about 80 years among females in First world countries, female postreproductive phase thus lasts on the average of 30 years. The potential maximum life span of recent *Homo sapiens* is even longer and is thought to be about 120 years. Considering this extraordinary long lifespan, we have to be aware that human females can spend more than half of their maximum life span potential with postreproductive period [23]. Such an extremely long postreproductive phase of life is unique in the animal kingdom and makes menopause to an extremely interesting event from an evolutionary point of view. If maximization of reproductive success is the ultimate goal of life, how can such a long postreproductive period be explained in evolutionary terms?

Since 1970s, several evolutionary scenarios of human menopause were proposed to explain the phenomenon of female reproductive senescence and in particular menopause; however, there is still no consensus about which of these hypotheses should be preferred [31, 45, 47, 48]. In general, two different types of evolutionary explanations of menopause can be distinguished: nonadaptive or by-product hypotheses and adaptive hypotheses [23]. Consequently, we have to ask that whether menopause is an adaption or an epiphenomenon [49].

At a first glimpse, the so-called by-product hypothesis seems comprehensible. The by-product hypothesis is based on the assumption that life expectancy increased dramatically during the last few centuries. In former times, however, the life expectancy was much shorter. Consequently, women did simply not live long enough to experience menopause for most time of our evolution and history. From a physiological point of view, menopause occurs when all oocytes are depleted. The maximum number of germ cells which is produced until fifth month in utero is adapted to a life expectancy of less than 50 years. According to the by-product hypothesis, it was assumed that in our past only few women lived until 50 years and beyond. Therefore, postmenopausal women did not exist. Consequently, menopause is not an adaptation, it is nothing else than a by-product of increased life span and therefore a very recent phenomenon [50, 51].

In contrast to by-product hypotheses, the adaptive hypotheses consider menopause itself as a fitness advantage [52]. The most important question is, how natural selection came to favor prolonged postreproductive phase in human life history? The antagonistic pleiotropy hypothesis—first proposed by Williams in 1957—suggests that if a gene caused both increased reproduction in early life and aging in later life, then reproductive senescence can be interpreted as adaptive. In case of menopause, it was assumed that follicular depletion may cause both more regular cycles in early life and loss of fertility in later life through menopause. Consequently, its early benefits may outweigh its late costs [53].

From the perspective of life history, the main question is, when in our evolution an extended postreproductive period occurred for the first time? At the moment, it seems that life circumstances of our ancestors changed dramatically about 2 or 1.8 million years ago at the time when *Homo erectus* lived [54]. At this stage of hominid evolution, new growth patterns and encephalization made a long dependency of offspring necessary and lead to life history patterns similar to those of recent *Homo sapiens,* such as introduction of childhood and also menopause and an extended period of postmenopause [54]. Consequently, it is assumed that menopause and prolonged reproductive senescence occurred first among *Homo erectus* about 2 million years ago [55]. Significantly associated with the existence of an extended postreproductive phase is the introduction with the life history stage of childhood between weaning and about 6 or 7 years of life. While weaned chimpanzees must forage for their own food, human children depend after weaning on older individuals for food and protection. This prolonged period of dependence during subadult phase of life makes an especially high parental investment necessary. Weaned children need extensive care because they are not able to use resources like adolescents and adults. Consequently, mothers have to provide a substantial fraction of their weaned children's diet [55]. Parents are often supported by the grandparents, first of all grandmothers, who provide a substantial investment in their grandchildren [56–58]. This is especially true for postmenopausal women with no young children of their own who help to feed and to take care of the offspring of their daughters and near relatives [55, 59]. This successful investment of postmenopausal women in related offspring, first of all grandchildren, suggests a solution to the riddle of prolonged postmenopausal period in humans. The so-called grandmother hypothesis as an evolutionary explanation of female menopause was a consequence of such ideas [60–62].

Human females are unable to reproduce after menopause; however, they invest in the offspring of their daughters and sons. In this way, a prolonged postreproductive span may have increased inclusive fitness of postmenopausal women. This point of view resulted in the introduction of the so-called grandmother hypothesis, which suggested increased fitness of women who stop reproduction and invest in their grandchildren [55, 61, 63–65]. The grandmother hypothesis is mainly based on the results of Kirsten Hawkes extensive fieldwork among Hadza hunter-gatherers northern Tanzania in eastern Africa [55, 60]. Nevertheless, the grandmother hypotheses have been criticized by several authors [66].

Beside the grandmother hypothesis, the so-called good mother hypothesis tries to explain the evolutionary benefit of an extended postreproductive phase in female *Homo sapiens*. The termination of reproductive capability independent of general senescence ensures that human females have a real chance to be young enough at their last birth to survive until their last offspring is able to survive without a biological mother [43, 67]. It is well documented that the survival of the mother during the rearing period is a major determinant of their children's survival. Considering subadult dependency in *Homo sapiens* mothers should survive until the last offspring reaches age of 7 years. According to Pavard et al. [52], menopause and subsequent postreproductive life are significantly advantageous when two conditions are satisfied: a marked increase in stillbirth and risk of birth defects as well as in maternal mortality with mother's age. Both the grandmother hypothesis and the "mother" hypothesis are the main adaptive explanations of human menopause. Female reproductive cessation seems to be a strategy that has been selected for during human evolution because women at older ages might maximize their fitness by investing resources in the survival and reproduction of their living offspring rather than by continuing to reproduce.

Recently, some new approaches to solve the evolutionary puzzle of menopause have been provided. According to the mate-choice hypothesis, male mating preference for younger females may lead to the accumulation of mutations deleterious to female fertility and thus lead to the evolution of an extended postreproductive period in human females [68]. Takahashi et al. [31] tried to explain the origin and evolution of menopause by combining a genetic basis, behavioral factors such as mating behavior, a life history perspective, and social changes in human evolution.

Although many different theories to explain the origin and evolution of menopause have been presented, human menopause remains as an unsolved evolutionary puzzle.

6. Climacteric syndrome from the viewpoint of evolutionary anthropology

As pointed out above, menopause is a common experience of all human females who lived until about 50 years of age and beyond [23, 46, 69]. From a biological viewpoint, menopause simply reflects reproductive senescence, the end of childbearing phase and is therefore a natural part of female life history [5]. Consequently, menopause is not pathology because all human females who live long enough experience menopausal transition and the cessation of reproductive capability. Despite this fact, menopause was increasingly interpreted as a pathological condition since early nineteenth century. This medicalization of menopause within biomedical practice has affected the way menopause is viewed within society until today. Of special importance in this case is the work of the British gynecologist E.J. Tilt, who introduced the phenomenon of menopause in British Gynecology in 1857 [70]. In continental Europe and North America, biomedicine practitioners began to think of menopause as a disease-like state by the 1930s. As endocrinology improved and as synthetic estrogens became readily available in the 1960s, menopause was treated as a hormone deficiency disease, comparably to diabetes [71]. As a consequence, the medical (pathological) viewpoint dominates menopause research for a long time.

Two different approaches to this medical viewpoint can be distinguished: on the one hand, menopause is interpreted as an own deficiency disease or endocrinopathy. According to this view, hormonal deficiency results in symptoms of the so called climacteric syndrome [6, 71, 72]. This medicalization of menopause is mainly due to the fact that many women experience a large variety of symptoms, such as hot flushes and night sweats, and also psychic problems such as depression, irritability, or insomnia during peri- and postmenopause. This symptom complex is commonly called climacteric syndrome, which make peri- and postmenopause very uncomfortable for many women. In western societies, 60–70% of menopausal women reported hot flushes and night sweats [46, 69]. Climacteric symptoms seem to be strongly related to the menopause-specific decline of estrogen levels [32, 33]. However, not all climacteric women suffer from climacteric symptoms and the interpretation of the individual symptoms varies between individuals according to culture and society [46, 73–76]. Quite different is the alternative approach: menopause is not seen as a disease by itself but menopause is interpreted as a major risk factor for the development of other diseases such as osteoporosis, cardiovascular disease, some cancers such as breast cancer, and also Alzheimer disease [4, 77]. Additionally, the decline of estrogen levels after menopause enhances the risk of cardiovascular disease such as hypertension [78].

Consequently, the risk of stroke, myocard infarct, and heart failure increases after menopause. Furthermore, menopause also seems to increase the risk of the development of certain cancers such as breast cancer [79, 80].

From the viewpoint of evolutionary anthropology, the so-called climacteric syndrome can be interpreted in an evolutionary sense. Of course, potential climacteric complaints cannot be reconstructed from fossil bones and it is not possible to search for climacteric complaints among nonhuman primates or other social mammals. However, different attitudes toward menopausal transition and climacteric symptoms are found in different cultural settings [73, 75, 76].

The climacteric syndrome, however, can also be interpreted from the viewpoint of evolutionary medicine [81, 82]. Evolutionary medicine was formalized in early 1990s, most notably by the evolutionary biologist George C. Williams and psychiatrist Randolph Nesse who tried to understand why natural selection has left the human body so vulnerable to diseases [83]. According to their concept, many medical conditions that are clearly pathological today have been adaptive in the ancestral environment in which *Homo sapiens* evolved. Evolutionary medicine is concerned with identifying and understanding these conditions in our environment of evolutionary adaptedness (EEA) [84]. Especially, the impact of changing living conditions during our evolution and also of more recent processes such as modernization and acculturation on health and disease is focused.

As pointed out above, we can assume that menopause and prolonged postmenopausal phase occurred first among members of *Homo erectus* about 2 million years ago [85]. In the first step, we have to look at the natural and social environment of our ancestors from about 2 million years ago up to 10,000 years ago when Neolithic transitions started. Ethnographic analyses of the few remaining contemporary forager populations such as the Hadza in Tanzania, the !Kung of Namibia and Botswana, Ache of Paraguay, or Efe of Central Africa provided information about diet and life style in recent foraging economy [8, 10]. The typical life style of foragers is highly mobile because high levels in daily activity in search of food, water, and sleeping sites are necessary. The diet consists mainly of lean meat, wild vegetables, tubers, berries, fruits, nuts, and roots, while excluding foods such as dairy products, grains, sugar, legumes, and fats. From a medical point of view, typical noncommunicable diseases such as hypertension, heart disease, cancer, type II diabetes, or obesity are rather unknown [86]. *Homo sapiens* is clearly adapted to an environment like this. With the emergence of agriculture in the area of the fertile crescent about 10,000 years ago, subsistence economy and life circumstances changed dramatically [87, 88]. Domestication of animals and plants allowed the production of a surplus of food, which resulted in population growth, and dietary changes [88]. Analyses of Neolithic skeletal remains indicated protein deficiencies and periodic food shortages, skeletal conditions which can clearly be interpreted as results of famine and starvation. Furthermore, the close proximity to domesticated animals exposed humans to a variety of new pathogens resulting in an increased frequency of infectious diseases [89]. Therefore, Neolithic transition has led to the so-called first epidemiologic transition [90]. A second epidemiologic transition occurred about 200 years ago during industrial revolution when a shift toward manmade diseases is observable.

During the twentieth and twenty-first century lifestyle changed again dramatically. Urbanization, technical advances, and general modernization resulted in a marked transition in human life style. Advances in medicine reduced human morbidity and mortality and lead to increased life expectancy. The daily energy effort to gather and prepare food is reduced nearly to zero, since only few individuals are working on food production. Mechanized transportation, sedentary jobs, and labor-saving household technologies reduce physical activity too. On the other hand, more than enough energy providing food, mainly consisting of sugar and fat is easily available [91, 92]. Consequently, a dramatic mismatch between current environment and human body evolved in the environment of our evolutionary adaptedness can be observed. In 99% of our evolutionary history, we have survived as foragers following a highly mobile life style in small groups. Obesity and noncommunicable diseases were quite unknown. Our gene pool was shaped by natural and sexual selection toward an optimal adaptation to these environments and life circumstances. Our recent environments, however, differ dramatically from that in which our ancestors evolved. There is no doubt that also some genetic changes had occurred since the Neolithic transition; however natural selection works slowly and our genome changed to a certain degree only. Therefore, we are still often adapted to a habitat that since more than 10,000 years no longer exists [83, 93–95].

Recent health problems such as climacteric complaints, cardiovascular disease, osteoporosis, or even postmenopausal breast cancer can be interpreted primarily as the results of a dramatic change in life style of women in contemporary societies. As pointed out above, the rapid decline in estrogen levels associated with menopause experienced by recent women in industrialized societies enhances climacteric symptoms such as hot flushes [23, 32, 33, 96]. These hormonal disturbances may be the result of our recent life style patterns. We have to be aware that life history patterns of contemporary women are unique within human evolution [65]. We can assume that female life history patterns in our environment of evolutionary adaptedness resemble those of contemporary hunter gatherer societies [65]. Recent female hunter gatherers reach sexual maturation quite late. Their reproductive span is characterized by many cycles of pregnancy, long periods of lactation, and early menopause. Consequently, the number of ovulatory cycles is quite low and about 100 ovulatory cycles are assumed during reproductive span. Therefore life-time estrogen levels were quite low [97]. These low levels of estrogens during adult life are caused by high levels of physical activity, a diet characterized by low fat contents, a low amount of body fat, and low body weight [79, 97]. Consequently, lifetime estrogen exposition was quite low in the environment of evolutionary adaptedness. Life history patterns of women in recent developed countries are quite different. Menarche occurs early and first pregnancy becomes late. In Austria, for example, first menstrual bleeding occurs at the age of 12 years on average, first birth, however, occurs at the age of 29.7 years [98]. This means a period of nearly 18 years between sexual maturation and first reproduction. Reproductive span of contemporary women living in First world countries is characterized by extremely few pregnancies, few births, and short periods of lactation. It can be assumed that a woman experiences about 400 cycles on the average. Menopause occurs late and hormone supply via hormonal contraceptives or hormone replacement therapy is usual. Consequently, life estrogen exposition is long and estrogen levels are high [99]. During menopausal transition, estrogen levels drop down very fast resulting in rapid hormone deficiency, which may lead to climacteric symptomatology [32, 33, 69].

Among recent traditional societies, following quite different life style patterns such as women in rural India or Maya women in Yucatan estrogen levels are very low during menopausal transition; nevertheless, climacteric symptoms are rarely reported. Traditional lifestyle is characterized by low life time estrogen levels. The decline of estrogen secretion during menopausal transition is therefore not as dramatic as among women in western societies. Sometimes, last lactational amenorrhea—characterized by low estrogen levels—switches to menopause [23]. Consequently, climacteric complaints as a reaction of a sudden drastic estrogen decline are prevented. The high prevalence of climacteric symptoms in western societies may therefore be interpreted as a result our recent life style.

Additionally, a high rate of physical activity and a traditional diet poor in fat reduce estrogen levels through reproductive phase and even during and shortly after menopausal transition. Estrogens are converted from androgens in adipose tissue. Consequently, a higher amount of body fat increase the estrogen levels during reproductive phase and even during menopausal transition. This positive association between body fat and estrogen levels increases also the probability to develop breast cancer during peri- and postmenopause. A sedentary life style, high fat contents in diet, high life time estrogen levels, and high rates of overweight and obesity during middle age increase the risk of several diseases associated with menopausal transition such as breast cancer, cardiovascular disease, and also osteoporosis [100].

7. Conclusion

From the viewpoint of evolutionary anthropology, menopause is a natural part of female life history and therefore not a pathology. Several theories have been proposed to explain the evolutionary basis of menopausal transition, although there is still no consensus. The climacteric syndrome—mainly caused by estrogen deficiency—may be interpreted as the result of a mismatch between recent life style and reproductive patterns and life circumstances in the environment in which our ancestors evolved.

Author details

Sylvia Kirchengast

Address all correspondence to: sylvia.kirchengast@univie.ac.at

Department of Anthropology, University of Vienna, Vienna, Austria

References

[1] Fernell RJ, Sowers MF. Longitudinal, epidemiologic studies of female reproductive aging. Annals of the New York Academy of Sciences 2010, **1204**:188-197

[2] Gold EB. The timing of the age at which natural menopause occurs. Obstetrics and Gynecology Clinics of North America. 2011;**38**:425-440

[3] World Health Organization (WHO). Research on Menopause in the 1990s. WHO Technical Reports Series No. 866. Geneva: WHO 1996

[4] Huber JC. Klimakterium – Diagnose und Therapie. Berlin: Berliner Medizinische Verlagsanstalt; 1995

[5] Melby MK, Lampl M. Menopause a biocultural perspective. Annual Review of Anthropology. 2011;**40**:53-70

[6] Utian WH. Overview of menopause. American Journal of Obstetrics & Gynecology. 1987;**156**:1280-1283

[7] Pavelka MSM, Fedigan LM. Menopause: A comparative life history perspective. Yearbook of Physical Anthropology. 1991;**34**:13-38

[8] Howell N. Life Histories of the Dobe !Kung. Food, Fatness and Well Being Over the Lifespan. Los Angeles: University of California Press; 2010

[9] Hill K, Hurtado AM. Ache Life History. The Ecology and Demography of a Foraging People. New York: de Gruyter; 1995

[10] Marlowe FW. The Hadza Hunter Gatherers of Tanzania. Los Angeles: University of California Press; 2010

[11] Voland E. Grundriss der Soziobiologie. Stuttgart: Fischer Verlag; 1993

[12] Hill K, Kaplan H. Life history traits in humans. Theory and empirical studies. Annual Review of Anthropology. 1999;**28**:397-430

[13] Bogin B, Smith H. Evolution of the human life cycle. American Journal of Human Biology. 1996;**8**:703-716

[14] Holland Jones J. Primates and the evolution of long-slow life histories. Current Biology. 2011;**21**:708-717

[15] Bogin B. Evolutionary hypotheses for human childhood. Yearbook of Physical Anthropology. 1997;**40**:63-89

[16] Kuzawa CW, Bragg JM. Plasticity in human life history strategy: Implications for contemporary human variation and the evolution of Genus *Homo*. Current Anthropology. 2012;**53**:S369-S382

[17] Carey JR, Molleman F. Reproductive ageing in tephritid fruit flies. Annals of the New York Academy of Sciences. 2010;**1204**:139-148

[18] Kenyon C. A pathway that links reproductive status to lifespan in Caenorhabditis elegans. Annals of the New York Academy of Sciences. 2010;**1204**:15-162

[19] Austad SN. Animal models of reproductive aging: What can they tell us? Annals of the New York Academy of Sciences 2010, **1204**:123-128

[20] Altmann I, Gesqiere L, Galbany J, Onyango PO, Alberts SC. Life history context of reproductive aging in a wild primate model. Annals of the New York Academy of Sciences. 2010;**1204**:127-138

[21] Hawkes K, Smith KR. Do women stop early? Similarities in fertility decline in humans and chimpanzees. Annals of the New York Academy of Sciences. 2010;**1204**:43-53

[22] Johnston RA, Cant MA. The evolution of menopause in cetaceans and humans: The role of demography. Proceedings. Biological Sciences. 2010;**22**:3765-3771

[23] Leidy-Sievert L. Menopause. A Biocultural Perspective. London: Rutgers University Press; 2006

[24] Walker MI, Herndon JG. Menopause in non human primates. Biology of Reproduction. 2008;**79**:398-406

[25] Ward EJ, Parson K, Holmes EE, Balcom KC, Ford JLB. The role of menopause and reproductive senescence in a long lived social mammal. Frontiers in Zoology. 2009;**6**:4-14

[26] Brent LJN, Franks DW, Foster EA, Balcomb KC, Cant MA, Croft DP. Ecological knowledge, leadership, and the evolution of menopause in Killer whales. Current Biology. 2015;**25**:746-750

[27] Moss CJ. The demography of an African elephant (*Loxodonta Africana*) population in Amboseli Kenya. Journal of Zoology. 2001;**255**:145-156

[28] Atsalis S, Margulis S. Primate reproductive ageing: From lemurs to humans. Interdisciplinary Topics in Gerontology 2008;**36**:186-194

[29] Thompson ME, Jones JH, Pusey AE, Brewer-Marsden S, Goodall J, Marsden D, Matsuzawa T, Nishida T, Reynolds V, Sugiyama Y, Wrangham RW. Ageing and fertility patterns in wild chimpanzees provide insights into the evolution of menopause. Current Biology. 2007;**17**:2150-2156

[30] Finch Ce, Homes DJ. Ovarian aging in developmental and evolutionary contexts. Annals of the New York Academy of Sciences 2010, **1204**:82-94

[31] Takahashi M, Singh RS, Stone J. A theory for the origin of human menopause. Frontiers in Genetics.2016, **7**:1-12

[32] Burger HG, Dudley EC, Robertson DM, Dennerstein L. Hormonal changes in the menopause transition. Recent Progress in Hormone Research. 2002;**57**:257-275

[33] Burger HG, Hale GE, Robertson DM, Dennerstein L. A review of hormonal changes during the menopausal transition: Focus on findings from the Melbourne Women's Midlife Health project. Human Reproduction Update. 2007;**13**:559-565

[34] Astrup A. Physical activity and weight gain and fat distribution changes with menopause: Current evidence and research issues. Medicine & Science in Sports & Exercise. 1999;**31**:S564-S567

[35] Douchi T, Yamamoto S, Yoshimitsu N, Andoh T, Matsuo T, Nagata Y. Relative contribution of ageing and menopause to changes in lean and fat mass in segmental regions. Maturitas. 2002;**42**:301-306

[36] Douchi T, Yamamoto S, Nakamura S, Ijuin T, Oki T, Maruta K, Nagata Y. The effect of menopause on regional and total body lean mass. Maturitas. 1998;**29**:247-252

[37] Tchernof A, Poehlmann ET. Effects of the menopause transition on body fatness and body fat distribution. Obesity Research. 1998;**6**:246-254

[38] Panotopoulus G, Ruiz JC, Raison J, Guy-Grand B, Basdevant A. Menopause, fat and lean distribution in obese women. Maturitas. 1996;**25**:11-19

[39] Messier V, Rabasa-Lhoret R, Barat-Artigar S, Elisha B, Karelis AD, Aubertin-Leheudre M. Menopause and sarcopenia: A potential role for sex hormones Maturitas. 2011;**68**:331-336

[40] Piche ME, Lapointe A, Weisnagel SJ, Corneau L, Nadeau A, Bergeron J, Lemieux S. Regional body fat distribution and metabolic profile in postmenopausal women. Metabolism – Clinical and Experimental. 2008;**57**:1101-1107

[41] Kirchengast S, Gruber D, Sator M, Hartmann B, Knogler W, Huber J. menopause associated differences in female fat patterning estimated by dual-energy-x-ray absorptiometry. Annals of Human Biology. 1997;**24**:45-54

[42] Dobzhansky T. Nothing in Biology makes sense except in the light of evolution. The American Teacher. 1973;**35**:125-129

[43] Sherman PW. The evolution of menopause. Nature. 1998;**392**:759-760

[44] Shanley DP, Sear R, Mace R, Kirkwood TBL. Testing evolutionary theories of menopause. Proceedings of the Royal Society B: Biological Sciences. 2007;**274**:2943-2949

[45] Pollycove R, Naftolin F, Simon JA, The evolutionary origin and significance of menopause. Menopause. 2011;**18**:336-342

[46] Palacios S, Henderson VW, Siseles N, Viaseca P. Age of menopause and impact of climacteric symptoms by geographical region. Climacteric. 2010;**13**:419-428

[47] Peccei JS. The origin and the evolution of menopause: The altriciality-lifespan hypothesis. Ethology and Sociobiology. 1995;**16**:425-449

[48] Wu JM, Zelinski MB, Ingram DK, Ottinger MA. Ovarian Ageing and menopause: Current theories, hypotheses and research models. Experimental Biology and Medicine. 2005;**230**:818-828

[49] Peccei JS. Menopause: Adaptation or epiphenomenon? Evolutionary Anthropology. 2001;**12**:43-57

[50] Washburn S. Longevity in primates. In: McGaugh JMJ, editors. Aging, Biology and Behaviour. New York: Academic Press; 1981. pp. 11-29

[51] Weiss KM. Evolutionary perspectives on human aging. In: Amoss PT, Harell S, editors. Other Ways of Growing Old. Stanford: Stanford University Press; 1981. pp. 25-58

[52] Pavard S, Metcalf CIF, Heyer E, Senescence of reproduction may explain adaptive menopause in humans. American Journal of Physical Anthropology. 2008;**136**:194-203

[53] Wood JW, O'Conner KA, Holman DJ, Bringle E, Barsom SH, Grimes MA. The evolution of menopause by antagonistic pleiotropy. Center for Demography and Ecology; 2001 (Working Paper)

[54] Bogin B. Patterns of Human Growth. Cambridge: Cambridge University Press; 1999

[55] Hawkes K, O'Connell JF, Blurton Jones NG, Alvarez H, Charnov AL. Grandmothering, menopause and the evolution of human life histories. Proceedings of the National Academy of Sciences. 1998;**95**:1336-1339

[56] Sear R, Mace R. Who keeps children alive? A review of the effects of kin on child survival. Evolution and Human Behavior. 2008;**29**:1-18

[57] Sear R. Kin and child survival in rural Malawi. Human Nature. 2008;**19**:277-293

[58] Coall DA, Hertwig R. Grandparental investment: Past, present, and future. Behavioral and Brain Sciences. 2010;**33**:1-59

[59] Sear R, Mace R, McGregor I A. Maternal grandmothers improve nutritional status and survival of children in rural Gambia. Proceedings of the Royal Society. 2000;**267**:1641-1647

[60] Hawkes K, O'Connell JF, Blurton Jones NG. Hadza women's time allocation, offspring provisioning and the evolution of long postmenopausal lifespans. Current Anthropology. 1997;**38**:551-577

[61] Hawkes K. Grandmothering of human longevity. American Journal of Human Biology. 2003;**15**:380-400

[62] Lahdenperä M, Lummaa V, Helle S, Tremblay M, Russell AF. Fitness benefits of prolonged post-reproductive lifespan in women. Nature. 2004;**428**:178-181

[63] Alvarez HP. Grandmother hypothesis and primate life histories. American Journal of Physical Anthropology. 2000;**113**:435-450

[64] Voland E, Chasiotis A, Schiefenhövel W. Grandmotherhood. The Evolutionary Significance of the Second Half of Female Life. New York: Rutgers University Press; 2005

[65] Blurton Jones NG, Hawkes K, O'Connell JF. Antiquity of postreproductive life. Are there modern impacts on hunter gatherer postreproductive life span. American Journal of Human Biology. 2002;**14**:184-202

[66] Peccei JS. A critique of the grandmother hypotheses: Old and new. American Journal of Human Biology. 2001;**13**:434-452

[67] Alexander RD. The evolution of social behaviour. Annual Review of Ecology and Systematics. 1974;**5**:325-383

[68] Morton RA, Stone JR, Singh RS. Mate choice and the origin of the menopause. PLoS One. 2013;**9**:e1003092

[69] Hunter M, Rendall M. Bio-psycho-socio-cultural perspectives on menopause. Best Practice & Research: Clinical Obstetrics & Gynaecology. 2007;**21**:261-274

[70] Van de Wiel L. The time of the change: Menopause's medicalization and the gender politics of aging. International Journal of Feminist Approaches to Bioethics. 2014;**7**:74-98

[71] McCrea FB. The politics of menopause: The discovery of a deficiency disease. Social Problems. 1983;**31**:111-123

[72] Bell SE. Changing ideas: The medicalization of menopause. Social Science & Medicine. 1987;**24**:535-542

[73] Beyene Y, Cultural significance and physiological manifestations of menopause: A biocultural analysis. Culture Medicine and Psychiatry. 1986;**10**:47-71

[74] Lock M. Encounters with Aging: Mythologies of Menopause in Japan and North America. Berkeley: University of California Press; 1993

[75] Kilaf E, Kirchengast S. Menopause between nature and culture: Menopausal age and climacteric symptoms among Turkish immigrant women in Vienna, Austria. Acta Medica Lituanica. 2008;**15**:313-329

[76] Pitkin J. Cultural issues and the menopause. Menopause International. 2010;**16**:156-161

[77] Worcester N, Whatley MH. The selling of HRT: Playing on the fear factor. Feminist Review. 1992;**41**:1-26

[78] Mayo JL. A natural approach to menopause. Applied Nutritional Science Reports. 1997;**5**:1-8

[79] Turner LB, A meta-analysis of fat intake, reproduction and breast cancer risk: An evolutionary perspective. American Journal of Human Biology. 2011;**23**:601-608

[80] Wu AH, Pike MC, Stram DO. Meta-analysis: Dietary fat intake, serum estrogen levels and the risk of breast cancer. Journal of the National Cancer Institute. 1999;**91**:529-534

[81] Froehle AW. Postmenopausal health and disease from the perspective of evolutionary medicine. Anthropology &Aging Quarterly. 2013;**34**:61-86

[82] Kirchengast S, Rühli F. Evolutionary medicine and its implications for endocrinological issues (e.g. menopause). Comparative Endocrinology 2013, **186**:145-149

[83] Nesse RM, Stearns SC. The great opportunity: Evolutionary applications to medicine and public health. Evolutionary Applications. 2008;**1**:28-48

[84] Bowlby J. Attachment and Loss. New York: Basic Books; 1969

[85] Henke W, Hardt T. The genus *Homo*: Origin, speciation and dispersal. In: Condemi S, Weniger G-C, editors. Continuity and Discontinuity in the peopling of Europe: One hundred fifty years of Neanderthal study, Vertebrate Paleobiology and Paleoanthropology. New York: Springer Press; 2011. pp. 17-43

[86] Eaton SB, Konner M. Paleolithic nutrition: A consideration of its nature and current implications. New England Journal of Medicine. 1985;**312**:283-289

[87] Maher LA, Richter T, Macdonald D, Jones MD, Martin L, Stock IT. Twenty thousand year old huts at a hunter gatherer settlement in eastern Jordan. PLoS One 2012;**7**:e31447

[88] Larsen C. Biological changes in human populations with agriculture. Annual Review of Anthropology. 1995;**24**:185-213

[89] Armelagos GI, Goodman AH,.Jacobs KH. The origins of agriculture: Population growth during a period of declining health. Population and Environment. 1991;**13**:9-22

[90] Barrett R, Kuzawa CW, McDade T,.Armelagos GI. Emerging and re-emerging infectious diseases: The third epidemiologic transition. Annual Review of Anthropology. 1998;**27**:247-271

[91] Popkin BM, Gordon-Larsen P. The nutrition transition: Worldwide obesity dynamics and their determinants. International Journal of Obesity. 2004;**28**:52-59

[92] Lieberman LS. Evolutionary and anthropological perspectives on optimal foraging in obesogenic environments. Appetite. 2006;**47**:3-9

[93] Trevathan WR. Evolutionary medicine. Annual Review of Anthropology. 2007;**36**: 139-154

[94] Vitzthum VI, Evolutionary models of women's reproductive functioning. Annual Review of Anthropology. 2008;**37**:53-73

[95] Wick G, Berger P, Jansen-Dürr P, Gerbeck-Loebenstein B. A Darwinian-evolutionary concept of age-related diseases. Experimental Gerontology. 2003;**38**:13-25

[96] Santoro N. The menopause transition: An update. Human Reproduction Update. 2002;**8**: 155-160

[97] Eaton SB, Pike MC, Short RV, Lee NC, Trussell J, Hatcher RA, Wood JW, Worthman CM, Nicolas GBI, Konner MJ, Bailey R, Hurtado AM, Women's reproductive cancers in evolutionary context. The Quarterly Review of Biology. 1994;**69**:353-3657

[98] Statistik Austria. Demographic Yearbook. Vienna, Austria. 2016

[99] Shaw LAM, Shaw SLJ, Menopause, evolution and changing cultures. Menopause International. 2009;**15**:175-179

[100] Strassmann BI. Menstrual cycling and breast cancer: An evolutionary perspective. Journal of Women's Health. 1999;**8**:193-202

Permissions

All chapters in this book were first published in AMLM, by InTech Open; hereby published with permission under the Creative Commons Attribution License or equivalent. Every chapter published in this book has been scrutinized by our experts. Their significance has been extensively debated. The topics covered herein carry significant findings which will fuel the growth of the discipline. They may even be implemented as practical applications or may be referred to as a beginning point for another development.

The contributors of this book come from diverse backgrounds, making this book a truly international effort. This book will bring forth new frontiers with its revolutionizing research information and detailed analysis of the nascent developments around the world.

We would like to thank all the contributing authors for lending their expertise to make the book truly unique. They have played a crucial role in the development of this book. Without their invaluable contributions this book wouldn't have been possible. They have made vital efforts to compile up to date information on the varied aspects of this subject to make this book a valuable addition to the collection of many professionals and students.

This book was conceptualized with the vision of imparting up-to-date information and advanced data in this field. To ensure the same, a matchless editorial board was set up. Every individual on the board went through rigorous rounds of assessment to prove their worth. After which they invested a large part of their time researching and compiling the most relevant data for our readers.

The editorial board has been involved in producing this book since its inception. They have spent rigorous hours researching and exploring the diverse topics which have resulted in the successful publishing of this book. They have passed on their knowledge of decades through this book. To expedite this challenging task, the publisher supported the team at every step. A small team of assistant editors was also appointed to further simplify the editing procedure and attain best results for the readers.

Apart from the editorial board, the designing team has also invested a significant amount of their time in understanding the subject and creating the most relevant covers. They scrutinized every image to scout for the most suitable representation of the subject and create an appropriate cover for the book.

The publishing team has been an ardent support to the editorial, designing and production team. Their endless efforts to recruit the best for this project, has resulted in the accomplishment of this book. They are a veteran in the field of academics and their pool of knowledge is as vast as their experience in printing. Their expertise and guidance has proved useful at every step. Their uncompromising quality standards have made this book an exceptional effort. Their encouragement from time to time has been an inspiration for everyone.

The publisher and the editorial board hope that this book will prove to be a valuable piece of knowledge for researchers, students, practitioners and scholars across the globe.

List of Contributors

Abdelhamid Benmachiche
Center for Reproductive Medicine, Clinique Ibn Rochd, Constantine, Algeria

Amel Dammene Debbih
Faculty of Medicine of Algiers, Bologhine University Hospital Center, Algiers, Algeria

María de Jesús Rovirosa-Hernández, Francisco García-Orduña and Abril de los Ángeles Aguilar-Tirado
Instituto de Neuroetología, Universidad Veracruzana, Xalapa, Veracruz, México

Marisela Hernández González and Miguel Ángel Guevara-Pérez
Instituto de Neurociencias, Universidad de Guadalajara, Jalisco, México

Abraham Puga-Olguín
Posgrado en Neuroetología, Universidad Veracruzana, Xalapa, Veracruz, México

Brisa Patricia Vásquez-Domínguez
Facultad de Medicina, Universidad Veracruzana, Zona-Xalapa, Veracruz, México

Simoni T. Bittar
Federal University of Paraíba, João Pessoa, Brazil

José O.R. de Macêdo
Patos Integrated Faculties, Patos, Brazil

Elisio A. Pereira Neto, Hidayane G. da Silva, Patrick A.S. Pfeiffer, Janine A. Padilha and Maria do S. Cirilo-Sousa
Federal University of Paraíba, João Pessoa, Brazil

Wagner V. dos Santos
Faculty of Medical Sciences, João Pessoa, Brazil

Juan Francisco Rodríguez-Landa and Jonathan Cueto-Escobedo
Laboratory of Neuropharmacology, Institute of Neuroethology, Universidad Veracruzana, Xalapa, Veracruz, México

Magdalena Wiecek
Department of Physiology and Biochemistry, Faculty of Physical Education and Sport, University of Physical Education, Krakow, Poland

Robert N. Taylor
Department of Obstetrics and Gynecology, University of Utah, Salt Lake City, UT, USA

Rosa Isela García-Ríos
Department of Biomedics, University Center of Tonalá, University of Guadalajara, Tonalá, Jalisco, México

Armando Mora-Pérez and Cesar Soria-Fregozo
Laboratory of Psychobiology and Molecular Biology, University Center of Los Lagos, University of Guadalajara, Lagos de Moreno, Jalisco, México

Iqbal Afridi
Department of Psychiatry & Behavioural Sciences, JPMC (Jinnah Postgraduate Medical Centre), Karachi, Pakistan
JSMU (Jinnah Sindh Medical University), Karachi, Pakistan
Pakistan Psychiatric Society, Pakistan
TAC (Technical Advisory Committee), PMRC, Islamabad, Pakistan JPMC, Pakistan

Preye Fiebai and Rosemary Ogu
University of Port Harcourt, Port Harcourt, Nigeria
University of Port Harcourt Teaching Hospital, Port Harcourt, Nigeria

Avwebo Ochuko Ukueku
University of Port Harcourt Teaching Hospital, Port Harcourt, Nigeria

Barriga-Pooley Patricio
Obstetrics and Gynaecology Department, School of Medicine, Finis Terrae and San Sebastian Universities, Santiago, Chile

Brantes-Glavic Sergio
Depto Ginecología y Obstericia, Universidad de Chile, Santiago, Chile

Erika Estrada-Camarena and Gabriel Sinhue Azpilcueta-Morales
Laboratory of Neuropsychopharmacology, Neuroscience Division, National Institute of Psychiatry "Ramón de la Fuente", Mexico, Mexico

Carolina López-Rubalcava and Brenda Valdés-Sustaita
Departamento de Farmacobiología, Centro de Investigación y de Estudios Avanzados del IPN, Mexico, Mexico

Eva María González-Trujano
Laboratory of Neuropharmacology of Natural Products, Neuroscience Division. National Institute of Psychiatry "Ramón de la Fuente", Mexico, Mexico

Olena Lutsenko
Department of Theory and Methods of Teaching of Natural Sciences, Hlukhiv National Pedagogical University of Alexander Dovzhenko, Ukraine

Courtney Marsh and Monique Monard
Department of Obstetrics and Gynecology, University of Kansas, Kansas City, KS, USA

Katelyn Schumacher
School of Medicine, University of Kansas, Kansas City, KS, USA

Warren B. Nothnick
Department of Molecular and Integrative Physiology, University of Kansas Medical Center, Kansas City, Kansas, USA
Department of Obstetrics and Gynecology, University of Kansas Medical Center, Kansas City, Kansas, USA
Center for Reproductive Sciences, Institute for Reproduction and Perinatal Research, University of Kansas Medical Center, Kansas City, Kansas, USA

Sylvia Kirchengast
Department of Anthropology, University of Vienna, Vienna, Austria

Index

www.ingramcontent.com/pod-product-compliance
Lightning Source LLC
LaVergne TN
LVHW081031210926
848485LV00004B/1000